Mometrix
TEST PREPARATION

SPEX®

Secrets Study Guide

Part 2 of 2

AF834548

Dear Future Exam Success Story

First of all, **THANK YOU** for purchasing Mometrix study materials!

Second, congratulations! You are one of the few determined test-takers who are committed to doing whatever it takes to excel on your exam. **You have come to the right place.** We developed these study materials with one goal in mind: to deliver you the information you need in a format that's concise and easy to use.

In addition to optimizing your guide for the content of the test, we've outlined our recommended steps for breaking down the preparation process into small, attainable goals so you can make sure you stay on track.

We've also analyzed the entire test-taking process, identifying the most common pitfalls and showing how you can overcome them and be ready for any curveball the test throws you.

Standardized testing is one of the biggest obstacles on your road to success, which only increases the importance of doing well in the high-pressure, high-stakes environment of test day. Your results on this test could have a significant impact on your future, and this guide provides the information and practical advice to help you achieve your full potential on test day.

Your success is our success

We would love to hear from you! If you would like to share the story of your exam success or if you have any questions or comments in regard to our products, please contact us at **800-673-8175** or **support@mometrix.com**.

Thanks again for your business and we wish you continued success!

Sincerely,
The Mometrix Test Preparation Team

Need more help? Check out our flashcards at:
http://mometrixflashcards.com/SPEX

Written and edited by the Mometrix Exam Secrets Test Prep Team
Printed in the United States of America

Table of Contents

Respiratory System

Infections

Acute Bronchitis

Acute bronchitis is inflammation of the **bronchial tree** usually caused by an **infection** (typically a virus) and this irritation causes the bronchial structures to secrete more **mucus**, resulting in a cough. Patients with acute bronchitis usually describe recent history of a URI (e.g., congestion, rhinorrhea, occasionally a fever), complain of a cough, which may be productive, and may describe some wheezing or substernal discomfort when breathing or coughing. The color of the sputum does not indicative whether it is due to a virus or bacteria. PE may reveal rhonchi and/or wheezing. *Diagnose* clinically; rule out other diagnoses like pneumonia or influenza. *Treatment* is supportive. Because acute bronchitis is usually caused by a virus, antibiotics don't help relieve symptoms unless there is a bacterial superinfection which only occurs about 10% of the time. Using a humidifier at night to moisten the air, mucolytics, drinking plenty of fluids to thin the mucus secretions, and resting should help to relieve the symptoms within a week. The cough of bronchitis may linger for 2-3 weeks as the bronchial tubes heal.

Acute Bronchiolitis

Acute bronchiolitis is a disease of the **lower respiratory tract** which is caused by a virus, typically **respiratory syncytial virus (RSV)**. This most often affects infants and young children (<2 years old) because older children and adults have larger airways that can accommodate the inflammation, epithelial necrosis, and edema associated with it. Bronchiolitis peaks in the fall, winter, or early spring months. More severe disease is common in the youngest patients (1-6 months old) and may require hospitalization; bronchiolitis is the most common reason children <1 are admitted. Incubation is 2-8 days, with a prodrome of 1-3 days and symptoms that range from a common cold to severe respiratory issues. Patients may remain contagious up to 4 weeks from the onset. Parents of patients with acute bronchiolitis may describe hearing their child wheeze and cough frequently, appearing short of breath, being fussy and irritable, and feeding poorly. A low-grade fever is usually present. Coughing and wheezing may continue for 2-3 weeks and rarely, severe respiratory symptoms can lead to respiratory arrest. Assess for wheezing, air exchange, respiratory rate, and retractions. *Diagnose* clinically (a rapid antigen RSV test is available but not routinely required). Since the cause is viral, *treatment* is supportive with nasal suctioning, antipyretics as needed, and plenty of fluids to prevent dehydration. Albuterol, racemic epinephrine, and steroids are no longer routinely recommended according to the AAP (American Academy of Pediatrics). A trial of nebulized albuterol may be used, but should not be continued of there is no improvement. If admitted, humidified oxygen and IV fluids are given. Premature infants born <29 weeks should receive palivizumab prophylaxis (a monoclonal antibody to RSV) during their 1st year of life.

Community-Acquired Pneumonia vs. Hospital-Acquired Pneumonia

Community-acquired pneumonia (CAP) is most commonly caused by *Streptococcus pneumoniae*. Other typical pathogens of CAP include *H. Influenzae, Moraxella catarrhalis*, atypical bacteria (e.g., *Legionella, Chlamydia pneumoniae,* and *Mycoplasma* species), and viruses.

Hospital-acquired pneumonia (HAP) occurs after ≥48 hours of being in the hospital and is most commonly caused by gram-negative bacteria (*Pseudomonas aeruginosa*) and *Staphylococcus aureus* (including MRSA) and are usually multi-drug resistant. Encourage influenza and pneumococcal vaccines for prevention.

Pneumonia

Pneumonia, which is an infection of the **lungs**, can be caused by bacteria, viruses, fungi, or parasites. Patients are at greater risk if they are >65 years old, <5 years old, are immunocompromised, have a chronic disease (e.g., CVD, DM, COPD, asthma), have had recent surgery, are asplenic, or smoke. CXR's are helpful, but findings vary greatly and so may not be used to diagnose a particular kind of pneumonia.

Patients with **bacterial pneumonia** typically present with a high fever, chills, a productive cough with purulent sputum, fatigue, pleuritic chest pain, SOB, dyspnea, elevated RR, elevated HR, and appear quite ill. Patients may have crackles, reduced breath sounds, and a lung consolidation present on chest x-ray (PA and lateral). Blood and sputum cultures/Gram stain may be obtained if other organisms are suspected that would change treatment. *Treat* bacterial CAP with empiric antibiotics (macrolide if previously healthy; a respiratory fluoroquinolone OR β-lactam plus macrolide if comorbidities, antibiotics within the past 3 months, or inpatient but not in ICU).

Review Video: Pneumonia
Visit mometrix.com/academy and enter code: 628264

Pathogens Typically Causing Bacterial, Viral, Fungal, and HIV-Related Pneumonias

Bacterial pneumonia is most commonly caused by *Streptococcus pneumoniae* (most common), *H. influenzae*, and *Moraxella catarrhalis. Staphylococcus aureus* can cause severe pneumonia after having influenza, and the gram-negative organism *Klebsiella pneumoniae* is more common in alcoholics and produces a currant jelly sputum. *Mycoplasma pneumoniae* is an atypical bacterium that causes a milder disease (e.g., "walking pneumonia"). Other atypical bacteria include *Legionella pneumophilia* and *Chlamydia psittaci* (pet birds).

Viral pneumonia is commonly caused by influenza A or B. RSV (especially if less than 1 year old), parainfluenza, human metapneumovirus, and adenovirus are other common causes. Herpes virus pneumonias like herpes simplex, CMV and varicella are rare in the immunocompetent patient.

Fungal pneumonia is usually caused by *Histoplasma capsulatum*, *Coccidioides immitis*, or *Blastomyces dermatitidis*. These may occur in healthy patients and are usually self-limited but may cause illness. Serious disease usually doesn't occur unless patients are severely immunocompromised.

HIV-related pneumonia is most often caused by *Pneumocystis jiroveci*, though the immunocompromised patient is susceptible to contracting any type of pneumonia. Opportunistic fungal pneumonias like *Aspergillus*, parasites like *Toxoplasma gondii,* and herpes viruses like CMV, EBV, and varicella-zoster are more common among HIV patients.

Symptoms and Empiric Treatments for Viral, Fungal, and HIV-Related Pneumonia

Viral pneumonia typically has a more gradual onset and presents with a low-grade fever, non-productive cough, a viral prodrome, myalgias, and a headache. Patients may be sick for several days before seeing a doctor. CXR is usually worse than the symptoms and typically shows diffuse interstitial infiltrates with hilar adenopathy. *Treat* influenza with oseltamivir or zanamivir if started within 48 hours of symptom onset; acyclovir for varicella-zoster. Otherwise, treatment is symptomatic. Secondary bacterial infections are common with influenza.

Fungal pneumonias have similar symptoms, but can also spread to become systemic. *Treat* with anti-fungals, depending on the infective organism.

HIV-related pneumonias have *symptoms* according to the type of pneumonia that's present; *treatment* depends upon the infective organism. Always follow local sensitivity patterns; patients should respond within 48-72 hours.

Pertussis

Pertussis, or whooping cough, is a highly contagious **respiratory infection** caused by the gram-negative bacterium *Bordetella pertussis*. Pertussis is becoming more common now because immunity from the DTaP vaccine tends to wear off by adulthood or because the vaccine was not received. Incubation is 4-21 days. The *symptoms* come in 3 stages:

- The **catarrhal stage (1st stage)** begins gradually with symptoms of a cold such as runny nose, sneezing, lacrimation/red eyes, mild cough, and low-grade fever. This lasts 1-2 weeks.
- The **paroxysmal stage (2nd stage)** is characterized by coughing spells that often leave the person breathless. These spells are followed by a loud inspiratory breath that makes a loud "whoop" sound. Posttussive vomiting is common. This stage may last 1-6 weeks or longer.
- The **convalescent stage (3rd stage)** lasts 2-6 weeks (sometimes months) as the chronic cough gradually fades.

Collect nasopharyngeal swab or nasal aspirates for PCR and culture before antibiotics are started. It is questionable whether antibiotics help to shorten the duration of symptoms of pertussis, but are given to reduce the spread of the disease. *Treat* with azithromycin for 5 days or erythromycin for 14 days. There are no proven effective treatments to treat the cough but try to not agitate the child. Prophylaxis is given to close contacts (same as treatment). Report suspected cases to the local health department who reports to the CDC.

Tuberculosis

Risk Factors

Tuberculosis (TB) is a disease caused by the aerobic bacillus *Mycobacterium tuberculosis*, is spread through air droplets, and can cause either a **latent** TB infection (LTBI) or an **active** form. TB is more prevalent in those who are at a high risk including those from countries with a high rate of TB, those in institutions/live in crowded conditions, the homeless, IV drug users, and those with weakened immune systems (HIV/AIDS). TB is seen more often in those frequently exposed to the disease like close family contacts or medical professionals. TB typically causes pulmonary disease but may also occur at other sites (extrapulmonary TB; lymphadenopathy is most common). After the primary infection (which is usually asymptomatic), the body encases the bacteria and forms granulomas (LTBI); both the primary infection and the latent stage are not contagious. This latent phase can be reactivated and become active (contagious).

Signs and Symptoms, Diagnosis, and Treatment

Symptoms of active TB may include night sweats, chronic cough, hemoptysis, dyspnea, low-grade fever, fatigue, loss of appetite, weight loss, and pleurisy. Those at high risk should receive a screening test of either a tuberculin skin test (PPD) or an interferon gamma release assay blood test (IGRA; use this if previous BCG vaccine, given in other countries). If either is positive (PPD [check for induration after 2-3 days]: ≥15mm if no risk factors, ≥10mm if some risk factors; ≥5mm if HIV+ or high risk factors) order a CXR and acid-fast bacilli (AFB) sputum smear and culture to confirm diagnosis. CXR (PA and lateral with apical lordotic view) may show cavitary lesions or multilobar opacities in apices and upper aspect of lower lobes. Firstline *treatment* includes multiple antibiotics: isoniazid (INH), rifampin (RIF), pyrazinamide (PZA), and ethambutol for 2 months; then, if susceptible, continue INH and RIF for 4 more months; but if resistant, instead use RIF, PZA, and ethambutol for 4 more months. Once diagnosed, patients with active TB should be kept in isolation, and the local health department should be notified. Latent disease is usually treated prophylactically with INH x 9 months.

Croup

Croup occurs because of inflammation around the **larynx and trachea** due to a **viral infection**. It occurs in children (especially age 6 months-3 years) and causes a **characteristic barking cough** that is seal-like and very distinguishable. It is most often caused by the parainfluenza virus (usually in the fall), though sometimes by adenovirus, RSV, or influenza. The barking cough associated with croup is usually worse at night and can wake a child up from sleep. Patients typically present with recent history of URI symptoms and fever, a barking cough, inspiratory stridor, hoarseness and some level of respiratory distress. More severe cases may have inspiratory and expiratory stridor at rest, retractions, and are distressed or agitated. Assess for hypoxia, tachypnea, and respiratory rate. *Diagnose* clinically; AP/lateral neck and chest x-rays may be ordered if indicated. *Symptoms* typically last <1 week and most cases can be *treated* at home with humidified air (cool mist vaporizer or sitting in the bathroom with steam from running a hot shower; however, there are no supporting research studies), keeping the child calm, cool drinks or popsicles to help to ease the inflammation in the throat, staying hydrated, and antipyretics. Also, oral steroids may be prescribed for a few days, or a one-time dose of IM dexamethasone (especially helpful if given in the first 4-24 hours of the disease; effective within 6 hours). If racemic epinephrine (nebulizer) is given in the emergency department for moderate or severe distress, patients must be observed for 3-4 hours due to a possible rebound effect from the medication. Occasionally, hospitalization is necessary with treatments including humidified oxygen, racemic epinephrine, steroids, or even intubation if very severe.

Asthma and COPD

Asthma

Asthma is a **chronic lung disease** in which the **airways** become inflamed and narrowed. In response to allergens or triggers, edema, inflammation, and mucus constrict airways producing breathing difficulties and the classic "asthma attacks." Risk increases with a positive family history and exposure to tobacco smoke. It can be aggravated by allergen exposure, aspirin, cold air, exercise, infections, and stress. The *symptoms* of asthma include wheezing, difficulty breathing, and chest tightness; symptoms may be worse during the night. Coughing spasms can also occur as the airways constrict and the lungs attempt to expel the extra mucus that is produced. *Diagnose* clinically and confirm with PFT if ≥5 years old to show obstruction and reversibility (spirometry before and after bronchodilator; FEV_1 is measured; airway obstruction = <70% FEV_1/FVC ratio; reversibility = ≥12% increase in FEV_1 or for adults, a >200mL increase in FEV_1 from baseline); obtain CXR and rule out other conditions. Asthma severity can be classified as **intermittent, mild persistent** (symptoms >2 days/wk needing rescue meds), **moderate persistent** (symptoms qd needing rescue meds), and **severe persistent** (symptoms qd and night, needs rescue meds several times/day). The goal of *treatment* is prevention which includes steps to reduce allergen exposure. Treatment can be divided amongst long-acting medicines and quick-acting "rescue" medications. The long-acting drugs used include inhaled corticosteroids (ICS), long-acting beta-2 agonists (salmeterol), leukotriene modifiers, theophylline, Cromolyn®, and sometimes immunomodulators (e.g., omalizumab). The short-acting medications are used when patients are having an acute exacerbation and include short-acting beta-2 agonists, ipratropium (Atrovent®), and systemic corticosteroids. A stepwise approach to treatment is best; intermittent asthma: use SA bronchodilators prn; persistent asthma: start with low-dose ICS and step up as needed (e.g., use medium-dose ICS or add a LA bronchodilator). The key is prevention by minimizing exposure to known allergens or triggers, using medications regularly, and not smoking.

Chronic Bronchitis

Chronic bronchitis is a type of **COPD** (chronic obstructive pulmonary disease) and occurs when the **bronchial tubes** are irritated and inflamed, causing hyperplasia of mucus glands, excess mucus secretion, and epithelial damage resulting in plugged airways and decreased oxygen flow. **Smoking** is the most common cause of chronic bronchitis; occasionally chronic exposure to dust and other irritants can cause chronic bronchitis. Patients usually complain of a chronic, productive cough, shortness of breath, dyspnea on exertion, fatigue, chest discomfort, and wheezing. PE may show rhonchi and wheezing. Patients have recurrent lung infections, and over time, signs of right-sided heart failure, cyanosis, and weight gain ("blue bloater"). *Diagnosis* is made by symptoms of a productive cough for at least 3 months during a 2-year period. Confirm with PFT's which show an increase residual volume, reduced FEV_1, and FEV_1/FVC ratio <70% which is not reversible with bronchodilators. CXR (PA and lateral) may show increased pulmonary markings and an enlarged heart; a chest CT may also be ordered. *Treatment* is symptomatic and usually includes bronchodilators (either short or long-acting depending on the severity), inhaled anticholinergics (ipratropium bromide is short-acting; tiotropium is long-acting), inhaled steroids, and possibly systemic steroids or antibiotics during exacerbations. Patients may require supplemental oxygen at home if hypoxia is severe. Patients should quit smoking to help decrease irritation to the lungs and should stay up to date on vaccines.

Emphysema

Emphysema, another type of **COPD**, occurs with lung damage past the **terminal bronchiole** causing alveoli to lose their elasticity, alveoli that incompletely empty air on expiration, and damage to the capillary bed. This causes **hyperinflation of the lungs** with difficulty drawing in the oxygen needed to take another breath. The most common cause of emphysema is **smoking**; a deficiency in alpha-1-antitrypsin protein can also lead to emphysema. Patients typically have a thin appearance with a barrel chest, are short of breath, easily fatigued, and may have a mild, usually non-productive cough. Patients often purse their lips when exhaling ("pink puffers"). On exam, patients may be tachypneic, hypoxic, may have decreased breath sounds, and a hyperresonant chest, but are not cyanotic. Over time, patients will develop fingernail clubbing and will increasingly use accessory muscles. *Diagnose* clinically and confirm with PFT's which show an increase residual volume, reduced FEV_1, and reduced FEV_1/FVC ratio; this is not reversible with bronchodilators. CXR shows hyperinflation, flattened diaphragms, increase retrosternal airspace, possibly bullae, and a small heart; a chest CT may also be ordered. Treatment consists of inhaled bronchodilators (short or long-acting), inhaled anticholinergics, inhaled steroids, and possibly systemic steroids or antibiotics during exacerbations. Quitting smoking is the best *treatment* to help prevent progression of the disease. Patients may require supplemental oxygen at home. Rarely, surgery may be done to remove the damaged tissue (bullectomy).

Congenital Disorders

Cystic Fibrosis

Cystic fibrosis (**CF**) is an **autosomal recessive genetic disorder** affecting the **exocrine glands** especially involving the lungs and GI tract. It causes **excessive mucus production** that leads to pulmonary obstruction, deficient pancreatic enzyme production, and infertility issues (especially in males). There is no cure for cystic fibrosis. The average life expectancy in the U.S. is to the late 30's or early 40's; and death usually occurs due to pulmonary complications or cor pulmonale. **Bronchiectasis** occurs which is a condition of the bronchial tubes caused by chronic inflammation and infection which causes dilatation and damage resulting in increasingly purulent sputum. The lungs become chronically infected with usually *Staphylococcus aureus* early on then *Pseudomonas aeruginosa* as the disease progresses. *Symptoms* may include recurrent lung/sinus infections with excessive congestion, bowel obstruction due to thickened feces (meconium ileus), and failure to thrive or poor nutrition because of decreased absorption of fat-soluble vitamins, fats, proteins, and carbohydrates. Check for clubbing, cyanosis, cough, increase AP chest diameter, HSM, and abdominal distension. The newborn screen now tests for CF and the *diagnosis* is confirmed with sweat-chloride testing and genetic testing. Still about 10% are diagnosed later on but usually by teenage or young adult years. Refer to a specialist team. Postural drainage and chest physiotherapy can be performed regularly to promote drainage of lung secretions. Pancreatic enzymes and multivitamins are taken orally to aid in digestion and nutrition. Bronchodilators, inhaled antibiotics, and mucolytics are given to decrease secretions and irritation in the lungs. In severe cases, lung transplantation can be performed to improve quality of life, though this still does not cure the disease.

ALPHA-1-ANTITRYPSIN DEFICIENCY

Alpha-1 antitrypsin deficiency is a congenital disorder in which the primary lung antiprotease (which prevent proteases from damaging lung tissue) is lacking, allowing the destruction of pulmonary tissue and leading to emphysema in adults in middle age and often to cirrhosis in children and adults. The condition is worsened if the patient smokes, as smoking increases protease activity as well. Pulmonary symptoms are consistent with COPD with dyspnea, wheezing, cough, and air trapping. The degree of pulmonary damage may vary from mild to severe. Some patients may develop panniculitis as well with indurated plaques/nodules on the lower trunk and thighs. Diagnostic tests include serum alpha-1 antitrypsin level, liver function tests, pulmonary function tests, and genotyping. Treatment includes supportive care as appropriate for the degree of COPD (bronchodilators) and alpha-1 antitrypsin replacement therapy. Smoking cessation is especially important. In severe cases, patients may be candidates for lung transplantation.

Cancers

CARCINOID TUMORS

Carcinoid tumors occur in the **neuroendocrine system** and are most frequently found in the small intestines, rectum, or appendix, but may also be found in the lungs, bronchi, or pancreas. They may be **benign** but are often **malignant** (especially if found in the ileum or bronchus) and metastasize to the liver, brain, or lungs. They are slow-growing tumors and may not be diagnosed right away. They most often present in adults and are often not diagnosed until patients are 50-60 years old. Patients with carcinoid tumors may be asymptomatic, but they may secrete hormones like serotonin and produce symptoms of **carcinoid syndrome** (flushing, diarrhea, wheezing, weight loss, loss of appetite). *Diagnose* with an imaging study (e.g., CT, bronchoscopy), plasma or urinary 5-HIAA, and biopsy. *Treatment* of carcinoid tumors consists of surgical removal of the tumor. Chemotherapy may be given if the tumor has spread to other locations in the body as well as radiation. Interferon- α may be given to help decrease the growth of the tumor, especially if metastatic or unresectable.

Lung Cancer

Lung cancer is the **most common cause of cancer death** for both men and women and **smoking** is the most common risk factor (~85%). There are 2 main types: **small cell lung cancer (SCLC)** and **non-small cell lung cancer (NSCLC)**. SCLC has the worse prognosis, is aggressive, and often already presents with metastases when diagnosed. 85% of all cases of lung cancer are NSCLC which can be adenocarcinoma, large cell, or squamous cell (bronchogenic). **Squamous cell** is typically found centrally in the bronchi, while **adenocarcinoma and large cell** are usually found as a peripheral mass or nodule. Symptoms of **bronchogenic carcinoma** include a progressively worsening cough, dyspnea, and chest pain, with or without hemoptysis. Weight loss and fatigue may be present as the disease progresses. Patients may be asymptomatic for a while. As the cancer spreads, it may encroach on the laryngeal nerve causing hoarseness or may cause **superior vena cava syndrome** (SVC; swelling in the face, neck, upper extremities, or trunk; cough; headache/head fullness) or may cause **Horner syndrome** (ptosis, miosis, anhidrosis). If metastases are present, patients may experience bone pain, abdominal pain, or confusion, depending on the location of the metastases. Some small cell tumors may serve as an ectopic source of hormone production, so *symptoms* that mimic an endocrine disorder may be evident. *Diagnose* with CXR, CT, sputum or fluid cytology, and biopsy (usually by bronchoscopy). Often, once diagnosed, prognosis is very poor with this disease. *Treatment* may involve surgery to resect (NSCLC), debulk a large tumor, or a lobectomy. This may be followed with radiation and/or chemotherapy depending on the location and type of cancer. New research shows promise with immunotherapy and targeted therapy for genetic mutations.

Pulmonary Nodules

Pulmonary nodules are **lesions** <3cm that are often found incidentally on CXR or CT scan that are surrounded by **aerated lung tissue**. If >3 cm, it is referred to as a mass. Pulmonary nodules may be benign (~90%) or cancerous. **Benign nodules** are slower growing and may have many causes including infection (abscess, TB, fungal, parasite), granulomas from a previous infection, hemangioma, cyst, lymph node, lipoma, or fibroma. Risk for a **cancerous nodule** increases with age, smoking, previous history of cancer, and larger size of the nodule. High risk patients >55 years old may be screened with a low-dose CT. Patients are usually asymptomatic but may have a cough. *Diagnosis* involves using imaging studies. Compare previous CXR or CT scans. Evaluate the nodule using CT. It is more likely benign if the nodule has not grown or doubled in 2 years, <1.5 cm, solid, and has a smooth edge. PET scan may be used to check for malignancy. Biopsy the nodule if malignancy is suspected. Rule out an infectious cause. *Treatment* is based on the findings and may include observation or resection. Growing nodules and those suspected to be cancerous should be resected. If the nodule is <1 cm, reevaluate in 3 months, 6 months, then annually for 2 years. If the nodule is confirmed to be benign, no further follow-up is necessary.

Obstructive Sleep Apnea and Obesity Hypoventilation Syndrome

Obstructive sleep apnea (OSA) is caused by partial or complete closure of the upper airway that leads to **apnea or hypoventilation** for >10 seconds during sleep. This may occur at any age and is more prevalent in men. In children this is usually due to hypertrophy of the tonsils and adenoids and in adults is often due to obesity, alcohol, or sedative use. Anatomical risk factors include a large neck, large tongue or uvula, and a crowded oropharynx. OSA can lead to many consequences including growth restriction, poor concentration and memory, poor performance at work or school, depression, weight loss or an increased BMI, HTN, and CHF. *Signs and symptoms* include snoring, difficulty staying asleep, fatigue, daytime sleepiness, and poor concentration/memory. *Diagnose* with an overnight polysomnogram (sleep study); OSA = ≥5 apnea/ hypopnea episodes per hour without symptoms or ≥15 episodes per hour with symptoms. *Treatment* includes modifying risk factors, using appliances, CPCP, or occasionally surgery to correct anatomic issues that cause OSA.

Obesity hypoventilation syndrome (OHS; aka Pickwickian syndrome) is a **breathing disorder** due to obesity that causes **hypercapnia and hypoxia**. This may lead to pulmonary HTN, cor pulmonale, erythrocytosis, and early death. This may or may not be associated with OSA.

Miscellaneous Pulmonary Disorders

Pleural Effusion

A **pleural effusion** is an accumulation of fluid in the **pleural space**. It has many causes, but is frequently caused by **infections** such as pneumonia, or by **chronic diseases** such as CHF or lung cancer. The effusion can be classified as a transudate (due to changes is hydrostatic and plasma osmotic pressure) or as an exudate (due to increased capillary permeability). **Transudates** are typically caused by CHF, cirrhosis, or nephrotic syndrome. **Exudates** are typically caused by pneumonia, PE's, TB, or malignancies. Patients may be asymptomatic or may complain of a cough, dyspnea, and pleuritic chest pain. On physical exam, there may be decreased breath sounds, pleural friction rub, reduced tactile fremitus, and dullness to percussion over the effusion. The effusion is evident on chest x-ray and may be better-examined by CT imaging. *Treatment* depends on the size and type of effusion. Small effusions may be watched and diuretics may be used to decrease the effusion if is it due to CHF. For a new or unexplained effusion, a thoracentesis and pleural fluid analysis may be done to draw the fluid off the lungs and to diagnose the type of effusion; a thoracentesis is both diagnostic and therapeutic. Check fluid pH, glucose, protein, LDH, cell count with differential, and Gram stain and culture. Treat the underlying cause. If the effusion is chronic, treat with pleurodesis or drain with an indwelling catheter. *Complications* include empyema, scarring, and pneumothorax.

Review Video: Pleural Effusions
Visit mometrix.com/academy and enter code: 145719

Pulmonary Hypertension

Pulmonary hypertension is a **rise in pressure within the pulmonary artery** carrying blood to the lungs. Pulmonary hypertension is now classified in 5 groups. **Group 1** involves narrowing of the pulmonary arterioles and includes idiopathic pulmonary arterial hypertension (PAH), familial, drug or toxin-induced, and PAH associated with medical conditions like portal HTN, sickle cell disease, scleroderma (connective tissue d/o), HIV, schistosomiasis, and congenital heart disease. It can be caused by left-sided heart failure (**group 2**; most common), especially as the ejection fraction decreases and left ventricular function decreases, or may be due to lung disease like COPD or hypoxia (**group 3**). **Group 4** includes cases due to chronic pulmonary thromboembolism; and **group 5** includes unclear, multifactorial causes. As resistance in the pulmonary vasculature increases, changes occur that can lead to **right-sided heart failure**. The symptoms of pulmonary hypertension include SOB, dyspnea on exertion which becomes progressively worse, fatigue, and chest pain. Patients may also complain of a cough, sometimes with hemoptysis, and may even have syncopal episodes. PE may show jugular venous distension, a right-sided heave, a split S2, and possibly a S3 in advanced cases. *Diagnose* with CXR (enlarged pulmonary arteries), ECG (right-axis deviation), and echocardiography and confirm with a right-sided heart catheterization. Management of pulmonary hypertension focuses on treating the underlying cause. *Treatment* may include oxygen therapy, diuretics (e.g., furosemide; avoid hypovolemia), digoxin, and anticoagulants which may be useful in treating symptoms and in preventing complications from this condition. Other advanced treatment: IV epoprostenol, prostacyclin agonists, or phosphodiesterase 5 inhibitors; and research continues.

Pulmonary Fibrosis

Pulmonary fibrosis (idiopathic) is a chronic and progressive condition in which the **alveoli** become damaged and are replaced by **fibrotic scar tissue**. This results in a thickening of the alveolar tissue, preventing the **transfer of oxygen**. The cause of pulmonary fibrosis is uncertain, but it is thought there is a genetic tendency for developing this disease. It is also thought that inhaled environmental agents, especially cigarette smoke, may increase the likelihood of developing pulmonary fibrosis. *Symptoms* develop over time and patients may complain of shortness of breath or dyspnea, especially during activity, may have a dry, hacking cough, and fatigue. Patients may also have a loss of appetite with significant weight loss. On exam, there may be fine inspiratory crackles (like Velcro) at both bases, clubbing, and a decrease in oxygen saturation on pulse oximetry. *Diagnose* with a high-resolution CT (diffuse subpleural and reticular opacities, subpleural honeycombing) and sometimes a biopsy. There is no cure for pulmonary fibrosis. Supplemental oxygen can be given to help with shortness of breath. Pirfenidone is a recently approved antifibrotic agent that may be used for treating idiopathic pulmonary fibrosis. In severe cases, a lung transplant may be performed. *Complications* include pulmonary hypertension, respiratory infections, and death.

Sarcoidosis

Sarcoidosis is an inflammatory disease that usually appears in the **lungs or thoracic lymphatics**, but may affect any organ system in the body causing **noncaseating granulomas** to form. It is often self-limited and resolves within a couple years, but in rare cases it may be fatal. It more commonly affects African Americans, 20-40-year-olds, and females. The cause of sarcoidosis is not known, but it is thought it may be due to an immune response after exposure to a certain bacteria, virus, or toxin. *Signs and symptoms* vary depending on the organ system affected and patients may be asymptomatic. With lung disease, patients may complain of shortness of breath with a chronic cough and crackles may be heard. A skin rash, arthralgias, weight loss, fatigue, and red or watery eyes (uveitis) may also be present. *Diagnose* with CXR (shows bilateral hilar adenopathy) and biopsy. Bronchoscopy is performed for granuloma samples and for confirmation of the diagnosis. Lab tests may reveal an elevation in ACE and calcium, but this is not definitive for diagnosis. *Treatment* may help to control some of the symptoms and involves NSAIDs and corticosteroids. Monitor with CXR's and pulmonary function tests every 6-12 months, and ECG's annually until resolved.

Chest Wall Disorders

Restrictive lung diseases are those in which the lung volume is altered because of disease within the lungs, neuromuscular functioning, or **chest wall disorders**.

Trauma (flail chest)	Occurs when at least 3 adjacent ribs are fractured, both anteriorly and posteriorly, so that they float free of the rib cage. In some cases, the sternum floats with ribs fractured on both sides. Results in failure of the chest wall to support changes in intrathoracic pressure so that paradoxical respirations occur with the flail area contracting on inspiration and expanding on expiration. Hypoventilation occurs because the lungs cannot expand properly.	Diagnosis is per physical examination and imaging (chest x-ray, CT) treatment includes analgesia, and respiratory physiotherapy. Surgical fixation is usually only indicated for those requiring thoracotomy for underlying injuries.
Masses	Benign (osteochondroma, chondroma, fibrous dysplasia) and malignant (sarcomas) primary tumors may occur in the bones or soft tissue of the chest wall. More than half of malignant tumors of the chest wall are metastatic. Symptoms vary depending on the size and location but most are asymptomatic until large.	Diagnosis is per biopsy and imaging (PET, CT, MRI). Treatment includes surgery and may also include chemotherapy and radiation.

Occupational Lung Disease

Occupational Asthma

Occupational asthma is triggered by contact with an agent (chemicals fumes, latex, dyes, drugs, plastics, plants, animal substances, enzymes, dust, powder, gas) in the workplace. The asthma may result from an allergic or immunological response or from direct irritation and damage to the respiratory system. Symptoms may be almost immediate or may be delayed for weeks or months until after repeated exposures. Symptoms are consistent with other types of asthma: wheezing, coughing, dyspnea, and feeling of tight chest. Patients may experience symptoms both in and out of the work environment. Those at greatest risk are patients with existing allergies and smokers. Diagnosis may include pulmonary function tests, allergy skin tests, and challenge test. Treatment includes avoiding trigger (even wearing a respirator may be ineffective once sensitized to a substance), inhaled corticosteroids, leukotriene modifiers, LABAs, combined inhalers, and SABAs.

High Altitude Sickness

At high altitude, oxygenation may be inadequate, especially if people ascend before their bodies are able to acclimate, leading to **high altitude sickness:**

- **Acute mountain sickness** (AMS). Usually occurs when ascending quickly to >9000 feet. Some may experience only mild to moderate shortness of breath but others may progress to more serious illness. Treatment is to descend and rest.

- **High altitude cerebral edema** (HACE) with swelling of the brain tissue and increased intracranial pressure. Onset is usually after a week or longer at high altitudes. The person may be confused, unable to walk, severely lethargic and experience seizures and coma. Without treatment, the condition is fatal. The person must descend to a lower altitude. Treatment includes hyperbaric treatment (usually in portable unit), oxygen administration, dexamethasone and benzodiazepine (for seizures).
- **High altitude pulmonary edema** (HAPE) with fluid buildup in the lung, resulting in severe shortness of breath, cough, and cyanosis, leading to respiratory collapse and death. HAPE may occur alone or along with HACE and is more common in males than females. The person must descend to a lower altitude. Treatment includes hyperbaric treatment, oxygen administration, nifedipine, and dexamethasone.

PNEUMOCONIOSIS

Pneumoconiosis is an occupational lung disease that is due to **inhaling particulate matter**. It can be due to inhaling the dust from coal, asbestos, silica (rock and sand), beryllium, iron, talc, and other materials. The specific type of pneumoconiosis will vary depending upon the material inhaled. For example, asbestos workers can develop **asbestosis** while those who work with silica develop **silicosis**. There is also **coal worker's pneumoconiosis (CWP)** or black lung disease. There should be workplace safety monitoring in place to help protect workers. Patients are often asymptomatic for years then typically complain of progressively worsening shortness of breath that is more pronounced during activities. They will also have a chronic cough that may be productive or nonproductive. On exam, there may be inspiratory crackles present. Chest x-ray or CT may show consolidated areas where the inhaled dust has damaged the lung tissue. CWP shows round, nodular opacities and fibrosis; Asbestosis shows reticular opacities usually in the lower lobes and pleural plaques; Silicosis shows ground-glass opacities. There is no known *treatment* for the pneumoconiosis diseases. Supportive treatment with supplemental oxygen may be necessary. Patients should avoid any future contact with causative substances and if they smoke, they should quit in order to prevent any further damage to the lung tissue to further exacerbate the illness. In very severe cases, lung transplantation can be performed. There is an increased risk of developing **lung cancer** (mesothelioma) with asbestosis.

Respiratory Emergencies

ACUTE EPIGLOTTITIS

Acute epiglottitis is a medical emergency that may result in the **epiglottis blocking the trachea** if it is not treated immediately. It can be caused by the *H. influenzae* bacterium, but is not seen as often due to the Hib immunization now available. Other causes are *H. parainfluenzae*, *Streptococcus pneumoniae*, or group A streptococci. Trauma to the throat can also cause inflammation of the epiglottis. Patients with epiglottitis usually have a muffled voice, throat pain, fever, difficulty swallowing, and possibly difficulty breathing. Patients lean forward in the classic tripod position to breathe and may even drool if swallowing is too difficult. If epiglottitis is suspected, one should NOT attempt to visualize the epiglottis directly with a tongue depressor during PE because this may cause more inflammation and could close the airway. Stridor, muffled voice, and a history of DM are indicators for the likelihood of airway intervention. Lateral neck x-rays will show an enlarged epiglottis (thumb sign). However, this is being replaced by nasopharyngoscopy/ laryngoscopy in the OR which allows for direct visualization and therefore, a rapid and accurate diagnosis. Treat with 3rd generation cephalosporins, like ceftriaxone (Rocephin), which are used due to the increasing resistance of ampicillin; amoxicillin/clavulanic acid is another option. If penicillin/cephalosporin allergic, chloramphenicol can be used. *Patients should be kept calm, should* *avoid swallowing or talking, and intubation and cricothyrotomy equipment should be kept on hand in case of airway obstruction.*

Primary, Secondary, Traumatic, and Tension Pneumothorax

A **pneumothorax** occurs when air invades the **pleural space** causing the lung to partially or completely **collapse**. *Symptoms* usually include sudden, sharp chest pain, dyspnea, and SOB, PE findings may include reduced breath sounds, asymmetric expansion of the lungs, tachypnea, and possibly respiratory distress. The main types include spontaneous, traumatic, and a tension pneumothorax. A **spontaneous pneumothorax** can be either primary or secondary.

A **primary pneumothorax** is not due to lung disease and usually occurs in young, tall males. This happens when a bleb ruptures on the lung, causing collapse of a portion of the lung. If small, it can be monitored with repeat chest x-rays and usually heals in 1-2 weeks. If large, hospitalization with a chest tube (tube thoracostomy) may be necessary.

A **secondary pneumothorax** is more serious than a primary and occurs due to chronic lung disease, such as COPD, cystic fibrosis, or TB. It can potentially be life-threatening and may require hospitalization and a chest tube for *treatment*.

A **traumatic pneumothorax** occurs when there is trauma to the chest wall that results in air entering the chest cavity. This can result in a small pneumothorax that can be monitored or it may be large enough to require a chest tube.

A **tension pneumothorax** is a medical emergency and can be fatal. It occurs when air becomes trapped in the pleural space and cannot escape (due to increased pressure within the pleural space compared to atmospheric pressure). This results in a worsening pneumothorax that will eventually cause hypotension, tachycardia, hypoxia, and the structures in the cavity to shift. It is life-threatening and should be *treated* immediately with a needle decompression (at the 2nd intercostal space and midclavicular line) before confirming with a CXR. Follow this with a chest tube.

Cor Pulmonale

Cor pulmonale is **right-sided heart failure**. This can occur because of **prolonged pulmonary hypertension** due to lung disease which causes an increase in pressure within the **right ventricle**. Chronic lung disease, such as COPD or cystic fibrosis, can lead to cor pulmonale or it may occur acutely due to a pulmonary embolus. Patients may complain of increasing shortness of breath and fatigue. They may have chest pain and dyspnea that is exacerbated with activity and not entirely relieved with rest as the disease progresses. On exam, patients may have jugular venous distention, hepatomegaly, ascites, or lower extremity edema. *Diagnose* with CXR and echocardiogram; a heart catheterization may be needed to confirm the diagnosis and assess the pressures. *Treating* the underlying cause is the focus of treatment with cor pulmonale. Patients may require anticoagulant therapy to prevent thromboembolism. Diuretics are sometimes used for chronic cor pulmonale but should be used with caution since they may worsen symptoms. Calcium channel blockers and vasodilators may be given to help optimize cardiac function if the right-sided heart failure is due to primary pulmonary hypertension. Oxygen therapy may be given to patients for home use in order to improve oxygenation of the blood; this is especially helpful in COPD patients.

Cor Pumonale

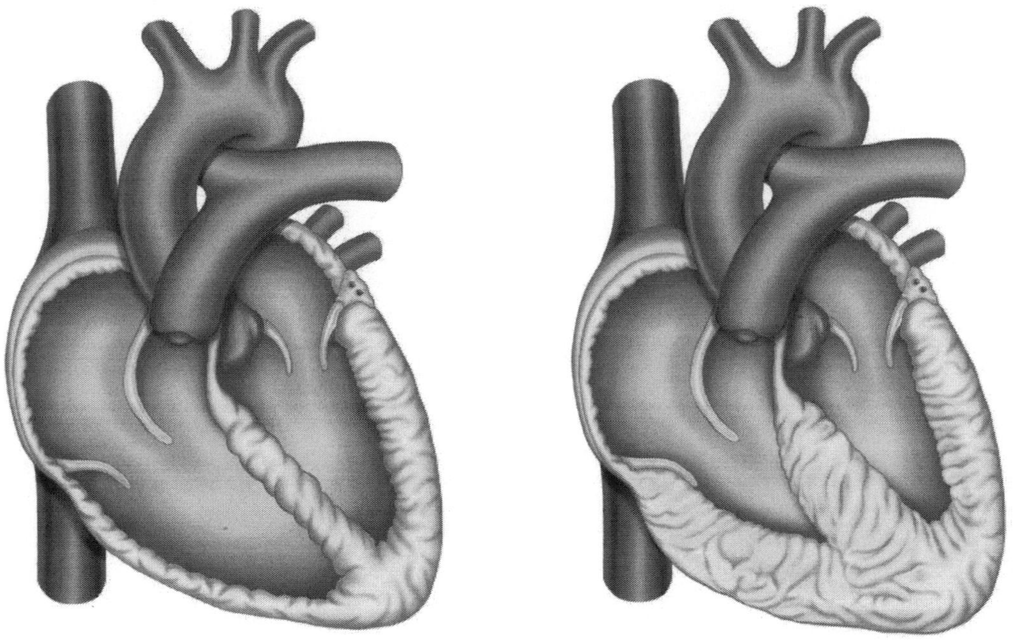

Normal Right Ventricular Hypertrophy

Pulmonary Embolism

A **pulmonary embolism** (**PE**) occurs when a **thrombus** travels to the **lungs** and causes obstruction of the airway. PE can be caused by a **deep vein thrombosis** (usually from the LE or pelvis) that travels to the lungs, by any conditions that cause the blood to be **hypercoagulable**, or by **cardiac dysrhythmias**. Patients at increased risk include those who are immobile, increased age, have cancer, heart failure, smokers, use oral contraceptives, postpartum, and recent surgery or trauma. Patients with a PE may be asymptomatic or may have gradual or sudden shortness of breath and may complain of pleuritic chest pain, shoulder pain, sweating, cough, or hemoptysis. On exam, patients may be tachypneic and tachycardic, with hypotension and there may be decreased breath sounds. Patients may become unconscious. Check oxygen saturations with a pulse oximetry. Those suspected of having a PE should receive a CXR and ECG. CT angiography is primarily used to confirm the presence of a PE. V/Q scans are also used but take longer and are sensitive but not as specific as CT angiography. Oxygen is given first to help patients. Anticoagulation is started, usually with heparin (typically SQ, fractionated LMWH) or fondaparinux; then switched to oral warfarin. Overlap with heparin therapy until therapeutic INR has been reached x 24 hours (2.0-3.0), Patients will need to stay on warfarin for 3 months or longer because of the risk of recurrent PE. "Clot buster" thrombolytic drugs may be given to break up large clots if the patient is hemodynamically unstable (e.g., hypotension). An inferior vena cava filter may be placed if anticoagulation is contraindicated or for recurrent DVT's/PE's. *Complications* include shock, cor pulmonale, and sudden death.

Pulmonary Embolism

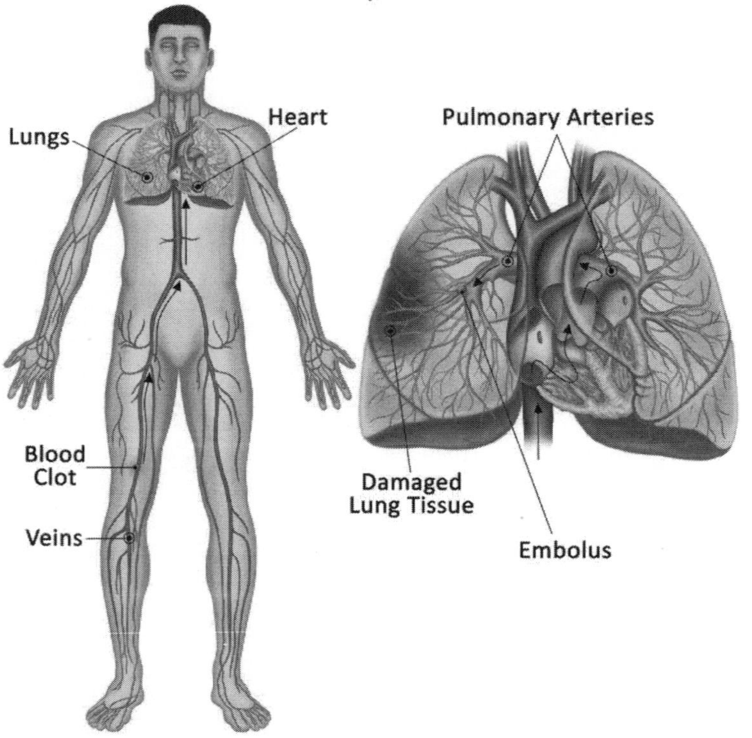

Acute Respiratory Distress Syndrome

Acute respiratory distress syndrome (ARDS) occurs when there is **acute inflammation and fluid accumulation within the lungs** that can quickly progress to **respiratory failure**. ARDS may be mild, moderate, or severe. ARDS can be caused by pneumonia, trauma, shock, aspiration, infection, sepsis, pancreatitis, chemical/gas inhalation, or burns/smoke inhalation. Damage occurs to the **alveoli and endothelium of the pulmonary capillaries** which results in ARDS. The onset of this condition is usually 1-2 days following the triggering event. *Symptoms* initially dyspnea on exertion that progresses to dyspnea at rest and anxiety. Patients usually have rapid respiratory decline with and multisystem organ failure to the point of becoming unconscious and respiratory arrest can occur. On exam, crackles may be heard in the lungs because of fluid accumulation and cyanosis is frequently present along with tachypnea, tachycardia, and hypotension (cardiogenic shock). *Diagnose* with imaging tests (CXR) and ABGs which show pulmonary infiltrates and hypoxia; rule out a cardiac source for the pulmonary edema. ARDS is life-threatening, and patients are treated by specialists in the ICU with supportive therapy as the lungs heal. Maintaining proper oxygenation is the mainstay of treatment and a prone position often helps with oxygenation. Patients are usually placed on ventilators until they can be weaned off and are able to breathe on their own. *Treat* the underlying cause; if an infection is present, appropriate antibiotics should be given. Diuretics may be given to decrease the fluid accumulation within the lungs. Mortality is about 30-45%.

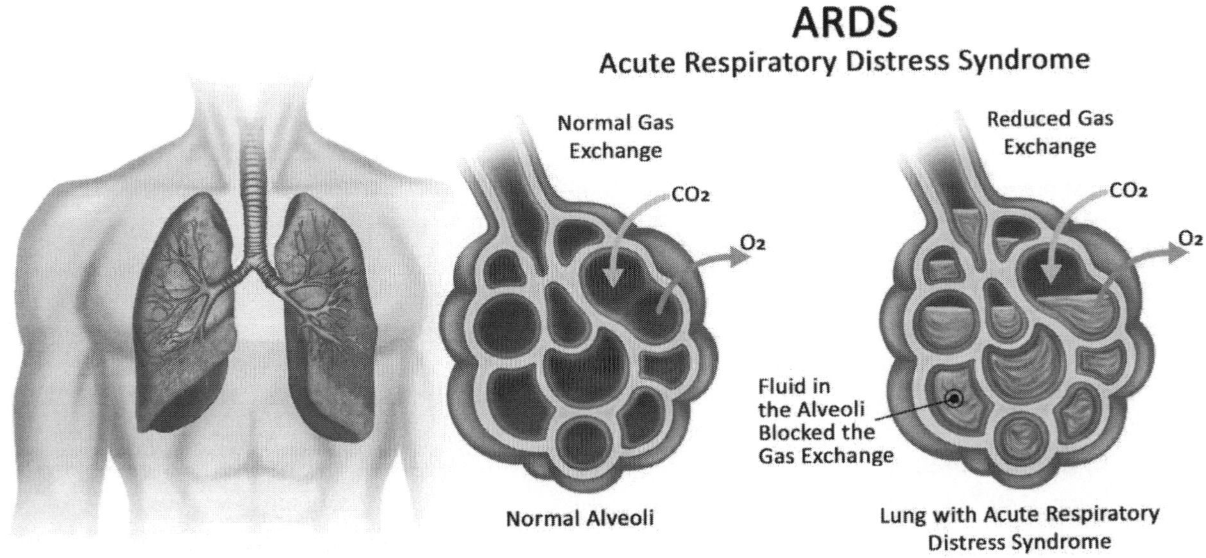

Fat Embolism Syndrome

With **fat embolism syndrome**, fat globules move from the bone marrow into the bloodstream where they can occlude small vessels. Risk is greatest with multiple fractures or fractures of long bones, ribs, or pelvis. Those 20-30 years and elderly adults with fracture of proximal femur are at increased risk. Onset of symptoms (hypoxia, tachypnea, elevated temperature, petechial rash, and tachycardia) is usually at 24 to 72 hours but may be delayed for up to 7 days:

- Occlusion of small vessels in the lungs may cause pulmonary edema and hemorrhage with PaO_2 of <60 mm Hg. X-rays may show "snowstorm" infiltrates. Early signs include respiratory alkalosis progressing to respiratory acidosis, leading to respiratory distress syndrome and congestive heart failure. Up to 75% of patients with FES have respiratory involvement.
- Fat emboli in the brain cause CNS abnormalities, such as headache and confusion leading to coma.
- Systemic embolization may cause widespread petechiae, elevated temperature (>39.5°C), and kidney failure.

Diagnosis is based on clinical presentation. Laboratory findings may include decreased hemoglobin, thrombocytopenia, increased ESR and fat macroglobulinemia. Treatment is primarily supportive and may include fluid resuscitation and mechanical ventilation (with ARDS).

Interstitial Lung Disease

Interstitial lung disease refers to a group of disorders (>200), all characterized by parenchymal lung abnormalities. Interstitial lung disease can be divided into inflammatory disorders and granulomatous diseases. Examples include idiopathic pulmonary fibrosis, sarcoidosis, Wegner's granulomatosis, bronchiolitis obliterans, Langerhans cell histiocytosis, hypersensitivity pneumonitis, and certain connective tissue disorders and autoimmune diseases. Risk factors for developing ILD include smoking, toxin exposure, and chronic exposure to high concentrations of oxygen, radiation, and chemotherapy. Patients present with shortness of breath and exercise intolerance. They may also have fatigue and weight loss. Symptoms tend to progress slowly. The diagnosis is made by clinical history, chest x-ray, CT scan, pulmonary function tests, bronchoscopy, and biopsy. A sweat chloride test should be performed to rule out cystic fibrosis. Treatment should address the underlying cause. Management can also include chest physiotherapy, immunosuppressive drugs, corticosteroids, and oxygen. Lung transplantation is sometimes and an option for severe cases.

Aspiration of a Foreign Body

Aspiration of a foreign body is commonly seen in children. Frequently patients will initially experience **choking** followed by a persistent **cough** and the feeling the something is "stuck" in their throats. Hoarseness, wheezing or stridor may be heard, depending on the location of the blockage within the airway. If severe, the airway may be completely blocked, and this could cause patients to collapse and go into respiratory arrest. On exam, decreased breath sounds may be present on one side due to blockage of the main bronchus. Wheezing may also be heard in any portion of the lungs. *Diagnose* using an AP and lateral CXR and endoscopy may be used to diagnose and treat the condition. *Treatment* is focused on removing the object. In severe cases with complete airway blockage, the Heimlich maneuver should be given to forcefully expel the object from the airway. In emergency cases, an emergency tracheostomy may be performed to create a new airway below the level of the obstruction. In patients who are stable, bronchoscopy can be performed to physically remove the object.

Gastrointestinal System

Esophagus

ESOPHAGITIS

Esophagitis is inflammation of the **mucosal tissues of the esophagus**. There are several forms including reflux, infectious, eosinophilic, pill, and radiation/chemoradiation induced esophagitis. **Reflux esophagitis** (the most common type) occurs when the lower esophageal sphincter (LES) becomes lax and does not remain closed properly, therefore, stomach acids reflux into the esophagus. This causes inflammation which can eventually lead to ulceration. Patients may complain of GERD-type *symptoms* with a burning or bad taste in the mouth/throat, pain over the chest/ into the throat (which may mimic cardiac pain), and possibly a mild cough. They may experience N/V. If esophageal ulceration occurs, patients will have severe pain. If the ulcer is bleeding, vomiting of blood may occur which may have a coffee-ground appearance, or the patient may have a positive stool guaiac. Patients may become anemic. Treat reflux with proton pump inhibitors (PPIs are first line; typically treat 4-8 wks) or histamine-2-receptor antagonists (H2RAs), sucralfate, or occasionally cisapride (associated with serious cardiac arrhythmias/death). Treat the underlying cause of infectious esophagitis (e.g., nystatin, acyclovir, etc.). *Treatment* of eosinophilic esophagitis involves elimination diets, steroids, and PPIs. Avoid offending meds and instruct patients on proper pill-taking methods (8 oz. of water). Radiation-induced inflammation may take several months to heal after treatment is stopped, and may be treated with viscous lidocaine and sucralfate. Lifestyle modifications may also help (avoid spicy foods, fried foods, caffeine, and alcohol. D/C smoking). Since the cause of esophagitis varies, diagnosis is often made clinically or with endoscopy and possible cytology or biopsy. *Complications* include erosive esophagitis leading to bleeding, strictures, Barrett esophagus, and aspiration pneumonia.

ESOPHAGEAL STRICTURE

Esophageal stricture is a **narrowing of the esophagus** due to intrinsic narrowing, extrinsic restriction, or lower esophageal sphincter (LES) /dysmotility issues. There are a variety of causes including reflux, infectious, caustic ingestion, congenital, medication or radiation-induced, and cancer. The majority of cases are caused by reflux-induced strictures due to LES issues or dysmotility issues that result in scarring. This scarring can cause the LES to be narrowed, which prevents food from passing into the stomach properly. Suspect achalasia if liquids are also an issue. Patients may complain of difficulty swallowing (dysphagia), odynophagia, a sensation that food is "stuck" in their throat, heartburn, and chest pain. *Diagnosis* is made with a barium esophagram or upper GI endoscopy. *Treatment* involves use of proton pump inhibitors (PPIs) and dilating the sphincter to widen it. This can be accomplished during an EGD (esophagogastroduodenoscopy) by passing dilators, which gradually increase in diameter, through the sphincter. A balloon procedure can also be performed during EGD to widen the sphincter. A risk with both of these procedures is tearing of the esophagus, requiring surgical repair. If these treatments fail to relieve the symptoms, surgery may be needed to correct the sphincter. *Complications* include perforation, bleeding, bacteremia due to endoscopy, Barrett esophagus, and recurrent strictures.

ESOPHAGEAL ACHALASIA

Esophageal achalasia is a disorder of the **esophagus** that affects **motility**. It may be primary or secondary to other conditions. Achalasia is most common in middle-aged and older adults and can also be a genetic trait. Achalasia can be present in esophageal tumors, Zenker diverticulum, Chagas disease, nutcracker esophagus, and diffuse esophageal spasms. Patients present with dysphagia with both solids and liquids. Other *symptoms* might include pain, chest pain, heartburn, cough, or a slight regurgitation of food. *Diagnosis* includes barium swallow to rule out a mass or tumor. Diagnosis is confirmed when there is incomplete lower esophagus sphincter relaxation and aperistalsis in the lower portion of the esophagus per manometry. Laboratory results may show anemia or malnutrition. The most effective *treatments* are pneumatic dilation and surgical myotomy. Other options are Botox injections, and medications aimed at esophageal sphincter relaxation.

Mallory-Weiss Tear or Syndrome

Mallory-Weiss tear or syndrome is a non-penetrating, longitudinal laceration of the **esophageal mucosa** that occurs in the distal portion of the esophagus or proximal portion of the stomach. The tear can be caused by forceful vomiting or coughing or chronic alcohol use. Patients may be light-headed and describe an episode of vomiting or coughing followed by hematemesis (vomiting bright red blood). They may report dyspepsia and pain in the chest or abdomen or, if this has been going on for a period of time, they may experience melena (dark, tarry stools from upper GI bleeding). An esophagogastroduodenoscopy (EGD) will be done to confirm *diagnosis*, and cauterization may be performed if the bleeding has gone on for more than a few hours. Esophageal clips or endoscopic band ligation may also be performed. Most tears do not need to be surgically corrected and heal spontaneously as early as 96 hours. Antacids can be given to prevent further irritation of the tear. If there has been significant blood loss, a transfusion may be necessary to correct a volume-depletion anemia. *Complications* include shock, anemia, need for a blood transfusion, and dehydration.

Esophageal Varices

Esophageal varices most often occur along with **cirrhosis of the liver**, but any form of **liver disease** can lead to their development. With liver disease, blood flow through the liver is obstructed and slowed. This causes portal hypertension, pressure that builds up in the portal vein, which causes collateral vessels to form to bypass the portal system. This causes veins around the esophagus and upper stomach to swell and engorge (varices). Bleeding varices may occur when the portal-systemic pressure gradient reaches 10-12 mm Hg and is fatal in approximately 20% of patients. If varices bleed, patient will present with sudden, painless and often massive vomiting of blood. If bleeding is less severe, melena can be present. Also, patients may be asymptomatic from the esophageal varices themselves but will show signs of liver disease (e.g., jaundice, ascites, edema, easy bruising, malaise). They may have a history of alcoholism though not all forms of cirrhosis are caused by alcohol. *Diagnose* with endoscopy. If varices bleed, immediate endoscopic banding along with administering IV octreotide (a somatostatin analog) is the *treatment* of choice. Sclerotherapy is second-line. If bleeding cannot be controlled or recurs, a TIPS (transvenous intrahepatic portosystemic shunt) procedure can be used. Nonselective β-blockers (e.g., propranolol) may be given to prevent rupture of varices. *Complications* include shock, uncontrolled bleeding, and death.

GERD

Gastroesophageal reflux disease (GERD) is a chronic condition in which gastric contents reflux into the **esophagus**, more than is physiologically normal, causing burning pain and possibly tissue damage. The esophagus, stomach, or lower esophageal sphincter (LES) dysfunctions, causing gastric and sometimes duodenal contents to reflux into the esophagus. Patients usually complain of experiencing heartburn ≥2 days a week along with regurgitation and dysphagia. Occasionally atypical *symptoms* of a hoarse voice, coughing, wheezing, or noncardiac chest pain are present which warrants further investigation. *Diagnose* clinically if symptoms are typical and respond to therapy. Endoscopy (EGD) and, if normal, 24-hour pH monitoring are also used to establish a diagnosis. Esophageal manometry is helpful when evaluating for surgery. *Treatment* includes lifestyle modifications, acid-suppressing therapy, and surgery. Lifestyle modifications include elevating the head of the bed, avoiding eating 2-3 hours before bedtime, avoiding causative foods (e.g., coffee, chocolate, alcohol, tomato-based foods) or medications (e.g., anticholinergics, β-agonists, calcium channel blockers), and weight loss. Antacids, H2-receptor antagonists (e.g., famotidine, cimetidine), and proton pump inhibitors (PPIs; e.g., omeprazole, lansoprazole) can be used for acid-suppression. The first two work better for mild and moderate symptoms respectively, and PPIs work best for severe symptoms and erosive esophagitis. Treatment is typically 4-8 weeks. Surgery (usually fundoplication) may be indicted for those with serious esophagitis not fully responding to PPIs and if extraesophageal issues (e.g., hiatal hernia, respiratory/ENT side effects of GERD). *Complications* include esophagitis (50% of patients), ulcers, strictures, and Barrett esophagus with an increased risk of adenocarcinoma.

Stomach

PUD

Peptic ulcer disease (**PUD**) occurs in the **stomach or duodenum** and has several causes. The most common causes are use of **nonsteroidal anti-inflammatory medications** (NSAIDs: ibuprofen, naproxen, aspirin), and infection with ***H. pylori* bacteria**. Excessive acid production in the stomach due to a tumor can also break down the gastric mucosa and cause ulcers. Patients may complain of a burning or gnawing epigastric pain usually right after eating if a gastric ulcer or 2-3 hours after eating if it is a duodenal ulcer. The pain may be relieved with eating as food coats the stomach; though spicy foods can aggravate the pain. Patients may also feel bloated, have nausea/vomiting, heartburn, and chest pain. With bleeding of the ulcer, stools may be tarry (melena), and there may be blood in vomitus (hematemesis). Further investigation is needed if patients have anemia, bleeding, early satiety, or weight loss. Confirm *diagnosis* through endoscopy and test for *H. pylori*. *Treatment* is focused on treating the underlying cause. Discontinue NSAIDs and treat *H. pylori* infections with a combination of antibiotics and a proton pump inhibitor (PPI). Dietary changes to reduce acid secretion are recommended (avoid alcohol, caffeine, tobacco). Acid production is suppressed through PPIs (e.g., omeprazole, lansoprazole) or H2RAs (e.g., cimetidine, famotidine). Surgery is necessary and recommended within 12 hours if the ulcer has perforated. *Complications* include perforation, hemorrhage, gastric outlet obstruction, and a future risk for gastric cancer if *H. pylori* was responsible for the ulcer(s).

Gastric Cancer

Gastric cancer is the fourth leading cause of **cancer death** in the world, according to the WHO (World Health Organization), as of 2015. It is highest in Eastern Asia and Central/Eastern Europe. The incidence increases with age and accounts for almost 30,000 new cases in the US per year. It can be caused by infection with ***Helicobacter pylori* bacteria** which causes chronic inflammation in the gastric mucosa, leading to development of cancerous cells (typically adenocarcinoma) in the **stomach lining**. Eating a diet high in salt (e.g., processed meats, smoked, and pickled foods) as well as smoking have been linked to stomach cancer. Alcohol use may also play a role in the development of gastric cancer. Most *symptoms* are similar to GERD-type symptoms (e.g., dyspepsia, N/V) and treated at home with antacids. Therefore, most patients are not aware they have stomach cancer until the disease has progressed to an advanced stage and other physical symptoms appear. Other symptoms include abdominal pain not relieved by antacids, unintentional weight loss, chronic feeling of fullness, and tarry stools if bleeding is occurring. *Diagnose* with endoscopy and biopsy. Tumor markers CEA and CA 19-9 may be elevated (in 45-50% and ~20% of patients respectively). *Treatment* is with surgical removal of the malignant tissue (partial or total gastrectomy) and possibly radiation and/or chemotherapy. *Complications* include a high rate of recurrence and death. 5-year survival rate is 30%.

Pyloric Stenosis

Pyloric stenosis occurs in infants when the **pylorus**, or opening between the stomach and duodenum, becomes **hypertrophied**. This inhibits the transport of food from the stomach to the small intestine and may cause almost complete obstruction. Though there is no definite known cause, it is thought it may be genetic in nature. This is more common in first born males and usually presents between 3-6 weeks of age. The infant will have gradually worsening vomiting after meals that becomes projectile. The child will act fussy and still hungry after eating. and may have a slower degree of weight gain. Dehydration will eventually develop as well as constipation. On exam, an olive-shaped mass can be palpated in the abdomen due to the enlarged pylorus. *Diagnose* with an ultrasound and check for metabolic alkalosis. *Treatment* is by surgical correction (pyloromyotomy) of the pyloric sphincter and correction of metabolic alkalosis with chloride and potassium. This is usually a very successful surgery that results in full recovery from the condition.

Gastritis

Gastritis is inflammation of the mucosal lining of the stomach. Gastritis can be acute or chronic. Causes include *H pylori* infection, chronic use of NSAIDs, excessive alcohol consumption, bile reflux, and other chronic illnesses. Patients typically present with dyspepsia, nausea, vomiting, weight loss, and a full or bloated feeling. Patients sometimes present with gastrointestinal bleeding. The diagnosis is usually made clinically, but can include *H pylori* testing and endoscopy. Treatment includes antacids, H2 blockers, proton pump inhibitors, and antibiotics to eradicate *H pylori*.

Acute Abdomen

Acute abdomen is defined as the acute onset of severe abdominal pain. There are many possible causes of acute abdomen. It often requires surgical intervention. Patients can present with abdominal pain, fever, nausea, vomiting, diarrhea, or constipation. The physical exam may be significant for a patient who appears ill and has a tender, rigid abdomen. The physical exam should check for guarding, rebound, and the presence and quality of bowel sounds. A rectal exam is an essential part of the workup. The workup should include CBC, electrolytes, BUN/creatinine, LFTs, amylase, and lipase. All women of childbearing age should have a pregnancy test. Chest x-ray, abdominal x-ray, ultrasound, and CT can all be helpful in making the diagnosis. Surgical consultation and exploratory laparotomy are sometimes necessary.

Acute GI Bleed

Acute GI bleeding is a medical emergency. Bleeding may arise from the upper or lower GI tracts. Upper GI bleeding usually presents with hematemesis and melena. Lower GI bleeds can present with blood-streaked stools if the bleed is distal (rectosigmoid to anus), maroon colored stools for bleeds in the right colon or small intestine, and melena if the bleed is proximal to the ligament of Treitz. Massive bleeding can present with hematochezia. Immediate management includes resuscitation and stabilization of the patient. Patients should be made NPO, aggressive IV rehydration should be started, and a nasogastric (NG) tube should be inserted. Blood work should include a CBC, type and cross-match. The location of the bleed should be determined by history, exam findings, and possibly endoscopy, colonoscopy or nuclear bleeding scan. Once the source is determined, appropriate therapy should be initiated to stop the bleed.

Gallbladder

Cholelithiasis, Biliary Colic, and Cholangitis

Cholelithiasis is the development of **gallstones** in the gallbladder from cholesterol (80%) and other bile byproducts (20% are pigment stones: black or brown). These can block the ducts leading from the gallbladder, causing **cholecystitis** (inflammation of the gallbladder) or **cholangitis** (infection of the bile ducts). Most patients with cholelithiasis are asymptomatic (~60-80%). *Symptoms* can vary depending on which duct is blocked by the stone. Ducts leading to the pancreas can cause acute pancreatitis with severe abdominal pain radiating to the back and vomiting. Blockage of ducts leading to the liver can result in jaundice (as in cholangitis). Generally, if a stone blocks the cystic duct, patients may experience **biliary colic**: N/V, RUQ abdominal pain that may refer to the right scapular tip (Collins' sign), and bloating until the stone falls back into the gallbladder and the pain subsides. Patients may have several flare-ups of pain/biliary colic and may be advised to have elective surgery. **Cholangitis** presents with the classic triad (Charcot triad) of fever, RUQ pain, and jaundice. *Diagnose* cholelithiasis with ultrasound. Medical *treatment* options include oral bile salt therapy (i.e. ursodeoxycholic acid) and extracorporeal lithotripsy, especially if stones are small (<1 cm) and cholesterol-based. Cholecystectomy to remove the gallbladder/gallstones or removal of a stone from a duct may be necessary. Patients who do not undergo surgery for correction of this condition should be advised to avoid fatty foods that can aggravate the problem and contribute to enlargement of the gallstones or development of new stones. Treat uncomplicated cholangitis with antibiotics, and if acute/severe, emergent ERCP or PTC (for biliary drainage) or emergent surgery. *Complications* of cholelithiasis include ascending cholangitis, cholecystitis, and pancreatitis.

Cholecystitis

Cholecystitis is an inflammatory condition of the **gallbladder** which can be **acute** or **chronic**. Bile normally passes from the gallbladder to the small intestine to aid in digestion, but there is a **disruption** in this flow with cholecystitis. This usually occurs due to a **gallstone** (≥95% of cases; 80% are cholesterol stones and 20% are pigment stones) in the **cystic duct** causing bile to build up, leading to inflammation, swelling, and possibly a bacterial infection (cholangitis). **Chronic cholecystitis** refers to long-standing inflammation and recurrent episodes of biliary colic that causes progressive fibrosis of the gallbladder. Cholecystitis risks include being older, female, pregnant, obese, taking HRT/birth control, or having rapid weight loss. Patients often have prior attacks of biliary colic (i.e. without abdominal PE findings) before presenting with cholecystitis. Cholecystitis usually begins with severe, constant epigastric pain that lasts longer than colic (usually >6 hours) and localizes to the RUQ, often occurring after a fatty meal. Patients may guard, have pain aggravated by taking a deep breath during RUQ abdominal palpation (+ Murphy sign), or complain of referred right shoulder pain. Also, there may be nausea, vomiting, and fever (usually no fever in chronic cholecystitis). *Diagnose* through transabdominal ultrasound which is 90-95% sensitive and about 80% specific. Scintigraphy is an alternative and a CT may be necessary to view other structures. *Treat* with a cholecystectomy, usually done laparoscopically. *Complications* include cholangitis, empyema of the gallbladder, gangrene, perforation/peritonitis, sepsis, and pancreatitis.

Sphincter of Oddi Dysfunction

The sphincter of Oddi is the sheath of smooth muscle about the ends of the common bile duct and pancreatic duct at the wall of the duodenum. The sphincter controls the flow of bile and pancreatic enzymes into the duodenum as part of the digestive process. **Sphincter of Oddi dysfunction** (most common in females after cholecystectomy) occurs when the sphincter cannot properly open and close, resulting in obstructed flow of bile and pancreatic enzymes. Symptoms include right upper abdominal pain and/or epigastric pain, aggravated by intake of fatty foods. Patients may also develop pancreatitis with nausea, vomiting, and severe abdominal pain. Diagnosis is per laboratory testing of hepatic and pancreatic enzymes, quantitative hepatobiliary scintigraphy, and endoscopic retrograde cholangiopancreatography. Treatment may include dietary modification (low fat), antispasmodics, analgesics, nifedipine, and/or nitroglycerine. Surgical interventions include injection of botulinum toxin to relax the sphincter (endoscopic procedure) or ablation of the sphincter.

Liver

Hepatitis A, B, C, D, and E

Viral hepatitis is an infectious disease that causes hepatic inflammation and includes hepatitis viruses A, B, C, D, and E. There are various routes of transmission: Hep A (fecal-oral), Hep B & C (blood), Hep D (needle), Hep E (water). Hep A and E both cause **acute** infections lasting <6 months. Hepatitis B, C, and D can become **chronic** (may take decades) and may also develop into cancer. Hep D only occurs with Hep B. Most of the hepatitis cases in the U.S. are from Hep A, B, and C. The *incubation period* varies from 15-180 days depending on the type (lowest incubation time for Hep A and E; longest for Hep B, C and D). The *prodromal phase* begins with anorexia, N/V, malaise, fever, and occasionally urticaria and arthralgias. Next, the *icteric phase* begins with dark urine, pale-colored stools, jaundice, and possibly RUQ pain with hepatomegaly. Finally, the *convalescent phase*, when jaundice/symptoms resolve and LFTs return to normal.

Symptoms and Treatments

Hep A is transmitted through the fecal-oral route by infected individuals and can be contracted through contaminated food (especially raw/undercooked) and water. *Symptoms* generally resolve spontaneously within 2 months. **Hep B** is blood-borne and is contracted through contact with blood and body fluids of infected individuals (often sexually transmitted). **Hep C** is also contracted through blood and body fluids. It is the most serious form of viral hepatitis, 75-85% develop chronic infection, and it is the leading cause of liver transplants. *Diagnose* acute disease through positive serology tests: IgM anti-HAV (= Hep A); HBsAG and IgM anti-HBc (= Hep B); anti-HCV (= Hep C); anti-HDV (= Hep D); anti-HEV (= Hep E). Chronic Hep B: IgG anti-HBc becomes +. Chronic Hep C: both the anti-HCV and HCV-RNA will remain + ≥6 months after the initial infection. *Treatment* involves supportive care. Treat chronic Hep B with pegylated interferon (PEG-IFN), entecavir, or tenofovir. Treat chronic Hep C with PEG-IFN and ribavirin. There are currently vaccines for Hep A, B, and E. *Complications* of Hep B, C, and D include fibrosis, cirrhosis, hepatic failure, and liver cancer.

Cirrhosis

Cirrhosis is a chronic, usually irreversible disease of the **liver** where, due to injury, normal tissue is replaced with **nodules and fibrotic tissue** (scarring). It is usually caused by **chronic viral hepatitis** (usually Hep C, but also Hep B with or without Hep D) or **alcoholic liver disease**. Often *signs and symptoms* are not present for years, until cirrhosis is in the late-stage. These include fatigue, weight-loss, jaundice, easy bruising and bleeding, pruritus, ascites, spider angiomas, gynecomastia, and confusion. *Diagnose* through liver function tests (LFTs), coagulation studies, serologic tests for hepatitis, imaging studies (e.g., U/S), and liver biopsy. *Treat* the underlying cause, treat complications as they arise, and offer supportive care. Lifestyle changes include discontinuing alcohol and drugs that harm the liver (e.g., NSAIDs, erythromycin, ketoconazole, etc.) and nutritional support (e.g., vit D, zinc, folate). Treat esophageal varices and portal hypertension with β-blockers, and a TIPS procedure (transjugular intrahepatic portosystemic shunt) may be necessary to control complications of portal hypertension. Screen patients with an U/S for hepatocellular carcinoma every 6 months. Assess the severity of the disease with the Child-Turcotte-Pugh and MELD (Model for End-Stage Liver Disease) scoring systems. A liver transplant may be necessary if disease is severe (in general, refer for a liver transplant evaluation if MELD score ≥15). *Complications* include portal hypertension, pulmonary hypertension, esophageal varices, ascites, spontaneous bacterial peritonitis, hepatorenal syndrome, hepatic encephalopathy, and liver cancer.

Hepatic Neoplasms

Hepatic neoplasms may be benign, malignant, or metastases from other primary tumors. Examples of **benign neoplasms** include hemangiomas (most common benign tumor), focal nodular hyperplasia, and hepatocellular adenoma (usually found in women of child-bearing age using estrogen-based OCPs). Many of these are found incidentally on U/S and usually require no treatment. However, when hepatocellular adenomas are ≥5 cm, they are usually resected due to the increased risk of hemorrhage and malignant transformation. **Primary malignant hepatic neoplasms** include hepatocellular carcinoma (HCC), cholangiocarcinoma, and hepatoblastoma (a rare tumor in infants or children). While uncommon, HCC is the most common primary liver cancer and is usually linked to hepatitis C infection. **Liver metastases** are by far the overall most common cause of hepatic neoplasms. They usually arise from the GI tract, breast, lung, pancreas, kidney, or skin. *Signs and symptoms* of hepatic neoplasms vary and may be absent or vague and nonspecific. They include weight loss, anorexia, fever, N/V, fatigue, ascites, edema, and possibly jaundice or abdominal pain. *Diagnosis* is through imaging studies (U/S, CT, MRI) and biopsy. *Treatment* is tailored toward the specific neoplasm and range from no treatment to resection, radiation, and chemotherapy. *Complications* include hemorrhage, liver failure, and death.

Additional Hepatic Diseases

Liver Abscess

Liver abscess may be pyogenic (polymicrobial), amebic (*Entamoeba histolytica)*, or fungal (*Candida* spp). Liver abscess is usually associated with biliary tract disease but can develop from penetrating trauma, systemic infection, or intraabdominal fistula. Multiple abscesses may occur. Liver abscesses are most common in neonates and in older adults. The disorder is characterized by fever, chills, anorexia, general malaise, and abdominal pain (RUQ, referred to right shoulder) and is fatal if untreated. Complications may include empyema, sepsis, and peritonitis. Diagnosis is per physical exam (hepatosplenomegaly often present), decreased basilar breath sounds, hepatic friction rub, and jaundice. Laboratory studies include CBC, liver function tests, blood cultures, abscess culture (needle aspiration), and enzyme immunoassay (if *E. histolytica* suspected*)*. Imaging may include CT, US, x-ray, and radionuclide scanning. Treatment includes identifying and treating underlying cause, antimicrobials, and percutaneous drainage and aspiration.

Hepatic Vein Thrombosis and Gilbert's Syndrome

Hepatic disease	Characteristics	Diagnosis and treatment
Hepatic vein thrombosis (AKA Budd-Chiari syndrome)	Obstruction of hepatic venous blood flow results in hepatosplenomegaly progressing to liver failure. Characterized by abdominal pain, peripheral edema, ascites, jaundice, and dilated collateral veins. Stasis ulcers may occur. The syndrome may be acute, subacute, chronic, or fulminant.	Diagnosis is per aspiration and testing of ascites fluid, which may show increased protein (>2 g/dL), WBC <500/mcL, and albumin gradient <1.1, and liver biopsy. Imaging may include US, CT, MRI, and venography. Treatment is with low sodium diet, paracentesis, portal decompression, angioplasty, anticoagulants, diuretics, and thrombolytics. Liver transplantation may be necessary.
Gilbert's syndrome	This autosomal recessive disorder is considered benign and is characterized by inability to adequately process bilirubin. Most people are asymptomatic or have only slight intermittent jaundice (usually beginning in adolescence).	Diagnosis is per evidence of hyperbilirubinemia without hemolysis or liver disease. No treatment is indicated.

Fulminant Hepatic Failure

Fulminant hepatic failure is a severe acute infection of the liver that can result in hepatic necrosis, encephalopathy, and death within 1-2 weeks. Most hepatitis is caused by infection with hepatitis viruses A, B, C, D, or E, but it can also be caused by numerous viruses, toxic chemicals (carbon tetrachloride) metabolic diseases (Wilson's disease) and drugs, such as acetaminophen. Fulminant hepatitis can result from any of these factors. Survival rates vary from 50-85%. Fulminant liver failure can be divided into 3 stages according to the duration from jaundice to encephalopathy:

- Hyperacute liver failure: 0-7 days.
- Acute liver failure: 8-28 days.
- Subacute liver failure: 28-72 days.

Symptoms	Diagnosis and treatment
Symptoms vary depending on the severity, but may present with: Poor feeding/anorexia. Increased intracranial pressure with cerebral edema and encephalopathy. Coagulopathies. Renal failure. Electrolyte imbalances	Diagnosis is per liver function tests, prothrombin time, CT or MRI, and liver biopsy. Treatment includes: Identify and treat underlying cause. Intracranial pressure monitoring and treatment. Diuresis. Liver transplantation may be necessary.

Workup for Cirrhosis of the Liver

The **workup** to determine the **cause of liver failure** includes laboratory examinations, such as liver function tests (LFTs), CBC, and albumin. Hepatitis screening should be performed. Ultrasound, CT, and MRI imaging may be helpful to assess the extent of disease. Liver biopsy is often needed to determine the cause. Cirrhosis is generally irreversible. Treatment is aimed at halting progression and alleviating symptoms. Alcohol use should be stopped. Treatments for hepatitis include interferon and other medications. Potentially hepatotoxic drugs like acetaminophen should be stopped. Ascites can be treated with paracentesis, which usually needs to be repeated. Patients with advanced disease should be considered for liver transplantation.

Pancreas and Appendix

Acute and Chronic Pancreatitis

Pancreatitis is inflammation of the **pancreas** and can be acute or chronic. The most common cause is **cholelithiasis** (gallstones causing duct blockage) and next is **excessive alcohol consumption** (in both binge drinkers and chronic alcoholics). Pancreatitis may occur after endoscopic retrograde cholangiopancreatography (ERCP). Certain drugs (e.g., ACE inhibitors, sulfa drugs, tetracycline), infections, cystic fibrosis, trauma, and high calcium or triglyceride blood levels can also lead to pancreatitis. Patients usually recover from the **acute** form within days/weeks. Smoking and alcohol use increase the risk of developing **chronic pancreatitis** which forms after repeated damage to the pancreas causing fibrosis, calcification, and ductal damage. The primary *symptom* of pancreatitis is constant, boring abdominal pain that radiates to the back which may be relieved by sitting upright and leaning forward. Other symptoms include N/V, anorexia, tachycardia, and fever. In the chronic form, diarrhea, weight loss, steatorrhea, and DM may develop later in the disease as pancreatic enzyme production declines. *Diagnose* pancreatitis clinically and with serum amylase and lipase levels (3 times the normal range for acute pancreatitis; generally lower in chronic pancreatitis and therefore not as helpful). Lipase is more sensitive and specific than amylase. Imaging studies (e.g., U/S, CT, MRCP) are helpful if diagnosis is unclear and to rule out cancer. *Treatment* of pancreatitis is mostly symptomatic. Early IV fluids (in the first 12-24 hrs.) and pain management are necessary. Enteral nutrition (nasogastric tube) usually begins within 48 hrs. Avoid TPN which has been linked to infectious complications. Sometimes the damage to the pancreas is severe enough to warrant surgical resection of a portion of the organ. Patients with chronic pancreatitis may require pancreatic enzyme replacement. *Complications* include pseudocyst formation, infection, hemorrhage, necrosis, perforation, SIRS (systemic inflammatory response syndrome), and organ failure.

Pancreatic Neoplasms

Pancreatic cancer is the 4th leading cause of **cancer deaths** in the U.S. for both men and women. There are 2 main categories: **exocrine** (most common, >95%; most aggressive) and **endocrine neoplasms. Adenocarcinoma** accounts for >90 % of exocrine tumors and usually arise from the duct cells vs. the acinar cells (produce digestive enzymes). Endocrine neoplasms, also termed **pancreatic neuroendocrine tumors (NET)** or **islet cell tumors**, are rare and can be functioning (produce hormones) or nonfunctioning. Both types of pancreatic cancer are usually *diagnosed* late in the disease process which partially accounts for the poor prognosis (5-year survival: <5% for locally advanced disease and <2% for metastatic pancreatic cancer). Risk factors for developing pancreatic CA include chronic pancreatitis, smoking, and obesity. *Signs and symptoms* include weight loss, pain radiating to the back, jaundice, dark urine, pruritus, and new onset DM. Physical exam may show a positive Courvoisier sign: the presence of a palpable pancreatic head tumor that can feel like an enlarged gallbladder. *Diagnose* with imaging studies (e.g., endoscopic ultrasound, CT, MRI, MRCP, ERCP) as well as with a biopsy. CA 19-9 can be used to track progress of the disease. Treatment depends on the stage and accessibility to the tumor(s). Options include resection (e.g., Whipple procedure also known as pancreaticoduodenectomy) although most are unresectable at the time of the diagnosis, radiation, and chemotherapy. *Complications* include metastases, malabsorption, biliary obstruction, liver failure, gastric outlet obstruction, bowel obstruction, and death.

Pancreatic Neuroendocrine Tumors

Pancreatic neuroendocrine tumors are islet cells tumors that may be functional (producing hormones) or non-functional (most common). Non-functional tumors are classified as nonfunctional islet cell tumors but functional tumors are classified according to the type of hormone that they produce: gastrinoma (gastrin), glucagonoma (glucagon), insulinoma (insulin), somatostatinoma (somatostatin), and VIPoma (vasoactive intestinal peptide). These tumors can be benign or malignant but tend to grow slowly. The pathophysiology is not clear. Functional tumors cause symptoms related to the type of hormone that is being over-produced. For example, glucagonoma may result in hyperglycemia, insulinoma in hypoglycemia, and gastrinoma in peptic ulcer, GI upset, and diarrhea. Diagnosis is by imaging (CT, MRI, PET scan) and tissue biopsy (FNA with endoscopic US). Blood tests include chromogranin A and pancreatic polypeptide as these are often elevated. Tests used to track whether the tumor is growing or responding to treatment include carbohydrate antigen 19-9 and carcinoembryonic antigen. Treatment includes surgical excision, chemotherapy, and/or radiation. Clinical trials may also be available.

Appendicitis

Appendicitis is inflammation of the **vermiform appendix** and is a medical emergency. This can occur due to an obstruction from lymphoid hyperplasia, impacted feces (fecalith), infection, or a foreign body (e.g., undigested seeds). Certain forms of cancer and parasites can also cause inflammation. Blockage of the appendix will lead to swelling, inflammation, infection, and possibly abscess formation. Patients may complain of periumbilical pain that gradually worsens and eventually migrates to the right lower quadrant (RLQ) at McBurney's point. Nausea, vomiting, anorexia, fever, diarrhea or constipation may also be present. On exam, patients have rebound tenderness, guarding, and may have a positive Rovsing, psoas, or obturator sign. *Diagnose* clinically and confirm with an ultrasound or CT scan. However, do not delay surgery for an imaging study if the patient presents with classic signs and symptoms. CT is preferred for atypical presentations. The WBC count will be elevated, often 11,000-15,000/μL. Appendicitis should be immediately *treated* with IV antibiotics (usually 3rd generation cephalosporins) and surgery to prevent eventual rupture and subsequent peritonitis. Appendectomy can usually be performed laparoscopically. *Complications* include abscess formation, rupture, and peritonitis.

Intestines

Celiac Disease

Celiac disease is an immune-mediated inflammatory response due to the inability to process dietary gluten, the storage protein of wheat, rye, and barley. This causes a delayed hypersensitivity reaction (48-72 hrs) that results in damage to the **small intestine villi** with villous atrophy which causes malabsorption. There is a genetic predisposition to developing this chronic condition and mainly affects those of Northern European descent. *Signs and symptoms* include abdominal pain and bloating, N/V, diarrhea, light-colored, very foul-smelling stool, steatorrhea, constipation, fatigue, weight loss, anemia, osteoporosis, muscle weakness and paresthesias, hormonal issues, and dermatitis herpetiformis. It may present as failure to thrive in infants or children. *Diagnosis* is made with immunoglobulin A anti-tissue transglutaminase antibody (IgA TTG). If younger than 2 years old, combine with the IgG-deamidated gliadin peptide test. Confirmation must be made through multiple biopsy sites of the of the duodenum. Supporting data are obtained through complete blood count (CBC), comprehensive chemistry panel, vitamin D, vitamin B-12, and bone density tests.

Treatment involves complete dietary restriction of gluten. Patients often improve within 1-2 weeks of being on a gluten-free diet. Correct vitamin deficiencies. Refer patients to a dietician, and regular follow-ups are recommended for monitoring symptoms. *Complications* include refractory disease, collagenous sprue, and intestinal lymphomas.

Diverticular Disease

Diverticula are outpouchings in the **intestine** that commonly develop during the aging process. True diverticula (e.g., Meckel diverticula) involve all layers of the GI tract which are the mucosa, submucosa, muscularis propria, and serosa/adventitia. However, **colonic diverticula**, which will be discussed here, are pseudo-diverticula and only involve the **mucosal and submucosal layers**. They can occur anywhere along the intestinal tract, but are most common in the sigmoid colon. **Diverticulosis** is asymptomatic diverticula. **Diverticulitis** involves inflammation of the diverticula and possibly occurs when digestive matter becomes trapped within these outpouchings leading to swelling and possible infection. Diverticula can rupture and bleed if the condition becomes severe. Patients will generally complain of left lower quadrant abdominal pain with changes in bowel habits. Bloating, gas, constipation, diarrhea, N/V, and fever may also be present. *Diagnose* clinically and confirm with a CT scan. Diverticulitis, if uncomplicated and mild, is generally treated with a clear liquid diet and possibly broad-spectrum oral antibiotics for 7-10 days (e.g., ciprofloxacin + metronidazole; trimethoprim/sulfamethoxazole + metronidazole; Augmentin®; or moxifloxacin). After symptoms improve in 48-72 hours, advance diet as tolerated. If severe or complicated diverticulitis, admit, keep NPO, and treat with IV fluids and IV antibiotics. Diverticulitis usually resolves without surgery, but resection of the affected portion of the intestine may be necessary in severe cases. Avoidance of small particulate matter in the diet, such as foods with seeds (sesame seeds, berry seeds, etc.) and popcorn, is no longer recommended. *Complications* of diverticular disease include GI bleeding, perforation, abscess or fistula formation, and peritonitis.

Irritable Bowel Syndrome

Irritable bowel syndrome (**IBS**) is a functional **GI disorder** causing abdominal pain, altered stool consistency, and/or altered bowel habits. It is very common and may affect up to 20% of Americans. The cause is unknown but it usually occurs in response to stressors, either psychological or physical, and can be severe enough to be debilitating. Chronic fatigue, dyspepsia, depression, and fibromyalgia are common comorbidities. Patients may complain of intermittent periods of bloating, painful gas, postprandial urgency, mucorrhea, diarrhea, and constipation. Some patients may have predominantly diarrhea (IBS-D) or constipation (IBS-C) while others alternate between the two (IBS-M, "mixed"). A pattern of *symptoms* may be discernible after people eat certain foods or during periods of stress. IBS used to be considered a diagnosis of exclusion. *Diagnosis* is made clinically following the Rome IV criteria: abdominal pain 1 day/week in the last 3 months with 2 or more of the following: related to defecation, associated with change in stool frequency, or associated with change in stool form. *Treatment* is directed at the symptom. Fiber supplements may help with constipation and diarrhea. Typically, a normal diet may be followed. However, patients may benefit from avoiding foods that lead to bloating (e.g., legumes, cabbage) and avoiding possible triggers like lactose or gluten. Some medications used in IBS include anticholinergics, antispasmodics, antidiarrheals, prokinetics, TCAs, and IBS agents (e.g., lubiprostone, linaclotide). *Complications* include interference with daily activities and work, hemorrhoids, and malnutrition.

Crohn's Disease

Crohn's disease is a **chronic inflammatory bowel disease** that can affect *any* portion of the digestive tract, from the mouth to the anus. It causes **transmural inflammation** in the mucosal lining of the GI tract, and patients usually experience periods of remission. It is usually diagnosed during the teens or 20's and there is no cure for Crohn's disease. The cause is not known, but it is proposed to be due to a bacterial infection, an autoimmune response, environmental factors like smoking, and predisposing genetic factors. Patients with Crohn's disease will complain of abdominal pain and chronic diarrhea with or without blood, fever, a poor appetite, and weight loss. Because Crohn disease can occur at any point in the digestive tract, *symptoms* may be more focused on a particular area. *Diagnose* through clinical assessment, endoscopy/colonoscopy with biopsy, imaging studies (e.g., CT), and inflammatory markers like CRP and ESR. During endoscopy "skip" lesions may be noted as well as granulomas (pathognomonic) on biopsy. *Treatment* is symptomatic with the goal being to reduce inflammation within the digestive tract. This can be accomplished with anti-inflammatory drugs (e.g., mesalamine, which is a 5-ASA or aminosalicylate), steroids, antibiotics (e.g., metronidazole, ciprofloxacin), immunomodulators (e.g., methotrexate), and biologics (e.g., infliximab). Antidiarrheals like loperamide are useful, but should be avoided in active colitis due to an increased risk of developing toxic megacolon. Surgery is usually necessary at some point in the course of the disease to treat complications. *Complications* include anemia, abscesses, fistulas, increased risk of cancer, bowel obstruction, and toxic megacolon.

Ulcerative Colitis

Ulcerative colitis (**UC**) is a **chronic inflammatory bowel disease** that *only* affects the **mucous membranes** lining the rectum and large intestine causing bloody diarrhea. It begins distally, typically in the rectum, and moves proximally in a continuous pattern with a clearly-defined margin. There are periods of flare-ups and remission. The etiology of UC is not understood, but it is thought to be due to multiple factors including environmental, genetic, and immune-mediated ones. Stress, NSAID use, and drinking milk may exacerbate or trigger UC. Unlike Crohn disease, cigarette smoking is actually protective in UC. Patients complain of abdominal pain and cramps with bloody diarrhea, sometimes with mucus/pus, and tenesmus. In severe cases fever, malaise, anorexia, and weight loss may be present. UC may have extraintestinal *signs and symptoms* which include uveitis, arthralgias, and aphthous ulcers. *Diagnosis* is made with sigmoidoscopy or colonoscopy with biopsy. However, caution should be taken in severe disease due to the risk of perforation from the endoscopy. Test stool for infectious cause. *Treat* with 5-ASA anti-inflammatory drugs (e.g., sulfasalazine, mesalamine) and steroids. 5-ASAs should be continued after steroids are tapered. There are immunosuppressants (e.g., cyclosporine, tacrolimus) and biologics (e.g., infliximab, adalimumab) available that may help if patients are steroid-resistant or have severe disease. Antidiarrheals and pain relievers may also be helpful. If mucosal damage is severe, hospitalization and surgery may be necessary to resect the damaged portion of the large intestine. *Complications* include anemia, perforation, colon cancer, ankylosing spondylitis, and toxic megacolon.

Review Video: Ulcerative Colitis
Visit mometrix.com/academy and enter code: 584881

Lactose Intolerance

Lactose intolerance develops in those individuals who are lacking in the enzyme **lactase** which breaks down the disaccharide **sugar** in milk. **Primary lactose intolerance** is an acquired lactase deficiency that occurs after the infant is weaned, and occurs in 75% of the world's population. It is especially high in the Asian, Hispanic, Native American, African American, and African populations reaching up to 98% in Southeast Asians. **Secondary deficiencies** occur due to damage to the mucosa of the small intestine and is common after viral gastroenteritis. Patients will regain lactase activity as the mucosa heals. Patients may complain of bloating, gas, abdominal pain, nausea, and cramping diarrhea usually within 30 mins. of consuming dairy. *Diagnosis* of true lactose intolerance can be accomplished several different ways, but the H_2 breath test is typically used. Hydrogen levels are measured in the breath at various intervals before and after patients are given a lactose-rich drink. These should remain low, but will become elevated if lactose intolerant. Another test is the lactose tolerance test which is rarely used. After fasting overnight, a baseline glucose level is measured, then the patient is given a dairy-rich drink and blood glucose levels are measured over two hours. If glucose levels remain low, there is a deficiency in lactase. *Treatment* is with dietary changes to avoid lactose-rich foods and beverages. Typically, yogurt and cheeses are tolerated better and most patients may ingest up to 375mL of lactose milk without symptoms. Lactose-free milk as well as OTC lactase preparations are available. Calcium supplementation is usually necessary. The primary possible *complication* is osteopenia.

Small Intestinal Diseases

Small intestinal diseases	Characteristics	Diagnosis and treatment
Bacterial overgrowth syndrome	Slow motility results in overgrowth of bacteria in small intestines, resulting in malabsorption. Characterized by abdominal cramping and distention, diarrhea, flatulence. Some may develop weight loss and malnutrition.	Diagnosis: 10^5 bacteria CFU/mL in aspirant from proximal jejunum, positive hydrogen and methane breath tests, and imaging. Treatment includes antibiotics and dietary modification (high fat, low carbohydrate and fiber).
Mesenteric ischemia	Results from impaired blood flow to the small intestines and may be acute (occlusion caused by a clot) or chronic, developing over time.	Diagnosis is per symptoms, ultrasound, and angiography.
	Acute: Severe abdominal pain, fever, nausea and vomiting, and urge to defecate.	Treatment: Acute (such as occlusion with a clot) requires immediate surgical intervention.
	Chronic: Abdominal pain one-half hour after eating, worsening, and then disappearing with one to 3 hours.	Chronic is treated with angioplasty or open surgical repair.

Short Gut (Bowel) Syndrome

Short gut (bowel) syndrome occurs when removal of part of the small intestine results in a malabsorptive condition. Symptoms relate to the amount of bowel removed and the area of resection:

- Resection of the terminal ileum interferes with absorption of bile salts and vitamin B12. If <100 cm removed, malabsorption of bile salts causes watery diarrhea. Treatment includes salt binding resins (cholestyramine 2 to 4 g three times daily). If >100 cm removed, steatorrhea with resultant malabsorption of fat-soluble vitamins occurs. Additional treatment includes low fat diet, vitamins, and calcium supplements to prevent oxalate kidney stone.
- Resection of >40-50% of small bowel results in weight loss, diarrhea, and electrolyte imbalance.

- If colon and 100cm of proximal jejunum are retained, a lowfat, high complex carbohydrate diet, and electrolytes may maintain nutrition, but if the colon is removed, 200 cm of jejunum is required for adequate nutrition. Otherwise, parenteral nutrition is required, and this can lead to liver failure and death or liver/intestine transplantation.

INTUSSUSCEPTION

Intussusception is a **telescoping of the intestine** inside an adjacent portion of intestine causing **bowel obstruction** and possible **ischemia**. It usually occurs in children between 6 months and 3 years, affects boys more often, and is fatal in 2-5 days if untreated. This is rare in adults, usually involves the colon, and is typically due to cancer. There may be a "lead point" or trigger found (e.g., Meckel diverticulum, polyp, lymphoid hyperplasia) usually in adults and older children that provides an explanation for the intussusception point. In 1998 the rotavirus vaccine, RotaShield, was introduced and was linked to an increased risk of intussusception. It was promptly removed from the market in 1999, and newer vaccines (RotaTeq and Rotarix) since released have not been linked with intussusception. *Symptoms* include vomiting, fever, intense colicky pain that may later become constant, and lethargy. They may have diarrhea with "currant jelly" stools because of the frank blood that is present, but this is a late finding. On exam, there may be a palpable abdominal mass. *Diagnosis* is made with ultrasound; either a target (donut) sign or pseudokidney sign may be noted. *Treatment* is usually successful with a barium or air enema. This forces the bowel to straighten and slides the telescoped portion of the bowel back to normal. Avoid enemas if a perforation is suspected. If there is damaged or dead tissue, surgery is necessary to resect the ischemic or dead portion of bowel. A laparotomy is usually necessary in adults due to the presence of a lead point. *Complications* include dehydration, bleeding, infection, gangrene, perforation, shock, and death.

Colon

Colonic and Anorectal Diseases

Colonic/Anorectal diseases	Characteristics	Diagnosis and treatment
Antibiotic colitis	Antibiotics alter the balance of bacteria, usually causing overgrowth of *Clostridioides difficile,* characterized by severe watery diarrhea, dehydration, fever, abdominal cramping, and nausea. Toxic megacolon, kidney failure, bowel perforation, and death may occur.	Diagnosis is per symptoms, multiple stool specimens for C&S, blood tests (increased WBC), and sometimes colonoscopy or imaging. Treatment may include stopping triggering antibiotic, and treating with effective antibiotic (metronidazole, vancomycin, fidaxomicin), or fecal microbial transplantation,
Radiation colitis	Inflammation of colon from radiation therapy involving the abdomen, rectum, or pelvis, resulting in nausea, vomiting, stomach cramps, and diarrhea, rectal bleeding, and/or rectal mucous discharge. Acute symptoms begin during treatment, and symptoms often persist for about 8 weeks after radiation has stopped. In some cases, a chronic inflammation can occur with symptoms persisting for months or years.	Diagnosis based on symptoms. Treatment may include antidiarrheals, analgesia, steroids, antibiotics and dietary modifications.
Neutropenic colitis	Injury to intestinal mucosa resulting from immunocompromise or chemotherapy (which can directly damage the mucosa). Characterized by colonic edema and intramural bacterial invasion resulting in nausea, vomiting, abdominal pain, fever, and diarrhea.	Diagnosis is per symptoms and CT. Treatment may include bowel rest, abdominal decompression, antibiotics, and TPN. Surgical intervention may be necessary with risk of perforation.
Lymphocytic colitis	Inflammatory cells in the colon cause inflammation, abdominal pain, joint pain, fatigue, and watery diarrhea. Trigger may be medications (NSAIDS, statins, antidepressants, diabetes medications, and acid reflux medications).	Diagnosis is per blood tests, tests for celiac disease, and stool specimens as well as colonoscopy. Treatment may include antidiarrheals, steroids, cholestyramine and dietary modifications, such as excluding caffeine, high fat foods, dairy foods, and artificial sweeteners.

Colonic/Anorectal diseases	Characteristics	Diagnosis and treatment
Ischemic colitis	Results from hypoperfusion of the colon, resulting in abdominal pain, GI bleeding, fever, and diarrhea.	Diagnosis is per colonoscopy and imaging. Laboratory tests may show increased WBC count and decreased serum bicarbonate. Treatment is supportive with bowel rest for mild to moderate disease, but severe ischemia may require surgical excision of damaged bowel.

Toxic Megacolon

Toxic megacolon is an acute, transmural **inflammation of the colonic mucosa** that causes dysfunction and severe, nonobstructive dilatation that can be life-threatening. This medical emergency usually occurs in patients who suffer from **inflammatory bowel disease (IBD)**, but may also be seen in Hirschsprung disease, infections, and pseudomembranous colitis due to antibiotic use. Patients may complain of abdominal distention, abdominal pain, diarrhea, usually have a fever, and may appear dehydrated. Toxic megacolon can progress to the development of symptoms of shock (e.g., hypotension, tachycardia, tachypnea, altered mental status). *Diagnosis* is made clinically and with abdominal x-rays which show the dilated colon (>6cm). This condition can lead to shock and death, so prompt *treatment* is necessary. WBCs may be elevated with a left shift, the patient may be anemic, and potassium may be decreased if patients are dehydrated. The colon is rested for 24 hours along with decompression (e.g., NG tube, rolling techniques) to try to reduce the distention. If this is not effective, surgery is usually performed to resect the affected section of the colon. Patients should be rehydrated with IV fluids and electrolyte imbalances should be corrected. IV steroids are given to reduce inflammation within the colon along with IV antibiotics. *Complications* include perforation, sepsis, and death.

Bowel Obstruction

A **bowel obstruction** can be caused by **improper function of the intestines** or by a **mechanical obstruction** (something is blocking the way). Improper functioning of the bowel is not caused by a mechanical obstruction, but is due to halted peristalsis, and is referred to as an *ileus* or *paralytic ileus*. It can be due to medications, infection, ischemia, injury, or manipulation during surgery. A mechanical obstruction is divided into **small (SBO)**, which is more common, or **large bowel obstruction (LBO)** and may be partial or complete. Mechanical obstruction of the bowel can occur from tumors, adhesions, volvulus, hernias, foreign objects, or impacted stool. With SBO, patients may complain of abdominal pain and cramping in the absence of regular bowel movements or gas (esp. if a complete obstruction). Patients may have vomiting and a full, bloated feeling. With a complete obstruction, a severe form of constipation (obstipation) ensues. On exam, bowel sounds may be high-pitched or tingling in nature early on, but eventually there may be absent bowel sounds. LBO's typically have milder symptoms that progress slower, but with marked abdominal distension. An ileus has diminished bowel sounds and usually less abdominal cramping. *Diagnose* with plain x-rays and further studies with CT may be necessary. CT's are the imaging choice for LBOs. *Treatment* involves bowel rest, NG tube suction to decompress the gut, IV fluids, antiemetics, and antibiotics (that cover gram neg. and anaerobic organisms). If the condition is severe (e.g., signs of ischemia/strangulation/volvulus) or does not improve with conservative management, surgery is necessary. Surgery should not be delayed if there is a complete obstruction. *Complications* include perforation, peritonitis, sepsis, bowel infarction, gangrene, and death.

Colonic Polyps and Colorectal Cancer, FAP, and Lynch Syndrome

Colonic polyps are slow-growing growths on the **colonic mucosa** that are common and increase with age. They have the potential for **malignant transformation** (<1%), and therefore, patients should be screened for colon cancer starting at the age of 50 and repeated every 10 years. The process of malignant transformation takes approximately 10 years and so this is a very preventable condition. **Colorectal cancer** is the 2nd leading cause of **cancer death** in the U.S. It usually arises from an **adenomatous polyp**. Risk factors for colorectal CA include eating processed or red meats, family history, sedentary lifestyle, obesity, and smoking/alcohol use. Patients with **familial adenomatous polyposis (FAP)** have hundreds of polyps resulting in cancer by the age of 40 and so a colectomy is performed when diagnosed. **Lynch syndrome** or **hereditary nonpolyposis colorectal cancer (HNPCC)** results in colorectal CA by the mid 40's; it is also linked with other CAs like uterine and ovarian). Patients with a FH of colon CA must be screened earlier (10 years before the age of the patient's 1st degree relative's diagnosis). There are typically no *signs or symptoms* of polyps or cancer until the neoplasm becomes large. However, there may be rectal bleeding, pain, cramps, changes in bowel habits, or signs of obstruction if the polyp or mass is large. *Diagnosis* is made with colonoscopy and biopsy, and further investigation with a CT as necessary. Also test for blood using a fecal occult blood test or fecal immunochemical test. *Treat* polyps by removal and cancer with resection and radiation and/or chemotherapy. Colorectal CA stages are as follows: Stage 0 = carcinoma in situ; Stage I = local involvement to the submucosal layer; Stage II = local involvement to the muscularis propria; Stage III = lymph node or regional involvement; Stage IV = distant metastases. Monitor progress with CEA levels. *Complications* of colorectal CA include bleeding, metastases, and death.

Anorectal Abscess and Fistula

An **anorectal abscess**, or localized infection in the **anal or rectal areas**, can have several causes. An **anal fissure** can become infected or an **anal gland** can become blocked, leading to abscess formation. Diverticulitis, Crohn disease, pelvic inflammatory disease, and anal intercourse can place a patient at risk for developing an anorectal abscess. These can be perianal (most common), ischiorectal, intersphincteric, or supralevator (least common) abscesses. An anorectal abscess will cause patients significant pain with the development of an indurated, inflamed area, and may feel like a hard, hot lump. Patients may have very painful bowel movements and may develop constipation because of the fear of having a bowel movement. If the abscess ruptures, pus may be discharged through the rectum. *Diagnosis* is made per clinical assessment/digital exam. A CT may be necessary if the lesion is located deep or high, toward the intestines. *Treat* with incision and drainage (I&D) and pack with iodophor gauze (remove after 24 hours). Sitz baths can help with some of the inflammation, and prescribe antibiotics if the patient is febrile, immunocompromised, or the infection is severe. If the abscess is deep or extensive, surgery may be necessary.

Anorectal fistulas are tracts that usually run between the **anus and the superficial skin**. This is a common complication of an anorectal abscesses and can also occur due to Crohn disease, diverticulitis, and trauma. There is usually a h/o recurrent abscesses followed by complaints of purulent discharge and sometimes pain. *Diagnose* clinically and with sigmoidoscopy. *Treat* with surgery. The main *complication* is fecal incontinence.

Anal Fissure

An **anal fissure** is a small, longitudinal tear in the **epithelial tissue** surrounding the **anal sphincter**. It is caused by excessive stretching of the anal sphincter, as with a large bowel movement. Patients will complain of pain at the anus, especially with bowel movements, usually with a history of constipation, and they may have noticed bright red blood in their stool or on toilet paper following a bowel movement. This can be extremely painful for patients, so a gentle perianal exam should be used to visualize and diagnose. The fissures are usually located in the midline and most are posterior. Anal fissures usually resolve with supportive *treatment*. If the fissures are very painful, warm Sitz baths may be soothing as well as a topical anesthetic which is helpful if the pain is preventing patients from having a bowel movement. To prevent recurrence, stool softeners and a diet high in fiber and fluids should be recommended to keep bowel movements regular and prevent constipation. Chronic anal fissures may be treated with nitroglycerine ointment, topical Ca^{++} channel blockers, or botulinum toxin injections. Occasionally surgery (lateral internal sphincterotomy) is necessary to correct the fissure. *Complications* include bleeding, infection, chronic anal fissures, fistulas, and fecal incontinence.

Pilonidal Disease

A **pilonidal disease** refers to either a hair-containing cyst, an acute abscess, or a chronic sinus that forms at the base of the **coccyx** that can become infected. It occurs at the superior end of the cleft between the buttocks, at the **sacrococcygeal area**. Pilonidal disease occurs more often in men than women. It is believed to occur due to **ingrown hair** in the region. The pilonidal cyst may form into a typical abscess with a red, indurated area at the base of the spine. Patients may or may not have a fever, but the abscess will be painful. If it opens, pus will drain from the abscess. *Diagnosis* is made per clinical assessment. No *treatment* is necessary if it is asymptomatic or there are no signs of infection. If an acute abscess does develop, treat with an I&D and pack with gauze, which should be removed in 24-48 hours. Once removed, start warm Sitz baths bid to tid. Antibiotics are typically ineffective. Surgical resection may be necessary if there is chronic disease or chronic sinus tracts. *Complications* include abscess recurrence, chronic sinus tracts, and rarely, squamous cell carcinoma has been reported in sinus tracts.

Hemorrhoids

Hemorrhoids occur when the **vessels surrounding the anus and rectum** become engorged and swollen. Hemorrhoids commonly occur with excessive straining with a bowel movement (e.g., when constipated), during pregnancy, and with prolonged sitting on the toilet due to the increased pressure applied to the pelvic floor. They can also occur as a result of anal intercourse, chronic diarrhea, obesity, and as part of the aging process. Hemorrhoids can be internal or external. **Internal hemorrhoids**, which originate above the dentate/pectinate line, are not painful, can bleed, can produce mucus, and will cause patients to have bright red blood on the toilet paper after a bowel movement. Internal hemorrhoids may prolapse causing itching and pain due to muscle spasms in the sphincter. Internal hemorrhoids are classified as follows: **Grade I**= in anal canal; **Grade II**= protrudes past anal verge with straining but reduce spontaneously; **Grade III**= protrudes past anal verge with straining but requires manual reduction; **Grade IV**= chronically prolapsed. **External hemorrhoids** are painful, may thrombose, and cause hygiene issues. *Diagnosis* is made per clinical exam and with anoscopy or sigmoidoscopy to evaluate bleeding. Most hemorrhoids will resolve on their own or with conservative, symptomatic treatment. Stool softeners are recommended. OTC topical ointments, creams, and suppositories are available to help relieve the swelling and pain (e.g., hydrocortisone). Sitz baths and witch hazel pads can also help. In office procedures include rubber band ligation (most common), infrared coagulation, and sclerotherapy. If severe or recurrent, surgery may be necessary to remove the hemorrhoids. *Complications* include infection, anemia, thrombosis, and strangulated hemorrhoids.

Acute Diarrhea

Acute diarrhea is the increased output of watery stool for less than two weeks duration. The most common causes are infectious, including viral, bacterial, and parasitic pathogens. Other causes include complications from certain medications, toxins, inflammatory bowel disease, and diverticulitis. The workup for acute diarrhea involves sending stool samples for culture (both bacterial and viral), fecal leukocytes, and ova and parasites (O&P). Stool should be checked for *Clostridioides difficile* antigen in patients with a recent history of antibiotic use. Endoscopy may be needed to rule out inflammatory bowel disease. Most cases of acute diarrhea are self-limited and do not require treatment. Patients must be given adequate fluid and electrolyte replacement and treated for dehydration if necessary. Antibiotic treatment is indicated for certain cases of bacterial diarrhea, including invasive *Salmonella*, *Shigella*, *Campylobacter*, and *Yersinia* septicemia. Diarrhea due to parasites usually requires treatment.

Chronic Diarrhea

Chronic diarrhea is the increased output of watery stool for more than two weeks duration. Chronic diarrhea has both infectious and non-infectious causes. Infectious causes include viruses, bacteria, and parasites. Non-infectious causes include inflammatory bowel disease, malabsorption syndromes, food allergies, and use of certain medications. Diagnosis should follow an organized approach dependent on the patient's history and physical exam. Diagnostic tests may include stool for culture, ova and parasite exam, and fecal leukocytes. Endoscopy may be considered to rule out inflammatory bowel disease. Studies for malabsorption syndromes include fecal pH, stool-reducing substances, breath hydrogen test, and stool for fecal fat. Treatment will depend on the cause of the chronic diarrhea.

Constipation

Constipation is defined as infrequent, hard or difficult to pass bowel movements. In general, passing a bowel movement fewer than three times per week is considered abnormal. Constipation is very common and affects both sexes and all ages. There are many causes of constipation:

- Acute
  - Medications such as narcotics
  - Spasm of the anal sphincter
  - Obstruction
- Chronic
  - Inflammatory bowel disease
  - Rectal abnormalities
  - Endocrine abnormalities (hypothyroidism)
  - Neurologic disorders (MS, spinal cord injury)
  - Inadequate fluid intake
  - Low fiber diet

Workup and treatment depend on the individual's history and physical exam. Most cases of constipation are benign and self-limited and are easily treated with dietary changes and stool softeners.

Hernias

Hernias are a protrusion of an organ through the **muscle or fascia** that usually contains it. There are several types. **Hiatal hernias** occur when the upper segment of the **stomach** protrudes through the diaphragm. **Ventral hernias** can occur anywhere there is a weakened area in the **abdominal wall** (e.g., epigastric, primary abdominal, incisional); they cause a section of bowel to protrude through the opening. These are most commonly due to **incisional hernias** which occur at the site of an **abdominal surgical incision** (more common if incision is vertical). **Spigelian hernias** are rare and occur on the outer edges of the **rectus abdominus muscle**. **Umbilical hernias** occur at the **umbilicus** due to a weakened area of the abdominal fascia, causing the bowel to protrude through the umbilical opening. **Inguinal hernias** are the most common hernia overall, are more common in males, occur through a weakened portion of the **lower abdominal wall**, and can be direct (weakness in the posterior wall of the inguinal canal/Hesselbach triangle) or indirect (more common; pass through the internal inguinal ring and into the inguinal canal). **Femoral hernias** are more common in women and occur below the **inguinal ligament** and bulge into the thigh. Hernias are *diagnosed* clinically and are *treated* surgically. Hiatal hernias may require a Nissen fundoplication procedure in which the lower esophagus is reinforced. Other hernias are repaired by surgical closure, sometimes using a mesh material at the site of the weakened area to strengthen the wall. *Complications* include bowel obstruction, incarceration, and strangulation.

Renal and Urinary System

Kidney Disorders

Nephrolithiasis/Urolithiasis

Nephrolithiasis (kidney stones or calculi) and **urolithiasis** (calculi anywhere in the urinary tract) are common in the U.S. There are 4 main types: **Calcium** (~75%; calcium oxalate and calcium phosphate), **struvite** (15%; infection), **uric acid** (6%), and **cystine** (~2%) stones. Nephrolithiasis affects men more often than women and there is a genetic predisposition to forming stones. However, struvite stones (due to UTI) affect women more often than men. Other risk factors include a high salt or protein diet, hypercalciuria, hyperparathyroidism, renal tubular acidosis, and cystinuria. *Symptoms* may include intense, sometimes radiating, intermittent flank pain causing the patient to constantly move around, diaphoresis, N/V, urinary urgency/frequency, and hematuria. *Diagnosis* is made clinically and with a noncontrast helical CT. A UA with culture, urine creatinine, and stone identification is also helpful. Usually stones <5mm pass on their own and may be *treated* with rehydration, analgesics, and medical expulsive therapy like α-receptor blockers (e.g., tamsulosin). If not able to pass in 4-6 weeks or with stones ≥10 mm (that cannot pass on their own), removal is required using various techniques (e.g., extracorporeal shockwave lithotripsy, ureteroscopy, percutaneous nephrostolithotomy). Stents may be placed in the ureter to help relieve symptoms while awaiting surgery. Treat infections with appropriate antibiotics and alkalinizing the urine (e.g., potassium citrate) can help dissolve uric acid or cystine stones. *Complications* of nephrolithiasis include UTI, scarring and stenosis of ureter, renal outflow obstruction, infective hydronephrosis, and loss of renal function.

Renal Cell Carcinoma

Renal cell carcinoma (**RCC**) is the most common **renal cancer** in the U.S. and is more common in men than women. This CA arises in the epithelium of the **proximal renal tubule**. Risk factors for developing RCC include obesity, smoking, exposure to chemicals, and some genetic disorders (e.g., von Hippel-Lindau syndrome, Birt-Hogg-Dube syndrome, hereditary papillary renal carcinoma). RCC may metastasize to the lungs (most common), bone, lymph nodes, liver, adrenal, and brain (least common). **Paraneoplastic syndromes** are common (20%) once it has metastasized. The classic signs and symptoms are flank pain, a flank mass, and hematuria, but may include fever (often FUO), weight loss, hypercalcemia, and HTN. Since *symptoms* often don't appear until the disease is advanced, RCC is often *diagnosed* incidentally. Diagnosis is confirmed and staged with a contrast CT (procedure of choice) or MRI. Include a chest x-ray or CT to look for possible thoracic metastases. For localized disease, surgical resection is the *treatment* of choice. RCC is resistant to radiation and chemotherapy; therefore, if found early before it has spread or metastasized, it can be treated by resection, otherwise the treatment is palliative (e.g., palliative surgery, immunotherapy, targeted therapy, experimental therapies). The primary *complication* is metastases which brings with it a poor prognosis (8% 5-year survival, according to the ACS) along with paraneoplastic syndromes.

Wilms Tumor

Wilms tumor, or **nephroblastoma**, is the most common **renal carcinoma** that affects children, usually ages 3-8. It is typically unilateral and affects males and females equally, except when bilateral, then it affects females more often. It is thought that Wilms tumors begin to form while *in utero* due to genetic mutations. The condition is usually diagnosed by age 1, though sometimes it may be as late as age 5. The prognosis is excellent with a 5-year-survival of 80-90%. Patients usually present with a painless abdominal mass. Wilms tumors can grow quite large before causing any symptoms in the child, so it may go undiagnosed until it becomes large enough to be palpable. Patients are usually asymptomatic but may experience abdominal pain/distension, hematuria, loss of appetite, N/V, constipation, or SOB. Often a mass can be palpated in the abdomen and in the back over the affected kidney. *Diagnosis* is made with an abdominal ultrasound, CT, or MRI and confirmed with surgical examination and biopsies for staging. 90% of patients have favorable histology which shows no anaplasia. *Treatment* comprises surgery and chemotherapy; and sometimes radiation, if the patient presents with a higher stage disease or has unfavorable histology. *Complications* include relapse, metastases, and treatment sequelae (e.g., CHF, renal insufficiency, liver damage, infertility, secondary neoplasms).

Acute Kidney Injury

Acute kidney injury (**AKI**), the new term for acute renal failure (ARF), occurs when the **kidneys** acutely become unable to function and the damage is either reversible or irreversible. This can be due to 3 main causes: **prerenal** (decreased blood flow to the kidneys); **intrarenal** (intrinsic inflammation or damage to the kidneys); or **postrenal** (urine blockage). Prerenal causes may include volume depletion (most common cause of AKI) due to hemorrhage, dehydration, or NSAIDS; intrarenal causes may include toxins such as some medications (e.g., aminoglycosides, methotrexate, imaging contrast), acute glomerulonephritis from infections or lupus, acute tubular necrosis, vascular diseases like malignant HTN, and systemic diseases like sarcoidosis; and postrenal causes may include tubular obstruction and obstruction of the ureter or bladder. *Signs and symptoms* may include peripheral edema, muscle weakness, muscle cramps, N/V, confusion, and possibly rashes or ecchymoses depending on the cause.

Diagnosis and Treatment

Acute renal failure is diagnosed with urine output, BUN, creatinine (Cr), UA, and renal ultrasound. Various groups have defined AKI including the RIFLE, AKIN, and the most recent, KDIGO (Kidney Disease Improving Global Outcomes). According to KDIGO, AKI is defined as: increase in serum Cr by ≥0.3 mg/dl in 48 hours, or increase in Cr ≥1.5 times the baseline within the last 7 days, or reduction in urine volume <0.5 ml/kg/hr for 6 hours. *Treatment* involves correcting the underlying issue (e.g., dehydration, etc.), diuretics for volume overload, and hemodialysis when K >6.0mmol/L or severe pH or electrolyte abnormalities that are unresponsive to treatment. Dietary treatment focuses on managing the patient with a low-sodium, low-potassium, low phosphorus diet, fluid restriction, and providing adequate protein. As the disease progresses, it brings more pronounced complications in fluid and electrolyte balances, anemia, and uremia. *Complications* include SOB, chest pain, permanent renal damage, and death.

Acute Renal Failure

Rhabdomyolysis

Rhabdomyolysis is a condition in which skeletal muscle tissue is broken down and releases myoglobin into the bloodstream. Myoglobin further breaks down into substances that are toxic to the kidney. Rhabdomyolysis may be caused by trauma or conditions that causes muscle damage, including crush injuries, infections (especially in children), diabetic ketoacidosis, seizures, muscle diseases, hyperthermia/hypothermia, electrical injuries, substance abuse (drugs/alcohol), ischemia, extensive burns, dehydration, hypophosphatemia, extended surgery, and excessive exercise/exertion. The typical triad of symptoms includes generalized weakness, dark urine, and myalgias. Other symptoms may include fever, nausea, and vomiting. Patients may complain of muscle pain/tenderness, especially in the lower legs and lower back. Laboratory findings may include abnormalities of electrolytes (hyperphosphatemia, hyperkalemia, hypocalcemia, and low levels of albumin but elevated uric acid. Creatine kinase levels increase within 12 hours of injury, peaking at 24 to 36 hours. Some patients may develop disseminated intravascular coagulation (DIC). Treatment includes identifying and treating underlying cause, IV fluid resuscitation, electrolyte corrections, and urinary alkalization. Some patients may require dialysis because of kidney injury.

Disseminated Atheroembolism

Disseminated atheroembolism (cholesterol embolization syndrome) is sometimes referred to as "blue toe syndrome" because discoloration typical of the disorder often appears on the toes and fingers. When an atheromatous deposit in a large artery (aorta or branches) ulcerates, lipid emboli may break loose and travels to small branches, resulting in occlusions in many different areas of the body (retina, liver, intestines), including the kidneys where it can result in acute renal failure. This embolization may occur spontaneously or be triggered by endovascular procedures or anticoagulants. Characteristics include fever, weight loss, myalgia, lethargy, fatigue, neurologic deficit, loss of appetite, and signs of acute renal failure (decreased urinary output, fluid retention, dyspnea, nausea, dysrhythmias, and confusion). Diagnosis may include findings of anemia, thrombocytopenia, increased ESR, increased C-reactive protein, eosinophilia, and observation of purpuric lesions. Renal biopsy confirms the disease. Treatment includes withdrawing anticoagulants (if using). For kidney failure, treatment may include IV fluids, antihypertensives, potassium lowering medications (calcium, sodium polystyrene sulfonate, calcium infusion, and/or dialysis.

Chronic Kidney Disease

Chronic kidney disease (CKD), previously termed chronic renal failure, refers to long-standing renal disease that leads to renal damage and decreased renal function. CKD is defined as **renal damage** (i.e. One of the following: albuminuria= albumin-to-creatinine-ratio, ACR, >30 mg/g or albumin excretion rate, AER, ≥30mg/24 hrs.; renal structure or histology abnormalities; urine sedimentation abnormalities; electrolyte or other abnormalities due to tubular disorders; h/o renal transplant) or a **reduced GFR** (glomerular filtration rate <60 mL/min/1.73 m^2) for ≥3 mos. The stages of CKD are: **Stage 1**-kidney damage with GFR >90 mL/min/1.73 m^2; **Stage 2**-GFR 60-89; **Stage 3a**- GFR 45-59; **Stage 3b**- GFR 30-44; **Stage 4**- GFR 15-29; **Stage 5**- GFR <15 or dialysis. Patients with stage 1-3 CKD are typically asymptomatic. *Signs and symptoms* appear as GFR decreases to <30 mL/min/1.73 m^2 (stage 4-5) and include fatigue, muscle weakness, HTN, edema, impaired cognitive function, restless leg syndrome, nocturia, N/V, diarrhea, pruritus and encephalopathy. *Diagnose* with labs using the above criteria: metabolic panel, CBC, UA with micro, and a lipid profile; and possibly a renal ultrasound. If possible, *treat* the underlying disease, and control HTN, hypercholesterolemia, anemia, and DM. To protect the kidneys, avoid combining ACE inhibitors and ARBs, and adjust doses or avoid certain medications as GFR drops (e.g., NSAIDS, IV contrast), especially when <30 mL/min/1.73 m^2. Avoid nephrotoxic drugs. *Complications* include CV disease, hyperkalemia, metabolic acidosis, anemia, and end-stage-renal disease requiring dialysis or transplant.

TREATMENT

Hemodialysis	Blood is filtered through artificial kidney to remove waste products and fluids from the blood. Access is per a tunneled catheter, AV fistula or AV graft. Dialysis is usually done for 4 hours 3 times weekly although some do more frequent treatments.
Peritoneal dialysis	Dialysate is instilled through a cannula to the peritoneum, which serves as a filter. The fluid is then withdrawn through gravity. While different protocols exist, exchanges typically take 30 to 40 minutes and are done 4 or 5 times in each 24-hour period.
Kidney transplantation	The only curative treatment for kidney failure is kidney transplantation in which a donor kidney is surgically inserted and begins to filter the blood and produce urine although the recipient must take lifelong medications to prevent the body from rejecting the organ.
Preventive measures	Most measure are intended to slow progression of disease (such as diabetes and hypertension) to kidney failure. Measures include smoking cessation, weight loss, taking medications and treatments as prescribed, monitoring health conditions, having routine checkups, maintaining target A1c and FBS, keeping BP below 140/90, and low salt diet.

HYPERTENSION SECONDARY TO RENAL ARTERY STENOSIS

Renal artery stenosis, a major cause of secondary renovascular hypertension, results from atherosclerotic occlusive disease (80-90%) or fibromuscular dysplasia. RAS is characterized by a greater than 75% narrowing of the main renal artery. When blood flow to the kidney is reduced, the kidney becomes ischemic, which in turn triggers activation of the renin-angiotensin-aldosterone system. The kidneys produce renin, which promotes angiotensin I, which is converted into angiotensin II, a vasoconstrictor, by the blood vessels. This in turns stimulates production of aldosterone, causing sodium and fluid retention, rapidly increasing hypertension. Risk factors include diabetes and smoking. Those most at risk for renovascular hypertension are younger than 30 or over 55. Signs and symptoms include sudden incidence of diastolic hypertension with increase of less than 30 or greater than 50 and hypertension that is refractory to treatment. Diagnosis may include CT, MRI, and/or per renal arteriogram (definitive). Treatment options include antihypertensives, percutaneous transluminal angioplasty, revascularization, or nephrectomy.

RENAL VEIN THROMBOSIS

Renal vein thrombosis is a condition in which one or two primary renal veins are occluded, leading to acute or chronic kidney disease. Renal vein thrombosis may be caused by various kidney diseases, including nephrotic syndrome (the greater the severity of hypoalbuminemia, the greater the risk) and membranoproliferative glomerulonephritis, as well as pregnancy, estrogen therapy, sickle cell nephropathy, renal vasculitis, allograft rejection, SLE, malignant tumors, aortic aneurysm, oral contraceptives, cocaine use, and amyloidosis. Onset of symptoms may be rapid or progressive but may include nausea and vomiting, pain in the flank area, decreased urinary output, and hematuria. Diagnosis may include CT angiography, magnetic resonance venography, and Doppler US, as standard venography may cause clots to break away. Treatment depends on identifying the underlying disorder but often includes anticoagulation (heparin) and percutaneous thrombectomy or thrombolysis. The need for nephrectomy is rare, but may occur if the kidney is not salvageable or if a tumor is causing the problem.

Obstructive Uropathy

Obstructive uropathy is a condition in which the flow of urine is obstructed either within the kidney or below because of anatomic abnormalities, compression (tumors, prolapse), functional abnormalities (neurogenic bladder), or mechanical obstruction (clots, urolithiasis, uric acid crystals). Pediatric obstructive uropathy is primarily associated with congenital disorders, such as posterior urethral valves and polycystic kidney disease. During young to middle adulthood, the most common cause is urinary calculi; however, in older adults, obstructive uropathy is most commonly associated with benign prostatic hypertrophy, cancer, or calculi. Obstructive uropathy may also be caused by some drugs, such as anticholinergics that impair bladder function. Signs and symptoms vary depending on cause but may include difficulty urinating, decreased urinary output, flank pain, abdominal pain, distended bladder, and/or hydronephrosis. Diagnosis is per urinalysis, BUN, creatinine, serum electrolytes, bladder catheterization, US, voiding cystourethrography, IVP, and imaging (such as CT, MRI, and radionuclide scans). Treatment depends on the cause but requires relief of the obstruction, such as by breaking up or removing calculi or surgical repair of BHP.

Pyelonephritis

Pyelonephritis is a severe infection of the **kidneys** and can be life-threatening if not treated promptly. Chronic renal damage or scarring can occur, especially without treatment. Usually pyelonephritis is caused by *Escherichia coli* from a urinary tract infection (UTI) that spreads upwards to the kidneys. It may also be caused by infection spreading through the bloodstream, and in cases of endocarditis or IV drug use, the causative pathogen is usually *Staphylococcus*. Pyelonephritis can be complicated by anatomical and functional abnormalities of the urinary tract (e.g., vesicoureteral reflux: diagnosed with VCUG and may require prophylactic antibiotics or surgery), immunity or metabolic issues (e.g., DM), antibiotic use, and recent urinary instrument use. The classic *symptoms* of pyelonephritis are a fever (usually high), N/V, and costovertebral angle tenderness. Also, similar to a UTI, patients may have urinary frequency, urgency, decreased stream, dysuria, lower abdominal pain, and foul-smelling urine. It is unusual for men to get UTIs/pyelonephritis, and therefore if present, should be considered complicated. Atypical presentations (e.g., failure to thrive, poor feeding, change in mental status) usually involve either the young or elderly patients. *Diagnose* clinically and with clean-catch UA with micro, gram stain, urine C&S, and CBC. Blood cultures and imaging may be needed. *Treat* immediately with appropriate antibiotics taking local resistance trends into consideration until susceptibility results are in. For outpatient cases start empiric therapy with fluoroquinolones x 7 days (1st line). If severe or the patient has a complicated UTI, hospitalize and start treatment with IV fluoroquinolones for 24-48 hrs (or until improving), switching to PO for a total of 10-14 days. *Complications* include recurrence, abscess, acute renal injury, chronic kidney disease, and urosepsis.

Acute Glomerulonephritis

Glomerulonephritis (GN) is inflammation of the **glomerular filters** within the kidneys. It is usually acute, but may be chronic, and can lead to permanent kidney damage if not treated promptly. There are many causes of glomerulonephritis including **infections** (e.g., poststreptococcal infection, viral, bacterial endocarditis), **systemic disease** (e.g., SLE), **primary renal disease** (e.g., IgA nephropathy, membranoproliferative GN), and **vascular disorders**. As damage to the glomeruli occurs, the GFR decreases which activates the renin-aldosterone system causing water and salt retention and therefore, HTN and edema. This causes a **nephritic syndrome** which is characterized by hematuria, proteinuria, oliguria, and HTN. Patients may note oliguria, dark, tea-stained urine due to hematuria, foamy urine due to a high protein level, and edema (especially limbs and face) that can be quite profound. Blood pressure is elevated due to the increased fluid load. *Diagnosis* is made clinically and with UA with micro, serum creatinine, BUN, ESR, and complement levels. The patient's age and history will help guide diagnostic tests and help disclose the most likely cause of GN. A renal biopsy may be needed to confirm the diagnosis. *Treatment* focuses on treating the underlying cause. If due to a recent *streptococcal* infection (antistreptolysin O is positive; peaks 3-5 wks. after strep) or bacterial endocarditis, appropriate antibiotic therapy should be prescribed. The condition will usually resolve on its own with management of the symptoms, such as ACE inhibitors to control HTN and diuretics to reduce edema. Some patients may need dialysis during the acute episode. *Complications* include CHF, pulmonary edema, AKI, chronic kidney disease, and end-stage renal disease.

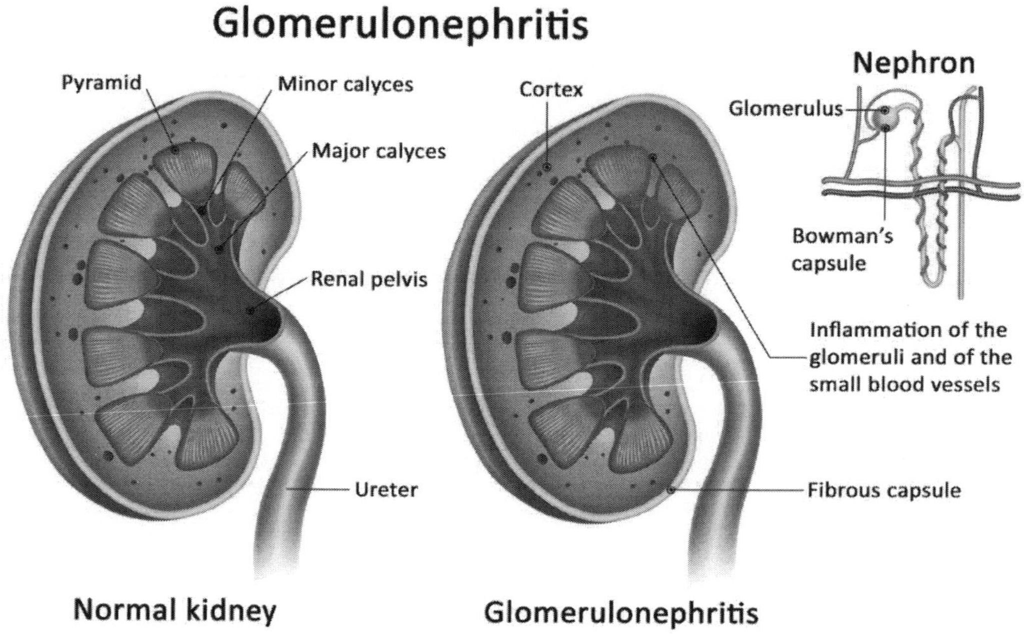

Nephrotic Syndrome

Nephrotic syndrome is a condition that occurs due to damage to the **microvascular system** within the kidneys which leads to excess excretion of protein in the urine, resulting in **hypoalbuminemia** which causes fluid to leak out of blood vessels (edema); high cholesterol is also part of this syndrome. There is an increased risk of developing blood clots and infections. Nephrotic syndrome can have primary and secondary causes. **Primary causes** include: minimal-change nephropathy, focal segmental glomerulosclerosis, and membranous nephropathy. **Secondary causes** include: diabetic nephropathy, SLE, viral infections, preeclampsia, amyloidosis, and drugs (e.g., NSAIDS, penicillamine, lithium). Nephrotic syndrome can cause a good deal of edema, especially in the extremities and face, and there may be noticeable weight gain or ascites due to this retained fluid. Patients may have a feeling of general malaise and note foamy urine due to proteinuria. *Diagnosis* is made in the presence of proteinuria ≥3 g/day, hypoalbuminemia, and high cholesterol. Order a UA with micro (usually followed by a 24-hour urine protein study), serum albumin, and cholesterol. Depending on the patient's history and PE, other tests and a renal biopsy may be needed to confirm the diagnosis. *Treatment* focuses on treating the underlying cause and controlling the symptoms of nephrotic syndrome. Diuretics to reduce the edema, ACE inhibitors can be given to control HTN, and anticoagulants may be necessary to prevent blood clot formation, and steroids for minimal change disease (most common in children). *Complications* include chronic kidney disease, infections, thrombi (renal vein thrombosis), emboli, hypercholesterolemia, CAD, and HTN.

Polycystic Kidney Disease

Polycystic kidney disease (PKD) is a condition in which groups of fluid-filled **cysts** form within the **kidneys**. This can lead to **high blood pressure** and even **renal failure**. Polycystic disease is not limited to the kidneys and can affect the liver and pancreas as well; and is associated with an increased risk of colonic diverticulitis, brain aneurysms, and heart-valve abnormalities. This is a genetic condition that can be autosomal dominant or autosomal recessive (rare). Patients with the autosomal dominant version usually don't start having symptoms or get diagnosed until they are 30-50 years old, and typically don't progress to renal failure until 60-70 years old. However, patients with the recessive version are diagnosed early, usually in utero, and progress to renal failure very quickly. Patients with the autosomal dominant form may complain of abdominal or flank pain, gross hematuria, and an increasing abdominal girth. HTN is an early sign of PKD and early signs of renal failure may be evident with elevated serum BUN and creatinine levels. *Diagnosis* is suspected with a family history of PKD and confirmed with multiple cysts on ultrasound (sometimes a CT, MRI, or genetic testing). *Treatment* of PKD is focused on treating the symptoms and preventing renal failure by using antihypertensives (e.g., ACE inhibitors, ARBs), diuretics, and being on a low-salt diet. Close monitoring and control of blood pressure is crucial to slow the progression of the disease. Treat infections and contact sports should be avoided. If the cysts become large, they may need to be surgically drained. Dialysis and a kidney transplant may become necessary. *Complications* include HTN, infection, preeclampsia, and end-stage renal disease.

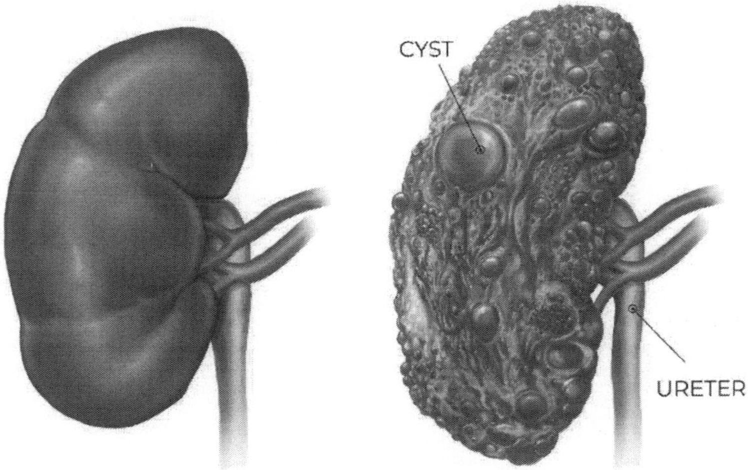

HEALTHY KIDNEY POLYCYSTIC KIDNEY

Electrolyte Imbalances

Hyponatremia

Hyponatremia is defined as a **serum sodium (Na^{+}) <135 mEq/L** and is the most common **electrolyte disturbance** in hospitalized patients, affecting up to 30%. Serum sodium represents the extracellular sodium concentration, which is used as an estimation of total body Na^{+}. Serum osmolality represents Na^{+} concentration in the body's fluids. Both of these reflect the body's state of water balance, which in hyponatremia is usually a state of **water excess**. The most common form is hypotonic or hypoosmolar (<280 mOsm/kg) hyponatremia. Hyponatremia can be divided into 3 categories: **hypervolemic** (due to CHF, renal or liver failure); **euvolemic** (due to SIADH, hypothyroidism, drugs); or **hypovolemic** (due to vomiting, diarrhea, diuretics, etc.). A pseudohyponatremia may be caused by hyperproteinemia, hyperlipidemia, or an increase in other osmoles like glucose (hyperglycemia). *Symptoms* vary and depend largely on the rate of sodium loss. Patients may be asymptomatic or have N/V, headache, malaise, lethargy, muscle weakness, and muscle pain. Severe hyponatremia (<125 mmol/L) causes changes in mental status, confusion, seizures, coma, and even death. *Diagnose* with serum Na^+ and determine the cause using serum and urine osmolality, and urine Na^+. If fluid overload (hypervolemia) is causing a dilutional hyponatremia, diurese and restrict fluid and salt intake. If SIADH is present or other euvolemic cause, treat the underlying disorder (e.g., cancer, infection, discontinue causative drug) and restrict water intake. *Treat* hypovolemic causes with isotonic saline. If hyponatremia is severe or chronic (>48 hrs), correct slowly with hypertonic saline IV fluids (3% NaCl). *Complications* include seizures, coma, and death.

Hypernatremia

Hypernatremia is defined as **serum sodium (Na^{+}) >145 mEq/L**. This reflects the body's state of **water deficiency** and is rarely due to Na^+ excess. This is common in the elderly and hospitalized patient. Hypernatremia can be caused by water loss (most common), a decrease in fluid intake (e.g., elderly who depend on others for water), an impairment in thirst, or not being able to concentrate urine as in diabetes insipidus (DI). Renal dysfunction can alter the excretion of sodium and result in higher levels within the blood stream. Hypernatremia can be divided into 3 categories: **hypervolemic** (rare & due to increased Na^+ intake with limited access to water, salt water or tablet ingestion, hemodialysis, Cushing syndrome); **euvolemic** (DI, fever, hypodipsia, nephrotoxic medications like lithium and phenytoin, mechanical ventilation); and **hypovolemic** (most common; due to GI losses, enteral feeding, burns, loop diuretics, osmotic diuresis). *Signs and symptoms* vary based on the cause of water loss and include thirst, N/V, diarrhea, fever, dry mouth, orthostatic BP changes, polyuria, and dementia. Effects due to brain cell shrinkage include changes in mental status with irritability, somnolence, nystagmus, increased deep tendon reflexes, and seizures. *Diagnose* clinically and with serum Na^+. *Treat* the underlying cause (e.g., dehydration, DI), discontinue any causative med, and replace free water deficit. How quickly water is replaced depends on if it is acute or chronic. Free water deficit may be corrected quickly (over 24 hrs) if hypernatremia has been present <24 hrs; and slowly (0.5 mEq/L/hr) if present >48 hrs. to avoid brain edema. *Complications* include cerebral edema, cerebral bleeding, coma, and death.

Hypokalemia

Hypokalemia is defined as a **potassium (K^+) level <3.5 mEq/L. K^+**. It is an essential **intracellular electrolyte** and involved in the sodium-potassium exchange pump of the cells. K^+ losses can be due to increased excretion (most common; renal or GI), decreased intake, or a shift to inside the cells. Increased excretion of K^+ can occur with diuretics, renal tubular acidosis, increased mineralocorticoid (e.g., aldosterone, cortisol), hypomagnesemia, and with dehydration from diarrhea and vomiting. Various medications can also cause hypokalemia (e.g., gentamicin, ampicillin, ephedrine, and bicarbonate). Intracellular shifts may be caused by insulin and albuterol. Inadequate intake may occur with dementia, eating disorders, and total parenteral nutrition (TPN). Hypokalemia can cause cardiac dysrhythmias, cardiac arrest, hypotension, muscle weakness and cramping, constipation, decreased respirations, reduced DTR, and even paralysis. Severe hypokalemia (K^+ <2.5 mEq/L) can occur in patients taking digoxin. *Diagnose* with a serum K^+. ECG (very important), and a urinary K^+ and serum magnesium are helpful in determining the cause. ECG changes include flattened T waves, ST depression, QT prolongation, and U waves. *Treatment* consists of discontinuing any causative agents and treating underlying cause of K^+ loss; give oral potassium (KCl) for mild hypokalemia. If K^+ <2.5 mEq/L, admit and use IV KCl with an infusion rate no greater than 10 mEq/hr. Patients must be closely monitored for signs and symptoms of hyperkalemia as potassium is replaced, especially cardiac effects. Other electrolyte levels (e.g., Na^+ and Mg^{2+}) should be closely monitored for abnormalities. *Complications* include digitalis toxicity, respiratory depression, rhabdomyolysis, paralysis, arrhythmias (VT, VF, torsades de pointes), and death.

Hyperkalemia

Hyperkalemia is defined as a **potassium (K^+) level >5.5 mEq/L**. This can be caused by decreased renal excretion (most common), increased K^+ intake, or a shift to outside the cells. K^+ is excreted through urine so any dysfunction resulting in decreased urinary output can cause increased serum K^+ levels (e.g., AKI, CKD, tubular defects, reduced aldosterone, adrenal insufficiency, meds). Increased intake can occur with salt substitutes (KCl), K^+ supplements, and any process that causes blood cell destruction, such as hemolytic anemia, can cause a rise in K^+ levels. Various medications (NSAIDS, heparin, ACE inhibitors, ARBs, K^+-sparing diuretics, pen VK) can also lead to hyperkalemia. *Symptoms* range from patients who are asymptomatic to those with cardiac arrhythmias or paralysis. Symptoms usually start when K^+ >6.0-6.5 mEq/L. The primary symptoms are neuromuscular and include weakness, lethargy, diminished reflexes, and paresthesias. Hyperkalemia can cause bradycardia, palpitations, and cardiac dysrhythmias (e.g., heart block, VF). GI symptoms of nausea, vomiting, and diarrhea may be present. *Diagnose* with serum K^+ and ECG. ECG changes are progressive and include peaked T waves, a long PR interval, wide QRS complex, loss of P waves, and eventually VF or asystole. If ECG changes or signs of cardiotoxicity, *treat* immediately with IV calcium gluconate or calcium chloride (cardioprotective). Also administer insulin with glucose, and albuterol as these redistribute K^+ back into the cell. Calcium is not recommended if digoxin toxicity is present. Discontinue any causative agents. Kayexalate, given PO or rectally, binds with K^+ to increase excretion of K^+ through the GI tract. Hemodialysis may also be used in those with renal failure. *Complications* include paralysis and cardiac arrest (K^+ >8.5 mEq/L).

Hypocalcemia

Hypocalcemia is defined as a **total serum calcium (Ca^{2+}) <8.8 mg/dL** (<2.2 mmol/L) or a **corrected total serum Ca^{2+} <8.5 mg/dL**. Correct calcium for changes in serum albumin (increase total serum Ca^{2+} by 0.8 mg/dL for every 1.0 g/dL albumin is below 4.0 g/dL). Hypocalcemia is frequent in hospitalized and chronically ill patients; Ca^{2+} is critical to the proper functioning of the body. It can be caused by under secretion of parathyroid hormone (PTH), resulting in more calcium remaining in the bones and less being circulated into the bloodstream. Ca^{2+} requires vitamin D to be absorbed in the GI tract, so a vitamin D deficiency can lead to hypocalcemia. It can also result from an alteration in renal function. *Symptoms* range from asymptomatic patients to tetany. With hypocalcemia there is excitability of the nervous system so patients may exhibit spasm of the facial muscles when tapped over the facial nerve (a positive Chvostek's sign), or a carpal spasm when a BP cuff is inflated for 3 mins. (positive Trousseau sign). Other signs and symptoms include paresthesias, muscle cramps, bronchospasms, weakness, poor teeth, dry skin, coarse hair, brittle nails, altered mental status, irritability, hallucinations, and seizures. Patients may be hypotensive, and have a prolonged QT interval on ECG. *Diagnose* with a total corrected serum or ionized Ca^{2+}; also check PTH, serum magnesium and phosphate, vitamin D levels, BUN, creatinine, and ECG. *Treatment* involves Ca^{2+} replacement (e.g., IV calcium gluconate or calcium chloride) if Ca^{2+} levels have dropped dangerously low (<7.0 mg/dL). Oral Ca^{2+} replacement for mild hypocalcemia. Treat any underlying condition. *Complications* include seizures, respiratory arrest, and tetany.

Hypercalcemia

Hypercalcemia is defined as a **total serum calcium (Ca^{2+}) level ≥10.5 mg/dL**. Ca^{2+} levels within the blood are controlled by many factors, but hypercalcemia is usually caused by **hyperparathyroidism** or **cancer**. Parathyroid hormone causes calcium to be reabsorbed by the bones if the Ca^{2+} level is too high, or causes Ca^{2+} to leave the bones and enter the blood if levels are too low. Tumors can cause paraneoplastic syndrome by elevating PTH levels, which results in elevated Ca^{2+} levels. Also, Ca^{2+} is excreted in the urine, so alterations in kidney function (e.g., CKD) can result in hypercalcemia. Patients may be asymptomatic if mild or may have many symptoms. The *signs and symptoms* of hypercalcemia can be remembered with the mnemonic *bones, stones, abdominal groans, and psychiatric moans*: bone pain; kidney stones; N/V, anorexia, constipation, and abdominal pain; muscle weakness, fatigue, lethargy, depression, confusion, and coma. There may be hypotonia, a decrease in the reflexes, hypotension, bradycardia, arrhythmias, and a shortened QT interval on ECG all due to nerve transmission malfunctions. Polyuria, nocturia, and decreased urinary output may occur due to kidney dysfunction. *Diagnose* with total corrected serum Ca^{2+} or ionized calcium. Use further labs to determine the cause (e.g., PTH, alkaline phosphatase, CXR, ECG, serum phosphate, serum protein, BUN, Cr). *Treatment* depends on the severity and the cause, and may consist of adequate hydration (1st line in severe hypercalcemia), loop diuretics, decreased intake, prednisone, bisphosphonates, or calcitonin. Treat the underlying cause. *Complications* include osteoporosis, kidney failure, arrhythmias, dementia, coma, and death.

Hypomagnesemia

Hypomagnesemia is defined as a **serum magnesium (Mg^{2+}) level <1.8 mg/dL**, and serum levels do not adequately reflect total body stores (stored in bones, muscles, soft tissues). It is seen more often than hypermagnesemia and can cause many issues throughout the body, including cardiac ones. Magnesium is an important **intracellular electrolyte and coenzyme** that is involved in many critical processes (e.g., cellular metabolism, protein synthesis, cell replication, neurotransmitter release, muscle contraction). Hypomagnesemia can be caused by decreased intake, decreased GI absorption or GI loss, endocrine causes, excessive renal excretion, and some medications (e.g., gentamycin, ticarcillin, PPIs, cisplatin, loop or thiazide diuretics). It is often seen in patients who are alcoholics, hospitalized, or have DM. *Signs and symptoms* include N/V, muscle cramps, positive Chvostek and Trousseau signs, hyperreflexia, nystagmus, paresthesias, seizures, ECG changes (e.g., prolonged QT, PVCs), and mental status changes (e.g., irritability, depression). *Diagnose* with a serum Mg^{2+} level; and check serum Ca^{2+}, K^+, and phosphorus levels since this can be associated with hypocalcemia, hypokalemia, and hypophosphatemia. *Treatment* of hypomagnesemia depends on the severity and includes IV or IM magnesium sulfate if severe (Mg^{2+} <1.25 mg/dL), and oral magnesium salts if the depletion is not as severe. Discontinue any causative agents; monitor often as Mg^{2+} is replenished, and replace Ca^{2+} and K^+ as needed. Meds used to decrease the amount of Mg^{2+} excreted in the urine include potassium-sparing diuretics and triamterene. *Complications* include osteoporosis, arrhythmias, digitalis potentiation, VF, torsades de pointes, hypokalemia, and hypocalcemia.

Hypermagnesemia

Hypermagnesemia is defined as a **serum magnesium (Mg^{2+}) >2.6 mg/dL** and is not very common. When it does occur, it is most often caused by **renal failure** and **excessive intake** (e.g., antacids, laxatives, enemas, cathartics). Hypermagnesemia can cause N/V, flushing, hyporeflexia, hypotension, muscle weakness, respiratory depression, and eventually cardiac arrest. *Diagnose* with serum Mg^{2+} levels. Also test for possible concurrent hypercalcemia and hyperkalemia. ECG may show a prolonged PR interval, widened QRS complex, and a tall T wave. When severe (respiratory depression or cardiac changes), *treat* immediately with IV calcium gluconate which will quickly reverse many of the symptoms. Also, discontinue any sources of magnesium. Other treatment options include furosemide to promote Mg^{2+} excretion and dialysis. *Complications* include respiratory depression, cardiac arrhythmias, neuromuscular paralysis, coma, and death.

Pregnancy, Childbirth, and the Puerperium

Preconception

Birth Control Methods

Various **methods of birth control** are available for both males and females:

- **Intrauterine devices** have an effectiveness rate of >99%. They do not prevent STDs. They are contraindicated in pregnancy, pelvic infection, gynecologic cancer, and breast cancer (hormone releasing IUD). Condoms are 85% effective with typical use and do provide protection against STDs.
- **Vaginal barrier methods** include the diaphragm, sponge, female condom, and cervical cap. They are all about 80% effective with typical use. The diaphragm and cervical cap must be fitted by a physician.
- The **female condom and sponge** are available over the counter.
- **Spermicides** are available over the counter and are generally used with a barrier.
- **Implants** (Implanon®) are a progestin containing rod that is implanted subcutaneously. It lasts for three years and is >99% effective.
- Both male and female sterilization procedures are available.
- Both **tubal interruption surgery and vasectomy** are >99% effective and considered permanent.

Oral Contraceptives

Oral contraceptive pills (OCPs) can be either combined estrogen and progestin or progestin only. Combined OCPs have a >99% rate of effectiveness if used perfectly and an estimated 92% success rate with typical use. Contraindications to the use of combined OCPs include history of thromboembolic disease, cardiovascular disease, uncontrolled hypertension, heavy smoking, breast cancer, migraines, chronic liver disease, or any condition that leads to prolonged immobilization. Combined OCPs are not recommended for breast-feeding mothers. Progestin only OCPs are also effective. The only absolute contraindication is breast cancer; however, caution should be observed if a patient has any of the above conditions. Progestin only pills are considered safe for breast-feeding mothers and babies.

Elective Abortion

Elective abortion is defined as the termination of pregnancy and removal of the embryo or fetus. First trimester abortion is usually accomplished with a dilation and aspiration procedure. Post procedure antibiotics should be administered and complications are rare. First trimester abortions can also be performed with medication. Mifepristone (formerly RU-486) is effective up to a gestational age of 9 weeks. The patient should be administered the first dose in the physician's office and a second dose is taken at home. Significant bleeding and cramping can occur. The patient should have a follow-up visit in approximately 14 days to confirm complete termination of the pregnancy. Second trimester abortions are performed by dilation and evacuation. There is an increased morbidity and mortality associated with later abortions.

Preconception Counseling and Workup

The goal of **preconception care** is to maximize the chances for a healthy pregnancy. The preconception assessment should include questions about the patient's medical history, diet, medications, possible exposure to toxins, substance abuse history, family history, and psychosocial history. Special attention should be given to the patient's reproductive history, including method of contraception, previous pregnancies, and any history of sexually transmitted diseases. A complete physical exam should be performed, including a pelvic exam. Laboratory tests should include CBC, blood type, rubella titer, hepatitis B antigen, rapid plasmin reagin (RPR), *Chlamydia*, and PAP test. Other lab tests that should be considered include HIV, *Varicella*, glucose, PPD, and toxoplasmosis titer. In some patients, genetic testing for a particular disease may be indicated. Patients should be counseled to stop any potentially harmful medications, refrain from alcohol and smoking, and to begin prenatal vitamins.

Pregnancy Assessment and Follow Up

Presentation and Diagnosis of Pregnancy

Pregnancy should be suspected in any woman of childbearing age whose menstrual cycle is disrupted. **Early symptoms** of pregnancy include nausea, vomiting, fatigue, and breast enlargement and tenderness. Physical exam findings include a blue discoloration of the cervix (Chadwick's sign), softening of the cervix (Goodell's sign), softening of the uterus (Ladin's sign and Hegar's sign), darkening of the nipples, and uterine enlargement. The *diagnosis* can be confirmed with urine beta-HCG assay. Pelvic ultrasound can also be used to confirm pregnancy. Assessment of gestational age and due date can be assessed by calculations using the date of the last menstrual period or by assessing fetal size using ultrasound.

Screenings Performed During Prenatal Visits

The **first prenatal visit** is usually between **8-10 weeks gestation** and includes a thorough history and ordering the initial labs. Measure initial height, weight, and calculate BMI. **Blood work** should include blood type, Rh factor, and antibody screen (Coombs test), CBC, rapid plasma reagin for syphilis (RPR), hepatitis B antigen (HBsAg), HIV, and rubella antibody. Also, a **pelvic exam** with a Pap smear (may test for HPV) and testing for gonorrhea and chlamydia. Offer **genetic screening/ testing** (especially if ≥35 years old). To check for **trisomy 18 and trisomy 21**: pregnancy-associated plasma protein-A (PAPP-A) PLUS β-HCG PLUS ultrasound for nuchal translucency (between 11-14 weeks). The **triple screen** (maternal serum alpha-fetoprotein level, β-HCG, and unconjugated estriol) and **quadruple screen** (same as triple screen but adds inhibin A) in the 2nd trimester screens for trisomy 18, 21, and neural tube defects. Other tests include a **chorionic villus sampling (CVS)** allows for early testing (11-13 weeks) of multiple chromosome anomalies like CF. Other tests include an **amniocentesis** (usually at 16-18 weeks' gestation), and **targeted ultrasounds**.

Initial Prenatal Consultation and Prenatal Visits

Feelings and expectations regarding pregnancy are explored at the **initial prenatal visit**, and careful questions regarding **personal safety and abuse** may be proposed. Smoking, alcohol, and recreational drug use should also be addressed. The major components of early prenatal care include identifying patients who are at risk for certain complications; anticipating problems and intervening when able; educating and communicating with the patient; getting early, repeated, and accurate measures of gestational age; and doing ongoing evaluations of the status of the fetus and mom. Visits are scheduled every 4 weeks until 28 weeks gestation, then every 2 weeks until 36 weeks gestation when weekly visits begin. Routine information to gather during a prenatal visit includes weight and blood pressure, urinalysis for blood, glucose, protein, and bacteria, fundal height, and fetal heart tones which can begin after 10 weeks' gestation.

Routine Prenatal Screens and Rh Incompatibility, Gestational Diabetes, and Group B Streptococcus

Routine prenatal screening includes: an ultrasound at 16-20 wks., a 1-hour glucose tolerance test at 24-28 wks. (screens for gestational diabetes), and Group B Streptococcus test of vagina/rectum at 36 wks.

Rh incompatibility: Moms with Rh negative blood can develop **Rh_0(D) antibodies** against their Rh-positive babies (risk increases after the 1st Rh positive baby). RhoGAM® is given to mom at 28 weeks and again within 72 hours of delivery if the baby is Rh+.

Gestational diabetes: This can lead to multiple issues like fetal macrosomia (large babies), shoulder dystocia, and preeclampsia. The 1-hour oral glucose tolerance test (OGTT) is normal if <130; if abnormal results, order a 3-hour OGTT (normal if <140-145 mmol/L). If abnormal, start insulin.

Group B Streptococcus: This bacterium is common in the vaginal flora. It may be passed on during delivery and may cause sepsis and meningitis in the newborn baby. If positive the mother is prophylactically treated: penicillin G or ampicillin. If penicillin allergic, use cefazolin for treatment.

Routine Second and Third Trimester Prenatal Care

Prenatal visits in the **second and third trimesters** are typically monthly until 28 weeks, bimonthly from 28 to 36 weeks, and then weekly until delivery. At each visit during the second and third trimesters of pregnancy, the following should be performed: fundal height measurement, blood pressure, auscultate for fetal heart rate, palpate and attempt to determine fetal position. The final visits in the third trimester should include a digital cervical exam for opening and effacement. Laboratory tests include urine dipstick for glucose and protein at each visit. At 15 to 18 weeks gestation, genetic screening should be offered. A 1-hour glucose tolerance test should be performed at 26 to 28 weeks and group B streptococcus testing should be performed at 36 weeks. Patients should be counseled regarding the onset of labor, when to call their physician, and anesthesia options in the delivery room.

Complications

Ectopic Pregnancy

An **ectopic pregnancy** occurs when a fertilized egg **fails to implant in the uterine lining**. It most often will implant within the **fallopian tube** but can implant within the ovary, abdomen, uterine cornu, or down low in the neck of the cervix. An ectopic pregnancy often occurs without any known cause, but risk factors include scar tissue, malformation of the tube, previous pelvic inflammatory disease (PID), IUD use, smoking, and history of infertility. Patients may or may not know they are pregnant. They usually present with gradually worsening abdominal pain, usually one-sided, with amenorrhea, and vaginal bleeding. **Rupture of the fallopian tube** can occur as the ovum enlarges, which causes severe stabbing pain on the affected side, guarding, and possible syncope and signs of hypovolemic shock (tachycardia, orthostatic hypotension). *Diagnose* with ultrasound and check β-HCG levels if the case is not urgent. *Treatment* includes watchful waiting if the patient is asymptomatic and β-HCG levels are declining; immediate surgical resection if hemodynamically unstable; and a single injection of methotrexate may be used if the ectopic pregnancy is confirmed, unruptured, <4cm, β-HCG <5,000 mIU/mL, and there is no fetal heartbeat. Follow β-HCG levels until 0. If rupture of the fallopian tube occurs, emergency surgery will be necessary to attempt to repair the tube or remove it.

COMPLICATIONS OF PREGNANCY

Pregnancy complications	Characteristics	Diagnosis and treatment
Asthma	Increases risk of pre-eclampsia, preterm birth, low birthweight, and poor growth. Symptoms (wheezing, cough, dyspnea) may improve or worsen during pregnancy, and heartburn may trigger symptoms. Should take usual medicines during labor and delivery.	Diagnosis per pulmonary function tests. Continue medications if diagnosed before pregnancy. May continue but not begin allergy shots during pregnancy.
Hyperthyroidism	Can lead to pre-eclampsia, low birthweight and preterm birth. Usually caused by autoimmune Grave's disease, may worsen after delivery. Estrogen and hCG can both increase thyroid levels, resulting in palpitations, loss of weight, nausea, and vomiting. Newborns may have transient neonatal hyperthyroidism.	Diagnosis: Thyroid tests. Treatment: Propylthiouracil during first trimester and methimazole in last two. In rare cases, thyroidectomy indicated.
Liver disease	Cholelithiasis common because of higher estrogen levels. Cholecystitis and pancreatitis associated with risk of fetal demise. May result in hyperemesis gravidarum (HG) (first trimester) or intrahepatic cholestasis of pregnancy (IHCP) (2nd and 3rd trimester), increase risk of fetal demise after 37 weeks.	Diagnosis: Liver function tests, US, MRI (2nd an 3rd trimester), ERCP. Laparoscopic cholecystectomy preferred to conservative treatment. HG treatment is supportive. ICHP requires UDCA therapy and early delivery.

INCOMPETENT CERVIX

Cervical insufficiency or an incompetent cervix refers to a cervix that **cannot maintain a pregnancy in the 2nd trimester in the absence of contractions** (ACOG definition). The cervix will not remain completely closed during pregnancy, placing the baby at risk for **premature birth**. This insufficiency can be due to past trauma to the cervix, such as from surgery, D&C, induced abortion, or cone biopsy, previous deliveries that were traumatic to the cervix, and genetic anomalies that cause a malformed cervix or reproductive tract (connective tissue disorder, Müllerian defects like a bicornuate uterus). Unfortunately, cervical insufficiency is often asymptomatic and not usually *diagnosed* until after a second or third-trimester pregnancy loss. Patients may have some bleeding in the second or third trimester, a feeling of vaginal pressure or fullness, increased discharge, or low back pain. The cervical dilation may be detected on pelvic exam. Those at risk should receive a **transvaginal ultrasound** at 15-16 weeks. If dilation or a short cervix is found (<2.5 cm), the cervix can be reinforced with a cerclage procedure, which involves placing purse string sutures in the cervix to draw it closed. This effectively sutures the cervix closed to prevent premature dilation. These sutures are usually removed in the last few weeks of pregnancy (about 37 weeks) when it is safe to deliver the baby. Risk of recurrent cervical insufficiency in future pregnancies is about 30%

MANAGEMENT OF HIV POSITIVE PREGNANT WOMEN

All pregnant women should be offered **screening for HIV infection**. All HIV positive women should be given antiviral treatment in order to decrease the likelihood of transmitting HIV infection to the baby. Antiviral treatment should be administered regardless of CD4 cell count and viral load levels.

The higher the maternal viral load, the more likely the transmission will occur. In general, it is recommended that HIV positive pregnant women receive aggressive antiviral treatment with multiple drugs. Most mother-to-child transmission occurs during delivery. Treatment with IV azidothymidine (AZT) during labor and delivery is recommended. C-section is recommended for women with a high viral load, or HIV positive women who have not received antiretroviral therapy. The newborn should be given anti-HIV therapy after birth. The mother should be counseled regarding breast-feeding and the risks of transmission. The usual regimen is six weeks of oral AZT. Both the mother and child should be seen by an HIV specialist.

Presentation of Urinary Tract Infection and Asymptomatic Bacteriuria During Pregnancy

Pregnant women are at increased risk for developing **urinary tract infections (UTIs)** due to ureteral dilation, increased bladder volume, and decreased bladder tone. Approximately 5% of pregnancies are complicated by urinary tract infections. The incidence of asymptomatic bacteriuria is as high as 10%. Routine screening for UTI should be performed at the first prenatal visit and repeated during the third trimester. The risk of progressing to pyelonephritis is high (up to 50%), so all positive cultures should be treated. Cystitis can be treated with appropriate oral antibiotics. Pyelonephritis necessitates hospital admission and IV antibiotics. Follow-up cultures should be obtained. All women with group B strep bacteriuria should be given intrapartum antibiotic prophylaxis.

First Trimester Vaginal Bleeding

Bleeding during the first trimester of pregnancy is not uncommon. Physiologic bleeding is usually light and self-limited. Causes include implantation and cervical changes or trauma following pelvic exam or sexual intercourse. The patient should be reassured, and generally, no further workup is needed. First trimester bleeding can also be a sign of a spontaneous or threatened abortion. The bleeding is usually moderate to heavy and is accompanied by uterine cramping. The workup should include a pelvic exam, ultrasound to assess the well-being of the fetus, and a CBC. If a spontaneous abortion is diagnosed, uterine evacuation may be indicated.

Hyperemesis Gravidarum

Hyperemesis gravidarum is defined as extreme, unrelenting vomiting that prohibits intake of adequate food and fluids, leading to weight loss and ketonuria. Hyperemesis gravidarum affects approximately 1 in 200 pregnancies and it usually starts by 10 weeks gestation. Patients present with persistent nausea and vomiting, weight loss of >5% of body weight, and signs of dehydration. Risk factors include a prior history of hyperemesis gravidarum, multiple pregnancy, first pregnancy, and molar pregnancy. The workup should include an ultrasound, electrolytes, CBD, LFTs, TFTs, and U/A. Once other causes are ruled out, the diagnosis can be made. *Treatment* may require hospital admission, IV fluids, NG feeds, or possibly total parenteral nutrition (TPN). Antiemetics can be used for severe cases. The condition usually resolves by the end of the first trimester.

Gestational Diabetes

Gestational diabetes is defined as glucose intolerance that occurs only during pregnancy. Gestational diabetes is very common, affecting up to 14% of pregnancies. Women at higher risk include those who are overweight, have a personal or family history of diabetes, and black, Hispanic, American Indian, and Asian women. Affected women are generally asymptomatic. Gestational diabetes is usually identified during routine screening. Gestational diabetes increases the risk of macrosomia, hypoglycemia, respiratory distress, jaundice, and subsequent development of type 2 diabetes in the fetus. Gestational diabetes also increases the risk of preeclampsia and polyhydramnios. *Treatment* options include dietary management and insulin if dietary measures do not control blood sugars. Close monitoring of blood glucose levels is essential.

Intrauterine Growth Restriction

Intrauterine growth restriction refers to a fetus whose weight is below the tenth percentile. There are many potential causes of IUGR. Placental abnormalities, maternal chronic disease, smoking, drug or alcohol abuse, as well as genetic anomalies of the fetus can all cause IUGR. IUGR is generally diagnosed at a prenatal visit when fundal height is not what is expected for gestational age. The diagnosis should be confirmed by ultrasound. *Treatment* options depend on the underlying cause. A full workup is needed to determine the etiology cause of IUGR. This may include a detailed ultrasound, fetal karyotype, and screening for maternal infection. Steroids are sometimes used to speed fetal lung development.

Hypertensive Disorders of Pregnancy

Preeclampsia, eclampsia, and HELLP syndrome are hypertensive disorders of pregnancy:

- **Preeclampsia**: This is new-onset HTN and proteinuria occurring after 20 weeks gestation and may even appear up to 6 weeks after delivery. This may be asymptomatic so screening for proteinuria and BP measurements at prenatal visits are important. Edema may be the only sign. Preeclampsia may become more severe with headaches, N/V, visual issues, and confusion. Close monitoring of patients is vital since this may progress to eclampsia. Delivery of the baby is the only cure.
- **Eclampsia**: Left untreated, this becomes fatal. It involves the same symptoms as preeclampsia but ADDS seizures. Immediate administration of high-dose magnesium sulfate is needed to treat seizures and this requires immediate delivery. Close postpartum monitoring is important.
- **HELLP syndrome**: HELLP stands for hemolysis, elevated liver enzymes, low platelets. This is a life-threatening disorder and can be a complication of preeclampsia. Signs and symptoms may include edema, headache, N/V, epigastric pain, hematuria, increased bilirubin, increased LFT's, and jaundice. Deliver immediately.

Abruptio Placentae

Abruptio placentae occurs when the **placenta** prematurely begins **separating from the uterine wall**. Blood collects between the placenta and the uterus and it can be a medical emergency that can place the unborn child and mother at risk. It usually occurs after 20 weeks and can be classified as **partial or complete** (*emergency*), **concealed** (no visible bleeding) or **revealed** (visible bleeding), and **central or marginal**. Frequently, the cause of the placental abruption is unknown; however, it can occur following some type of trauma, such as a bad fall or car accident in which there is some degree of trauma to the mother. Risk factors include maternal HTN, previous abruption, cigarette, alcohol, or cocaine use, chorioamnionitis (intra-amniotic infection), and premature rupture of membranes (PROM). Patients may present with vaginal bleeding (80% of cases), decreased fetal movements, abdominal, back pain, or uterine tenderness with uterine contractions that are very close together, usually one after another, pain between contractions, and possibly signs of hypovolemic shock. *Diagnose* clinically and with an ultrasound; check fibrinogen level and for a coagulopathy. *Treatment* depends on the severity of the abruption: Admit, manage, and observe; or an emergent C-section may be required. If the mother is preterm and ultrasound determines that the placental abruption is chronic, minor, and the baby is stable, the mother may be closely monitored on bed rest. Monitor signs of maternal or fetal distress. If symptoms should worsen, however, treatment is to deliver the baby as quickly as possible, via emergency C-section. Consult a maternal-fetal-medicine specialist; and a pediatrician/NICU if preterm delivery is inevitable.

Placenta Previa

Placenta previa occurs when the **placenta** forms **very close to the cervical os** or may partially or completely **cover the cervix**. Placenta previa is classified as **marginal** (edge of placenta is within 2 cm of the cervical os) or **complete** (covers the cervical os). The cause is not fully understood, but risk factors include scarring of the lining of the uterus from previous surgery or trauma, malformation of the uterus or fibroids, multiple gestation, and smoking or cocaine use. Painless bright red bleeding during the 3rd trimester is the most common presenting symptom with placenta previa. The amount and duration of bleeding late in pregnancy will depend upon how much of the cervix is covered by the placenta. There is a risk of massive bleeding and danger to the unborn child if the cervix begins to dilate, causing the placenta to tear prematurely. *Diagnose* and follow progress of a marginal placenta previa with ultrasound(s); rule out abruption. Low-lying placentas usually move to a safe location by 28 weeks as the uterus grows. *Treatment* depends upon the severity of symptoms. Patients without bleeding can be monitored closely as an outpatient. If bleeding occurs, hospitalize and monitor. The goal is to reach 36-37 weeks before delivering. If bleeding is persistent, the baby should be delivered via C-section as soon as possible, even if premature, to prevent fetal distress, maternal complications, or death. If preterm delivery is inevitable, give corticosteroids if <34 weeks to help promote fetal lung maturity. Placenta previa may be associated with hemorrhage, abruption, and placenta accreta (placenta implants deeply into uterine wall).

Labor

Normal Labor

Normal delivery progresses in 3 stages:

- **Stage 1** begins with regular contractions (every 2-3 minutes), until fully dilated to 10 cm (nulliparous women usually progress <1 cm/hour and multiparous usually dilate <1.5cm/hour. This has 2 phases: **latent**, which is the slow progression of contractions and dilation; and **active**, which is a time of increased dilation and fetal descent.
- **Stage 2** begins when fully dilated until the baby is born.

- **Stage 3** is the delivery of the placenta (usually occurs in ~ 10 minutes; should occur within 30 minutes post-delivery). Dystocia is diagnosed clinically when these stages last longer than predicted (e.g., dilated 6 cm with rupture of membranes and no cervical change after 4-6 hours depending on the adequacy of contractions). *Treatment* may involve Pitocin (oxytocin), assisted vaginal delivery (e.g., forceps, vacuum extraction), or C-section.

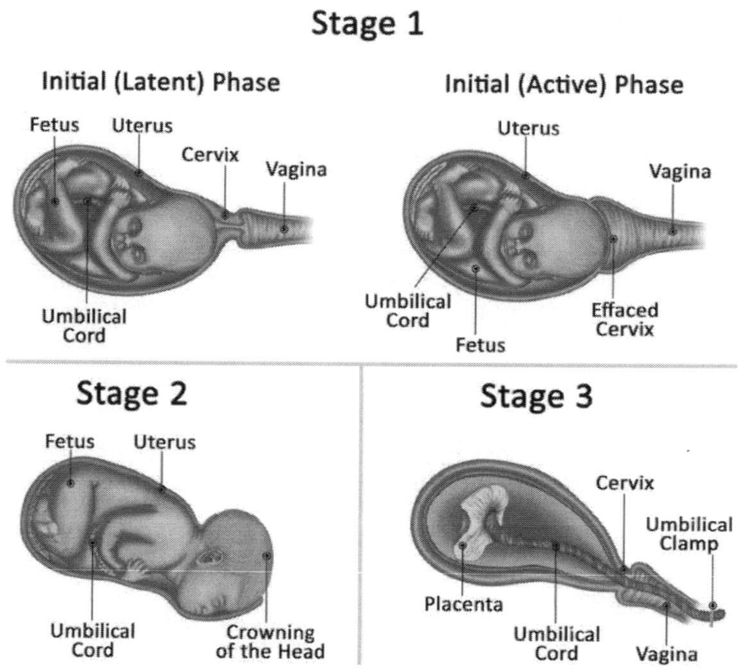

PROM

Premature rupture of the membranes (PROM) is a condition in which the **amniotic sac ruptures** before labor begins. This refers to situations in which the female is at least at 37 weeks' gestation. If this occurs earlier (<37 weeks), it is called **preterm premature rupture of the membranes (PPROM)** and is the leading cause of **preterm birth**. Premature rupture of the membranes can occur because of infection, increased amniotic fluid, a multiple gestation pregnancy, smoking, history of PROM or amniocentesis, previous surgery or cervical cone biopsy, and abruptio placentae. Patients will experience a trickle or a sudden gush of **amniotic fluid** from the vagina. *Diagnose* with a sterile speculum exam (shows vaginal pooling of amniotic fluid) and evaluate fluid (amniotic fluid shows a ferning pattern when dried on a microscope slide; and has an alkaline pH = Nitrazine paper turns blue). *Treatment* depends on the gestational age and may consist of bed rest and close monitoring, or if term, delivery of the baby. Vaginal delivery can be performed if the baby and mother are stable. Pitocin may be needed to start contractions if they have not started within 24 hours after rupture. Delivery should occur within 24 hours of PROM to decrease the chance of infection.

INDUCTION OF LABOR

Induction of labor should be considered when there is evidence that continuing the pregnancy puts the mother, fetus, or both at risk. The most common reasons for inducing labor include post-dates pregnancy (>42 weeks gestation), signs of fetal distress, or maternal illness (e.g., preeclampsia). The method and likely success of different induction methods depends on several factors. These factors can be evaluated using the Bishop score. A cervical exam is performed and a score of 0 to 3 is given in the following areas: cervical position, consistency, effacement, dilation, and station. If the Bishop score is >6, IV Pitocin alone is sufficient. If the score is <6, a cervical ripening agent should be used in addition to Pitocin to increase the likelihood of success. During induction procedures, continuous fetal monitoring is indicated.

Pain Management Options During Labor

There are several nonpharmacologic methods for **controlling labor pain**. They include relaxation techniques often taught in childbirth education classes, the presence of a specialized labor coach (doula), water therapy, changing positions, acupuncture, and reflexology. During stage I of labor, pharmacologic pain management options include narcotics given IV or IM, epidural or spinal anesthesia. Epidural and spinal anesthesia may slow progress and prolong labor. They may also lead to maternal hypotension and fetal heart rate decelerations. During stage II of labor, anesthesia options include a pudendal block and local perineal anesthesia, especially prior to an episiotomy. Epidural and spinal anesthesia are not generally initiated during stage II.

Parameters for Dystocia

Dystocia is defined as **difficult, prolonged childbirth or failure to progress**. This is a condition that occurs in approximately 10-15% of pregnancies and is more common in nulliparous/obese women, those with gestational diabetes, and in those with a small pelvic diameter. This can be due to uncoordinated uterine contractions, abnormal fetal presentation or fetal size, or cephalopelvic disproportion (referred to as the 3 P's: power, passenger, or pelvis).

A common form of dystocia is **shoulder dystocia**, in which the infant's shoulders are difficult to deliver after the head has already been delivered due to the size of the infant. This can lead to **brachial plexus injury** or **clavicular fracture** in the newborn.

Degrees of Perineal Lacerations

Perineal lacerations are a very common complication of vaginal delivery. Risk factors for developing perineal lacerations include first delivery, precipitous delivery, use of forceps or vacuum, shoulder dystocia, malpresentation, and fetal macrosomia. Lacerations are categorized as follows:

- **First degree** – Laceration of vaginal mucosa.
- **Second degree** – Laceration extends deep into vaginal tissue.
- **Third degree** – Laceration extends into the external rectal sphincter muscle.
- **Fourth degree** – Laceration goes through rectal mucosa.

Surgical repair is indicated depending on the degree of the tear. *Complications* of perineal lacerations include hemorrhage, chronic pain, difficulty passing bowel movements, urinary or fecal incontinence, and fistula formation.

Postpartum Care

Postpartum and postnatal care involves **monitoring the mother and baby** in the hours after delivery. Special care for the mother includes monitoring for signs of hemorrhage and for a fever. It is also important to discuss and provide aid for breastfeeding and to discuss the importance of maternal rest, good eating habits, and signs of postpartum depression.

Endometritis

Endometritis is an infection of the uterus following childbirth (most common in the 1st 24-72 hours; late endometritis may not appear until 6 weeks postpartum), usually due to bacteria ascending from the vagina or from retained placental fragments. It can be life-threatening if not promptly treated and should be considered as a diagnosis in any woman who develops a fever after childbirth. Incidence increases in patients with a C-section, especially if unscheduled, or with PROM, but may also occur after a vaginal delivery. *Signs and symptoms* include a fever (>38° C) with chills, lower abdominal or pelvic pain, and N/V. The uterus will be tender on palpation and vaginal discharge present will have a foul odor. The cause is polymicrobial and IV antibiotics (usually clindamycin and gentamycin) should be started immediately and continued until afebrile x 48 hours. If not improved, consider a pelvic abscess.

POSTPARTUM HEMORRHAGE

Postpartum hemorrhage is a leading cause of **maternal mortality** and is usually due to **atony of the uterus**; other causes include lacerations, uterine rupture, and chorioamnionitis. After delivery the uterus should be massaged to help it contract which should slow down bleeding; also, any retained placenta should be removed. If massage is not sufficient, oxytocin should be given. Fluid resuscitation is important and a blood transfusion may be necessary. If blood loss is severe, surgery may be necessary (artery ligation or hysterectomy).

Female Reproductive System and Breast

Cervical Disorders

Cervical Dysplasia

To help **screen** for **cytology changes on the cervix**, a **Pap smear** is recommended every 3 years if ≥21 years old until about 65-70 years old (not needed if patient has had a non-cancer-related total hysterectomy); starting at 30 years old another option is a Pap smear PLUS HPV testing every 5 years.

Cervical dysplasia is also referred to as cervical intraepithelial neoplasia refers to these changes and can be classified as **mild dysplasia** (CIN I; low grade intraepithelial lesion, LSIL), **moderate dysplasia** (CIN II), or **severe dysplasia** (CIN III; high grade intraepithelial lesion, HSIL). Severe dysplasia has the highest risk of transforming into invasive cancer (>12%). Follow-up tests for cervical dysplasia include colposcopy, biopsy, endocervical curettage, a cone biopsy (loop electrosurgical procedure, LEEP aka large loop excision of the transformation zone, LLETZ; cold-knife cone biopsy). The LEEP or LLETZ are also used for treating dysplastic changes. Treatment depends on the level of dysplasia; 5-fluorouracil (5-FU) may be applied topically for CIN II.

Cervicitis

Cervicitis is **inflammation or infection of the cervix**. This usually occurs due to **sexually-transmitted diseases**, such as chlamydia or gonorrhea. Chemical irritation from lubricants, spermicides, or douching may also cause cervicitis as well as trauma or malignancy. **Bacterial vaginitis** may also cause a bacterial infection of the cervix. Patients may be asymptomatic or complain of lower pelvic pain that is aggravated during sexual intercourse as well as bleeding after intercourse or between menses. They may have noticed an increase in vaginal discharge that is yellow or grayish in color with a foul odor. Frequent, burning urination may also be present. Fever may or may not be present depending on the severity of infection. Perform a full pelvic exam (speculum and bimanual); the cervix may appear erythematous, inflamed, or friable. Note type of cervical discharge which is usually thick and yellowish-green. Perform a Pap smear as needed (e.g., every 3-5 years if ≥21 years old) and HPV testing every 5 years starting at 30 years old. Obtain gonorrhea and chlamydia cultures for a definitive *diagnosis* as well as urine testing. Appropriate empiric antibiotics should be started to prevent spreading the infection (Chlamydia: azithromycin + doxycycline; Gonorrhea: ceftriaxone + azithromycin), which could lead to pelvic inflammatory disease, a pelvic abscess, or spreading to the patient's sexual partner. Treat sexual partners at the same time as the patient. Adjust antibiotics when culture results are obtained. If the irritation is chemical in nature, patients should stop using the causative agent.

Cervical Cancer

Cervical cancer is usually **squamous cell carcinoma** (followed by adenocarcinoma) caused by HPV; it is the **3rd most common cancer in women**. Risk factors for cervical cancer includes HPV infection, multiple sex partners, early age at first intercourse, smoking, and being immunocompromised. This is usually caught on Pap smears, but bleeding after sexual intercourse is a common finding by patients. Once the cancer is staged, *treatment* may involve surgery or radiation and chemotherapy.

Ovarian Disorders

Ovarian Cysts

Ovarian cysts are relatively common and occur in or on the surface of the **ovary**. Most do not produce symptoms, but some women have significant symptoms from these cysts. Functional cysts may be either follicular or corpus luteum cysts. **Follicular cysts** occur in the follicle when the egg does not release from the maturing follicle and continues to grow, leading to a cyst; these generally resolve without treatment. A **corpus luteum cyst** occurs after the egg ruptures, and the follicle becomes the corpus luteum. It seals itself off and begins to expand as fluid accumulates in it to form a cyst. The follicular cysts generally do not cause symptoms. The corpus luteum cysts, however, can grow to be >4 cm wide and may cause significant abdominal pain. **Dermoid cysts** (teratoma), which are germ cell tumors that may contain teeth or hair, can grow quite large. Cysts can also rupture, which causes sudden, severe abdominal pain, or even syncope. *Diagnose* with an ultrasound and rule out cancer. Cysts may be followed by ultrasound for several cycles. Oral contraceptives may prevent cyst formation by regulating hormones. If symptoms are persistent, surgery may be necessary to remove the cyst. If a cyst ruptures, removal of the ovary may be necessary.

Ovarian Torsion and Ovarian Cancer

Ovarian torsion is fairly uncommon but may occur with ovarian cysts/tumors that are usually benign. This occurs more often in cysts >4 cm and on the right side. It typically causes severe, sudden pain, and N/V. *Diagnose* with an ultrasound or CT; rule out cancer. *Treat* with immediate surgical detorsion (try to preserve the ovary) or ovarian removal if the tissue is nonviable.

Ovarian cancer has a poor prognosis since it is often not *diagnosed* until in an advanced stage when it has already spread. The main risk factor is a positive family history of breast or ovarian cancer. CA 125 is increased in ovarian cancer. Surgery is used to stage and *treat* this, as well as chemotherapy.

Polycystic Ovarian Syndrome

Polycystic ovarian syndrome (**PCOS**) involves dysfunction of the **hypothalamic-pituitary-ovarian axis**. It causes menstrual irregularities, anovulation, infertility, and signs of increased androgens. This is the most common cause of **infertility** within the U.S. and usually starts affecting women in adolescence. *Signs and symptoms* may include increased weight (in half of patients), hirsutism, acne, acanthosis nigricans, irregular menses, amenorrhea, and insulin resistance/metabolic syndrome. *Diagnose* clinically and confirm with a transvaginal ultrasound which shows multiple (>25) cysts or follicles; rule out other causes of the symptoms. *Treatment* includes lifestyle changes (exercise, weight loss), oral contraceptives (help with menstrual irregularities, acne, hirsutism), metformin for insulin resistance, and infertility treatment for those who desire to have children.

Uterine Disorders

Abnormal Uterine Bleeding

Abnormal uterine bleeding (Dysfunctional uterine bleeding) is **irregular uterine bleeding** that is not due to pregnancy or other gynecologic issues. This is common in adolescent and perimenopausal women, and this is usually associated with **anovulation**. Bleeding may be heavy or light and long or short. Patients present describing their irregular bleeding and usually do not have any premenstrual symptoms. Perform a thorough history and PE with a Pap smear. This is a *diagnosis* of exclusion. Rule out pregnancy, bleeding disorders, PCOS, pituitary issues, thyroid issues, and endometrial hyperplasia or cancer. *ANY bleeding in a post-menopausal woman is a red flag and diseases like cancer should be ruled out. Treatment* involves low-dose oral contraceptives.

ENDOMETRIOSIS

Endometriosis occurs when the **endometrial tissue** that makes up the uterine lining is also present **outside the uterus**. This can occur on areas like the fallopian tubes, the ovaries, on the outside of the uterus, peritoneum, bowel, or the bladder. The **ectopic tissue** will thicken with the hormonal changes that occur during the menstrual cycle and can shed, causing irritation to the surrounding structures. When severe, endometriosis can cause scarring, adhesions, and severe pain. The severity of the endometriosis does not correlate to the amount of pain and the cause of endometriosis is unknown. Risk factors include a positive family history in a 1st degree relative, early menarche, a menstrual cycle <27 days that is heavy and long, and nulliparous women. Patients may be asymptomatic but the most common presenting symptom is cramping pain (usually starts a few days before menstruation), along with dysmenorrhea, dyspareunia, pain with bowel movements, and low back or inguinal pain. **Infertility** may occur as scar tissue and adhesions form. The physical exam is usually non-specific and may only reveal pelvic pain. *Diagnosis* begins with clinical suspicion and is confirmed with laparoscopic surgery which can be used to *treat* it at the same time as the diagnosis; the endometrial tissue is laparoscopically removed and this may decrease symptoms and increase chances of pregnancy. Medications include NSAIDs for pain, oral contraceptives to help maintain hormone levels and possibly reduce excessive symptoms, and meds to prevent the secretion of hormones by the ovaries like danazol and GnRH agonists (leuprolide). As a last resort, hysterectomy may be considered, especially if the patient is finished having children. Endometriosis tends to improve during pregnancy and after menopause.

Review Video: Endometriosis
Visit mometrix.com/academy and enter code: 278236

LEIOMYOMA

Leiomyomas, or **uterine fibroids**, are very common **benign uterine tumors**. They are formed in the **uterine smooth muscle** and can be **submucosal** (under the inner lining of the uterus), **intramural, subserosal** (under the outer lining of the uterus), or **pedunculated**. They usually form during childbearing years, incidence increases with age (until menopause), and most women are unaware they have them since they are frequently asymptomatic. Leiomyoma risk factors include a positive family history, increased weight, African American women, and increased estrogen. When they do produce symptoms, patients may complain of heavy and prolonged menstrual bleeding, and bleeding that may not be associated with menstrual periods, abdominal or pelvic pain, and if large enough those applying pressure to the bowels or bladder may produce constipation and urinary frequency or incontinence. *Diagnosis* is made by ultrasound. *Treatment* may involve medication like GnRH agonists to decrease the size of the fibroids, androgenic agents like danazol to reduce symptoms, NSAIDs for the pain, and surgery like laser ablation, myomectomy, or fibroid embolization. A hysterectomy can be performed to remove the uterus if the symptoms are severe and the woman is not planning to have any more children.

CYSTOCELE AND RECTOCELE

When the vaginal wall becomes weakened, the bladder or rectum may protrude into the vaginal canal and a cystocele and/or rectocele result. Muscle weakness can result from straining during childbirth, chronic constipation, coughing, or heavy lifting. In some women, the decrease in estrogen that occurs after menopause may cause laxity of these connective tissues, leading to a cystocele or a rectocele.

- A **cystocele** or **prolapsed bladder** results when the weakness occurs on the side against the bladder. Patients might present with complaints of pressure within the vagina, a feeling of discomfort when sitting, pain when bearing down, having intercourse, coughing, or lifting, multiple urinary tract infections, or urine leakage.
- A **rectocele** is a weakness on the **posterior wall of the vagina** against the rectum and results from the same types of injuries. There may be a complaint of vaginal fullness, discomfort when sitting, difficulty passing stool, the sensation that the rectum is not completely emptied following a bowel movement, and possibly chronic constipation. Occasionally, patients may experience episodes of fecal incontinence. However, patients may or may not experience symptoms from a cystocele or rectocele, depending on its severity.

Diagnose these by physical exam while the patient is straining. *Treatment* involves Kegel (pelvic floor) exercises and a pessary can be inserted to support the vaginal wall and prevent the bladder or rectum from bulging into the vagina. If symptoms are very bothersome, surgery may be necessary to strengthen the connective tissue and support of these structures.

Urethral Prolapse, Uterine Prolapse, and Vaginal Prolapse

Urethral prolapse or a **urethrocele** is the protrusion of the **distal urethra** into the **urethral meatus** and presents as a urethral mass with vaginal bleeding. This is fairly uncommon, but usually occurs in prepubertal girls or in postmenopausal women. *Diagnosis* clinically per PE (the urethral prolapse looks like a donut). *Treatment* involves topical estrogen cream and if necessary, surgical repair.

Uterine prolapse occurs when the **uterus** protrudes into the **vaginal canal** and possibly further. They are more common with increasing age, increased weight, and in those who have had multiple births or a hysterectomy. They can be classified as **1st degree** (upper vaginal canal), **2nd degree** (introitus), **3rd degree** (cervix is outside the introitus), and **4th degree** (cervix and uterus are outside the introitus). This also may or may not occur with **vaginal prolapse**. Patients may experience fullness and pressure that increases with straining, and a sensation that their insides are coming out. Other *symptoms* include constipation and urinary issues like incomplete emptying of the bladder. Smaller prolapses may be asymptomatic. *Diagnose* per clinical exam and an ultrasound may be ordered to assess comorbid conditions (e.g., UTIs, bladder outlet obstruction). *Treat* with estrogen or surgery.

UTERINE DISORDERS

Uterine disorder	Characteristics	Diagnosis and treatment
Fibroids	Benign tumors (fibromas, myomas, leiomyomas) in or on the uterus. Fibroids may be intramural (most common), subserosal (on outside of uterus), pedunculated (subserosal tumors on a stem), or submucosal (myometrial) (least common). Cause unclear but may be associated with hormone production, genetics, or pregnancy. Characterized by abdominal pressure, bleeding, menstrual cramping, abdominal distention, and pain during intercourse.	Diagnosis is per US and MRI. Treatment may include leuprolide to lower estrogen level and shrink tumors or birth control pills to control symptoms. Definitive treatment is surgical excision.
Endometrial cancer	Uterine cancer involving the endometrium. Characterized by vaginal bleeding and pelvic pain. Associated with increased estrogen level (but not progesterone), prolonged years of menstruation, older age, obesity, tamoxifen treatment for breast cancer, and HNPCC.	Diagnosis is per pelvic examination, endometrial biopsy, US, and hysteroscopy. Treatment includes salpingo-oophorectomy and hysterectomy, radiation, hormone therapy, and/or chemotherapy.

Breast Disorders

GALACTORRHEA

Galactorrhea refers to an **abnormal milky discharge** that is **not related to lactation** from the nipple of one or both breasts in either a male or female. This condition is more common in women, but it may occur in men or infants. This condition can be brought on by excessive breast stimulation, side effects of certain medications (oral contraceptives, H2-blockers, antidepressants, BP medications, and some herbal supplements), or pituitary adenomas. It can occur spontaneously or be produced by manual manipulation and can be continuous or intermittent. Patients presenting with this complaint may also be experiencing dysmenorrhea, headache, or vision changes. If the discharge is other than a milky substance, it may indicate a more significant underlying disease state such as cancer. Obtain prolactin levels. Discontinue the causative medication or *treat* the underlying cause.

MASTITIS

Mastitis is a condition in which **bacteria** enter the **breast tissue** through a milk duct or a break in the skin causing **inflammation, erythema and pain**. This is usually due to *Staphylococcus aureus* and caused by breastfeeding; but rarely, occurs in women who are not breastfeeding. Patients present with a painful, erythematous, warm, tender area of the breast and may be accompanied with fever generally >101°F. fatigue, and an ill appearance. The location of the infection may be indurated and feel hard due to a blocked milk duct. *Treat* with antibiotics (e.g., dicloxacillin, cephalexin, Augmentin®) with attention to the safety of the antibiotic while breastfeeding. Encourage patients to continue breastfeeding and apply warm compresses to the infected area.

Fibrocystic Disease

Fibrocystic disease (or fibrocystic breast changes) is a common condition in which women develop **bilateral lumps or thickened areas in their breasts.** It is most common in women 20-45 years old, but can appear earlier. There is no increased risk of breast cancer in patients who have this condition; it is thought that the fibrocystic masses may be due to **changing hormone levels** during the menstrual cycle. Patients usually complain of breast masses that may change in size, and become more painful especially during the menstrual cycle; nipple discharge may also be present and patients may describe their breasts as feeling full or heavy. These bilateral changes can be described as lumpy, bumpy, ropelike, or having an uneven texture of tissue (e.g., nodular). The lumps are most noticeable in the upper outside area of the breast and maybe into the axillae. Ultrasound exam will show cystic masses within the breasts. There is no definitive cure for fibrocystic changes. It is thought that caffeine may worsen the condition, so limiting caffeine in the diet may help. These changes are considered a normal deviation and not indicative of any actual disease. However, it is important to emphasize monthly self-exams (best 1 week after a period when lumps are smallest) and mammograms because these textures can mask the development of abnormal lumps. *Symptoms* and palpable changes tend to disappear after menopause.

Fibroadenomas and Breast Abscesses

Fibroadenomas are **benign breast masses** that are painless, round, mobile masses that tend to appear during child-bearing years (usually <30). They usually appear as solitary lumps. An ultrasound and biopsy may be used for *diagnosis*; and *treatment* includes leaving or removing it.

Abscesses are **loculations of infection**. They can be *treated* with fine-needle aspiration or incision and drainage if necessary, plus antibiotics for 10-14 days (e.g., dicloxacillin, cephalexin, TMP-SMX).

Breast Cancer

Breast cancer is the **2nd leading cause of cancer death in women** after lung cancer. They are classified as either **carcinoma in situ** or **invasive breast cancer**. Approximately 5-10% of breast cancer is connected to a genetic mutation (BRCA1 or BRCA2) that can be passed on. Other risk factors include a positive family history, increasing age, early menarche, late menopause, or first birth >30 years old, use of HRT, overweight, smoking, and alcohol use. **Screening mammography** starts at 40-50 years old (depends on the organization) and repeats every 1-2 years until 75 years old. Monthly self-breast exams are vital to early *diagnosis* and treatment. Indications of breast cancer include changes in the appearance or texture of the breast and nipple, dimpling of the skin, a retracted nipple, bloody nipple discharge, an obvious lack of symmetry between breasts, and lymphadenopathy. When assessing for signs indicating breast cancer, the practitioner should feel for a painless, hard, fixed (sometimes to the skin), irregular mass in the breast or surrounding tissue. Sometimes MRI's are used by clinician to asses those with mutation instead of by PE. The most common locations are directly beneath the nipple and the outer-axillary portion of the breast. Workup of a suspicious mass usually begins with an ultrasound to determine if it is solid (possible cancer) or cystic (less likely). If it is solid, next a fine-needle aspiration or biopsy and mammogram are performed. Once the cancer is staged, *treatment* may include surgery (lumpectomy), mastectomy, radiation, hormone therapy (tamoxifen) or chemotherapy. Breast cancer most commonly metastasizes (Stage 4) to the bone, liver, brain, and lung. Breast cancer patients face issues associated with body changes – loss of femininity and loss of sexual appeal and function.

Menstruation

Menstrual Cycle Phases and Premenstrual Syndrome

Premenstrual syndrome (**PMS**) is a condition affecting women during the **luteal phase** of their cycles. This is quite common and usually starts in adolescence, but can be particularly bad when patients are in their 40's. However, PMS completely goes away after menopause. The exact cause is not known, but risk factors include smoking and obesity. The **menstrual cycle** (average 28 days) typically has several phases: **follicular phase** (FSH stimulates the ovary to prepare a follicle; FSH & LH are low); **ovulatory phase** (about Day 13-14 there's a hormonal surge in estrogen, FSH, and LH; LH has the largest surge; ovulation takes place); **luteal phase** (progesterone surges; estrogen and progesterone remain elevated until they both drop suddenly around Day 24 then menses begins, about Day 28). Patients present describing symptoms starting in the luteal phase including cravings, anxious feeling, depressive symptoms, sleep issues, bloating/edema, dysmenorrhea, bowel changes, acne, nausea, and mastalgia. *Diagnose* clinically and treat symptoms with NSAIDs, diuretics, diet and exercise, SSRI's for severe mood issues, and possibly oral contraceptives.

Premenstrual Dysphoric Disorder

Premenstrual dysphoric disorder is a severe and chronic condition, with **symptoms** occurring during most menstrual cycles. Symptoms of premenstrual dysphoric disorder include but are not limited to mood lability, depressed mood, increased tension and anxiety, poor concentration, and anhedonia. Vegetative symptoms may also be present, including appetite changes, sleeplessness, lethargy, and muscle pain.

A depletion in serotonin is known to accompany hormonal changes during menses. As such, the pharmacological treatment for premenstrual dysphoric disorder consists of **selective serotonin reuptake inhibitors (SSRIs)**, which are effective for treating the physical and emotional symptoms of premenstrual dysphoric disorder. Treatment recommendations also include dietary changes, exercise, and smoking cessation.

This is *treated* with a variety of methods including diet and exercise, light therapy, relaxation techniques, cognitive-behavioral therapy; and meds like NSAIDs, SSRI's, anxiolytics, oral contraceptives, and diuretics.

Treatment of Amenorrhea

Amenorrhea refers to the **absence of menses** and may be primary (no menses by 16 or 2 years after puberty onset) or secondary (menses stops after cycles have started). If **primary amenorrhea** the work up includes: checking for hypothalamic-pituitary axis for abnormalities, ruling out genetic disorders like Turner syndrome, ruling our ovarian insufficiency like PCOS, and uterine outflow issues like an imperforate hymen. For **secondary amenorrhea**; rule out pregnancy (most common), Asherman syndrome, PCOS, prolactinomas, and possible causes like excessive weight loss or stress, hypothyroidism, and Cushing syndrome. *Diagnose* with appropriate tests (e.g., β-HCG, FSH, LH, prolactin, TSH; and imaging studies as needed like ultrasound, MRI); and *treat* the underlying cause.

Dysmenorrhea

Dysmenorrhea refers to **painful menstruation** and may be primary (not due to pelvic abnormalities) or secondary (due to pelvic abnormalities). This can be quite painful and incapacitating and may lead to absence from school or work. **Primary dysmenorrhea** usually starts within 6 months of menarche. Those at increased risk include those with a positive family history, early menarche, long or heavy menstrual bleeding, and smoking. **Secondary**

dysmenorrhea usually starts in the 20's-30's after having cycles without major pain, and has an increased incidence in those with fibroids, endometriosis, PID, and tubo-ovarian abscesses. **Elevated prostaglandins** play a role in both primary and secondary dysmenorrhea. Patients (with primary) present describing cyclical lower abdominal or low back pain (may radiate to the thigh) surrounding their menses. *Diagnose* primary dysmenorrhea clinically; use imaging studies (e.g., ultrasound, hysterosalpingography, CT) to determine the underlying cause of secondary dysmenorrhea; rule out infections and pregnancy. Further studies may include hysterosalpingography, laparoscopy, D&C. *Treat* symptoms with NSAIDs by starting them 24-48 hours before menses and continuing them 1-2 days into menses; sometimes OC's are used. For secondary, treat any underlying causes.

MENOPAUSE

Menopause is a natural part of a woman's life when **menstruation** stops and **ovarian function** decreases. Menopause is reached after menses have stopped for 12 months. Most *symptoms* occur in the perimenopausal phase when hormone levels are greatly fluctuating; usually about 45 years old. Perimenopausal symptoms vary between patients and may last on average 3-8 years. Patients may describe irregular menses, hot flashes/night sweats, weight gain, mastalgia, moodiness, headaches/menstrual migraines, vaginal dryness, urinary symptoms like dysuria and frequency, and sleep issues. This is a clinical *diagnosis*; however, may confirm with FSH (>25 mIU = perimenopause/ menopause). Certain changes take place with menopause and managing patients after menopause includes protecting against osteoporosis and CVD, screening for breast, cervical, and colorectal cancer, and receiving annual influenza vaccines. Hormone replacement therapy (HRT) may be offered to women to help relieve symptoms and to protect from osteoporosis and CAD (may be protective if given early in the course of menopause). HRT should not be started if >60 years old and >10 years since the onset of menopause. Contraindications to HRT include unexplained vaginal bleeding, liver disease, thrombosis, and a history of breast cancer.

Male Reproductive System

Penis

Micropenis

Micropenis is also called microphallus. Micropenis is a disorder that is characterized by an unusually small penis. Lee *et al.* characterized micropenis by a common criterion of "dorsal erect penile length of at least 2.5 standard deviations smaller than the mean human penis size." The micropenis disorder is typically diagnosed shortly after birth. Micropenis is associated with diminished androgen production or androgen effect in the prenatal period. Multiple conditions are affiliated with micropenis. Some of the associated conditions include Klinefelter syndrome, Leydig cell hypoplasia, testosterone or dihydrotestosterone synthesis defects, and androgen insensitivity syndromes.

Hypospadias

Hypospadias is a disorder wherein the urethral meatus is positioned on the ventral aspect of the penis proximal to the glans penis. The urethral meatus may even be located in the scrotum or the perineum. Hypospadias is congenital and is thought to happen to the embryo during weeks 8 through 20 when the urethra is formed and developed. Also often linked with hypospadias is chordee of the penis. Chordee of the penis is a ventral curvature of the penis. Hypospadias is classified by the location of the urethral opening. Classifications are anterior, middle, and posterior.

Epispadias

Epispadias is a disorder wherein the urethral meatus is positioned on the dorsal aspect of the penis and is considered a rare genetic defect. Epispadias is rarely an isolated condition, and more severe forms involve the urethra and/or the bladder and are distinguished as the exstrophy-epispadias complex. Chordee of the penis is often also involved; however, it is a dorsal curvature of the penis in this case. Epispadias is congenital and is thought to occur embryonically at five weeks' gestation. Epispadias is classified as well by the location of the urethral meatus on the penis. Classifications are glanular, penile, and penopubic.

Premature Ejaculation

Premature ejaculation is classified as either primary or acquired. Primary premature ejaculation is characterized by the International Society for Sexual Medicine by the following: "ejaculation that always or nearly always occurs within one minute of vaginal penetration; the inability to delay ejaculation on all or nearly all vaginal penetrations; and negative personal consequences, such as stress, frustration, or the avoidance of sexual intimacy." Acquired premature ejaculation is overall similar to primary premature ejaculation but has one important difference. The important difference is that the patient has had previous sexual encounters without exhibiting ejaculatory problems.

Erectile Dysfunction

Erectile dysfunction (ED) is a disorder that is characterized by the lack of erection or by the inability to sustain an erection. There are numerous causes of ED, including medications, spinal cord and brain injuries, renal failure, tobacco use, Peyronie's disease, surgery and radiation treatment, psychological factors, mental illnesses, circulatory diseases, diabetes, multiple sclerosis, and aging. ED does not have any formal laboratory tests for establishing the diagnosis; however, lab tests may be indicated to rule out forms of other medical conditions that may be causing or contributing to the disorder.

Spermatocele

A **spermatocele** is a common disorder and is also known as a spermatic cyst. Spermatoceles typically occur in the epididymis and are benign and painless. The spermatocele usually is comprised of fluid that may contain sperm. The actual causes of spermatoceles are not well known but can include an obstruction in the spermatic cord, as a result of trauma, or as a result of inflammation. Risk factors for spermatoceles include diethylstilbestrol (DES) exposure in the prenatal period, age between 40 and 60 years, and von Hippel–Lindau disease. Diagnosis may be made by physical exam, ultrasound, or MRI. Treatment includes surgery or sclerotherapy.

Peyronie's Disease

Peyronie's disease is also called chronic inflammation of the tunica albuginea. This disorder is the result of connective tissue disease, trauma, or certain antihypertensive medications. Peyronie's disease is characterized by proliferation of fibrous plaques with deposition in the tunica albuginea and results in pain, curvature of the penis, indentations on the penis, loss of penile width and length, and impotence. It is most often exhibited in white males older than age 40. Peyronie's disease is usually isolated to the penis; however, some males may also exhibit concomitant connective tissue issues in the hands and the feet.

Phimosis and Paraphimosis

Phimosis, or the inability to retract the **foreskin** in uncircumcised males, is physiologically normal in male children and usually resolves by 5 years old. If not, circumcision is the treatment of choice. **Paraphimosis** is a condition that occurs in the uncircumcised or partially circumcised males and can develop into a medical emergency. It occurs when the **foreskin** of the penis becomes trapped behind the **glans**. The foreskin can normally be retracted manually and will slide back over the glans on its own or with little effort. With a paraphimosis the foreskin and glans become red, edematous, and patients will complain of pain from the constriction. This can compromise the blood flow and may lead to gangrene if untreated. Various techniques (e.g., lubricant, ice, osmotic agents) can be used to assist in manually sliding the foreskin over the glans to its normal position. More invasive techniques, like the Dundee technique (a small gauge needle is used to create punctures in the foreskin and then the edematous fluid is then compressed from the tissue so the foreskin can be slid down) or aspiration of the glans can also be used. If these procedures fail, surgery may be necessary to create a vertical slit in the foreskin to enable it to slide back to its normal position. A circumcision may be performed in these patients to prevent reoccurrence. *Complications* include recurrence, infection, necrosis, gangrene, and autoamputation.

Cancer of the Penis

Cancer of the penis is a rare disease that involves a malignancy of the penile skin or of the tissues of the penis. 90% of cancer of the penis is squamous cell carcinoma, which typically originates in the glans penis or in the foreskin of the penis. Penile cancer primarily occurs in men over the age of 60. Symptoms of cancer of the penis may include erythema or irritation of the penis that may progress to a wartlike lesion or ulcer; a foul-smelling penile discharge or a bloody penile discharge may also occur.

The exact etiology of the causes of cancer of the penis is not known; however, risk factors have been identified. Risk factors identified include human papillomavirus infection, phimosis, males older than 60, inadequate personal hygiene, tobacco product use, smegma, AIDS, psoriatic treatment with UV light, and possibly lichen sclerosis. Jackson's staging of penile carcinoma is as follows: Stage 1 involves the glans penis or foreskin; Stage 2 cancer has spread to the penile shaft; Stage 3 penile cancer involves operable lymph nodes; and Stage 4 involves inoperable inguinal lymph nodes or distant metastatic spread.

Prostate

Benign Prostatic Hyperplasia

Benign prostatic hyperplasia, or **BPH**, is a benign enlargement of the **prostate gland**. Incidence increases with age and there is no definite known cause; however, it seems to be familial and related to hormone changes. The prostate gland is located at the base of the bladder, surrounds the urethra, and is responsible for producing seminal fluid. Whenever there is a change in the size of the prostate gland, a complete assessment should follow to rule out a malignancy. Patients may complain of urinary frequency or urgency, straining, decreased force of urination, incomplete emptying, dribbling, and nocturia. Patients may have recurrent urinary tract infections. A combination of history, PE, and labs are used to make *diagnosis*. The prostate gland will feel smooth and enlarged on digital rectal exam. The PSA may be mildly elevated, and order a UA with culture to rule out infection. It is important that other diagnoses be ruled out, especially carcinomas, bladder outlet obstruction, strictures, and overactive bladder. All men with BPH should be advised on the following behavioral modifications: reduce alcohol and caffeine, avoid antihistamines, decongestants, and opioids, avoid fluid before bedtime or certain activities, and practice double voiding to try to fully empty the bladder. Alpha-adrenergic blockers help relax the smooth muscles (e.g., Cardura®, Flomax®, Hytrin®) and can help with voiding issues. Medications that help slow the growth of the prostate, the 5 α-reductase inhibitors, include Proscar® and Avodart®. If symptoms of upper urinary tract injury develop, surgery may be necessary to remove a portion of the prostate (e.g., TURP or laser ablation). *Complications* include urinary retention, hematuria, UTIs, bladder and kidney dysfunction, and bladder calculi.

Prostatitis

Prostatitis is inflammation or infection of the **prostate gland** and may be classified as: **acute or chronic bacterial prostatitis** (both usually caused by *E. coli*); **chronic prostatitis/chronic pelvic pain syndrome, CP/CPPS**, (most common; 90-95%); or as **asymptomatic inflammatory prostatitis**. Chronic prostatitis/CPPS can be either noninflammatory or inflammatory and is possibly caused by blockage of urine flow or spasms of the urinary sphincters. Patients with acute or chronic bacterial prostatitis may complain of urinary urgency/ frequency, decreased stream (and other obstructive symptoms), lower abdominal/back or perineal pain, but a fever, systemic symptoms, and pain are much more pronounced with acute prostatitis. CP/CPPS is characterized by pain for ≥3 months, and can have pain on ejaculation as well as voiding symptoms. On exam, the prostate may feel boggy and enlarged, and is usually tender. *Avoid* prostatic massage with acute bacterial prostatitis. *Diagnose* clinically, with UA (before and after prostate massage, unless contraindicated); urine C&S and gram stain can help guide therapy. For acute or chronic bacterial prostatitis, TMP/SMX or a fluoroquinolone are the usually the drugs of choice, but check local susceptibility patterns; treat for 4-6 weeks, or longer if needed. Chronic prostatitis may benefit from α-blockers, muscle relaxants, and anti-inflammatory agents. Surgery is rarely needed. *Complications* include acute urinary retention (will need bladder drained by urethral or suprapubic cath), recurrent UTIs, abscess, sepsis, infertility, and epididymitis.

Prostate Cancer

Prostate cancer is the third most common **cancer** diagnosed in the U.S. according to 2017 statistics. It is typically diagnosed in 65-74-year-old men, and in the second leading cause of **cancer**

death in men. However, 5-year survival is close to 99%; and when caught early (localized or regional), is 100%. Controversy surrounds the topic of screening. According to a 2017 draft by the USPSTF, if the patient desires and is expected to live for >10-15 years, screening for prostate cancer should occur at 55-69 years old with a PSA and is usually accompanied with a digital rectal exam. There can be many false positives since PSA may also be elevated in with other disorders like BPH. This should occur earlier, 40-45 years old, if at higher risk (e.g., African American or 1st degree relative diagnosed with prostate CA). Patients are usually asymptomatic, but *symptoms* may include difficulty urinating, urinary retention, blood in semen or urine, sexual dysfunction, and back pain. Urination difficulties can include difficulty starting or stopping the flow of urine, decreased force of urine stream, or dribbling. Bone pain in the lower back or pelvis may indicate metastasis. Use screening to guide workup: rectal exam reveals a palpable prostate that is enlarged, hardened, with a lumpy or uneven surface, and PSA blood levels may be elevated. *Diagnose* with a biopsy. *Treatment* varies according to the stage at diagnosis and includes surgery, radiation, and sometimes hormonal therapy for localized CA or palliative therapy if it has moved outside the prostate. *Complications* include metastases, incontinence, urethral strictures (may need dilatation, stent, or surgery to correct), erectile dysfunction, and death.

Testes

Cryptorchidism and Testicular Cancer

Cryptorchidism occurs when one (most common) or both of the **testicles** fail to descend into the **scrotum**. This can be due to prematurity, low birth weight, or hormone imbalance. In most boys, the undescended testis will descend spontaneously within the first 3-4 months of life. Cryptorchidism resolves in most infants by the first birthday, but about 1% of infants don't resolve. Patients should be referred by 6 months of age if not descended by then to help reduce complications. The initial newborn exam includes palpating the scrotum to feel that both testes are there. They may be palpable a little further up the inguinal canal on one or both sides. Repeated checks should be done at follow-up visits to ensure the testes descend. Some testicles will descend and then temporarily retract again. This condition is not true cryptorchidism. *Diagnose* by physical exam. Further testing is required if hypospadias or epispadias is also present to rule out a disorder of sex development. If the testicle is not descended by 6 months of age, surgical intervention (orchiopexy) where the testicle is sutured or fixed to the scrotum will be needed as it is very unlikely to spontaneously descend after that time. Hormonal treatments are no longer recommended. *Complications* of untreated cryptorchidism include testicular torsion, infertility, testicular cancer, and inguinal hernia. **Testicular cancer** usually affects males between 15-35 years old and presents as a painless testicular mass that does not transilluminate. Therefore, it is important to encourage monthly self-exams, especially in young men.

Testicular Torsion

Testicular torsion is a medical emergency and occurs when the testicle **rotates** and causes **strangulation of the blood vessels**. This can be seen in 7-10-day-old males since many times the testes haven't descended yet and so haven't attached to the tunica vaginalis. Also, the testicle is usually posteriorly held in place by the **tunica vaginalis**, which allows little movement. Some males have a congenital anomaly, where the tunica vaginalis is fixed too high, which allows the testicles to move easily and rotate horizontally on the spermatic cord. This leaves them susceptible to developing testicular torsion, where a testicle can twist on the spermatic cord, causing obstruction of blood flow to the testicle. Peak incidence is between 12-18 years old and is infrequent over 30. Patients will complain of sudden, severe testicular pain with nausea and vomiting. The affected testicle may appear swollen or discolored, may appear elevated when compared to the other, and the cremasteric reflex is usually missing. *Diagnose* per clinical exam and use a color doppler ultrasound if the diagnosis is unclear. *Treatment* should be emergent (≤6 hours from initial symptoms) due to the risk of tissue death from decreased blood flow. The torsion may be resolved by manually manipulating the testicle by rotating it outwardly, back into a normal position, but emergent surgery may be necessary. With tissue death, an orchiectomy is performed. *Complications* include infertility, testicular infarction, and tissue death/loss of the testicle.

Testicular Tumor Types and Staging

There are two types of **testicular cancer**. The two types are seminoma and nonseminoma.

- **Seminomas** typically may occur in all male age groups and tend to be not as aggressive as nonseminomas. Seminomas are generally radiation-sensitive tumors.
- **Nonseminomas** usually occur at an earlier age and are more aggressive tumors. Several forms of nonseminomas exist: choriocarcinoma, embryonal carcinoma, teratoma, and yolk sac tumor.

Chemotherapy is generally effective, as is radiation, for nonseminomas. Testicular cancer has three stages: Stage 1 is confined to the testicle; Stage 2 has spread to the periaortic lymph nodes; and Stage 3 has distant metastases—typically to the lung, liver, bone, and brain.

Testicular Trauma

Trauma to the testicles is rare and has three categories: blunt, penetrating, and degloving. Trauma to the testicles typically occurs in males from ages 15 to age 40.

- **Blunt** testicular trauma is much more common than penetrating testicular trauma and is typically unilateral in nature. An example of blunt testicular trauma includes being hit or kicked in the groin.
- **Penetrating** testicular trauma involves sharp objects or missiles: examples include gunshots or stabbing.
- **Degloving** injuries to the testicles are also known as avulsion injuries and may be the result of shearing from heavy machinery, for example.

Epididymitis and Orchitis

Epididymitis is inflammation of the **epididymis**, which is located on the posterior surface of each testicle and functions to store **sperm**. Epididymitis is most common in males under age 35 and is frequently due to a bacterial infection from a STD (e.g., chlamydia or gonorrhea). **Orchitis** is inflammation of the testes and when it occurs along with epididymitis, is termed **epididymo-orchitis**. Orchitis is typically due to a bacterial STD or the mumps virus (orchitis will appear 4-7 days after parotitis). *Symptoms* are usually unilateral. Patients may complain of pain that begins on the back of the affected testicle that spreads. They may also have dysuria, urgency, and frequency along with referred, lower abdominal pain. Fever and chills may also be present (high fever with mumps). On exam, the testicle may feel warm and swollen with a palpable enlarged and tender epididymis. With orchitis, the testis is tender and enlarged, and the scrotum is swollen and erythematous. *Diagnose* clinically and confirm with U/S. If the patient complains of acute testicular pain, it is important to rule out testicular torsion with a color Doppler ultrasound (because a positive Prehn sign is not as reliable for diagnosing epididymitis). If urethritis/STD suspected, rule out a STD with NAA testing, and obtain a UA and urine culture. *Supportive care* includes analgesics, scrotal elevation, rest, and ice. *Treat* bacterial STDs (e.g., gonorrhea or chlamydia) with ceftriaxone plus doxycycline, OR if enteric organisms suspected (e.g., *E. coli*), use levofloxacin or ofloxacin. Follow proper reporting protocol for patients who are positive for *C. trachomatis* or *N. gonorrhoeae,* evaluate partners, and counsel on condom use to prevent future STDs. *Complications* include a scrotal abscess, testicular atrophy (mumps), infertility, and rarely testicular infarction.

Scrotum

Hydrocele

A **hydrocele** is a painless collection of fluid in the **scrotum**, surrounding the testicles. In the U.S., this is most common in infant boys (6%) due to a patent processus vaginalis and usually resolves within the first year of life. Occasionally, the fluid does not reabsorb because it is not able to flow back into the abdomen. A hydrocele can also occur in adult males, usually over 40, due to an injury or infection. In the developing world, the most common cause of hydroceles is **filariasis** caused by a parasitic roundworm that enters the lymphatic system. Patients do not usually have any pain in the scrotum when a hydrocele is present. Pain will be present if an infection is the cause, or if there has been an injury to the scrotum. *Diagnose* per PE. To help differentiate a hydrocele from hernia, mass, or hematocele, the hydrocele will make the scrotal sac transilluminate due to the fluid, and also, this fluid will lie anterior and superior to the testis. Rule out an inguinal hernia, and an ultrasound can be used if further investigation is needed. Most of the time, a hydrocele will resolve spontaneously. Rarely, surgery may be necessary to remove the hydrocele from the scrotum. Aspirating the fluid is not recommended since it is not curative and may introduce infection. *Complications* are rare, but large hydroceles may cause ischemia and infertility. The main concerns are usually cosmetic issues.

Varicocele

A **varicocele** is an engorgement of the **veins of the pampiniform plexus**. This plexus is part of the **spermatic cord** that travels through the inguinal canal, terminating in the testes. A varicocele is more likely to occur in the left testis (90%) because the veins from there run vertically into the renal vein while the veins from the right testis empty into the inferior vena cava. A varicocele is usually idiopathic in nature but can be caused by compression preventing the veins from draining. This condition can occur as early as adolescence, but usually occurs in males ages 15-25. A malignant tumor (e.g., renal tumor) should be considered in patients who develop a varicocele after the age of 40. Patients may be asymptomatic or may complain of a heavy, aching, fullness in the affected side. On exam, the scrotum may appear visibly enlarged with engorged veins and when palpated, it may feel like a "bag of worms." The swelling may increase with a Valsalva maneuver and may decrease when the patient is recumbent. If asymptomatic and there are no fertility issues, watchful waiting is the usual approach. If mild, a scrotal support may be used to try to resolve the condition on its own. If this is not effective, embolization or surgery (e.g., ligation) may be necessary. *Complications* include infertility and atrophy.

Scrotal Cancer

The **staging of scrotal cancer** is similar to the staging of other nonmelanotic skin cancers. Lowe's staging of cancer of the scrotum includes the following stages: A1, A2, B, C, and D.

- **Stage A1** is cancer that is confined to the scrotum.
- **Stage A2** is locally extensive and may involve the testicle, spermatic cord, penis, pubis, and perineum.
- **Stage B** involves metastasis to the inguinal lymph nodes.
- **Stage C** involves metastasis to the pelvic lymph node.
- **Stage D** includes distant metastases.

Treatment of cancer of the scrotum includes extensive local excision and bilateral lymphadenectomy.

Other Male Reproductive Disorders

Hypogonadism

Hypogonadism is a disorder in which insufficient amounts of testosterone are produced. Hypogonadism may be either primary or secondary. Primary hypogonadism is also called primary testicular failure and is due to a testicular defect. Secondary hypogonadism is due to a defect in either the hypothalamus or the pituitary. Both types of hypogonadism may be either congenital or may be acquired. Some causes of primary hypogonadism include Klinefelter syndrome, cryptorchidism, testicular injury, orchitis, radiation/chemotherapy treatment, and hemochromatosis. Secondary causes of hypogonadism include medications, aging, obesity, HIV, inflammatory diseases, pituitary abnormalities, and Kallmann syndrome.

Fournier Gangrene

Fournier gangrene is a necrotizing fasciitis that involves the soft tissue of the genitalia. The causes of Fournier's gangrene include perianal gland infections that result from a colorectal injury or as a consequence of colorectal malignancy, appendicitis, diverticulitis, or inflammatory bowel disease. The urogenital causes of Fournier's include urinary tract infection, injury to the urethra, or as a consequence of urethral manipulation during surgery. Other causes include skin popping, skin piercing, bone marrow malignancies, lupus, HIV, and perineal injury. Some risk factors for Fournier's are diabetes, obesity, immune suppression, cirrhosis, and pelvic vascular diseases.

Balanitis

Balanitis is the result of inflammation of the foreskin of the penis. The condition typically affects males who are uncircumcised and can be the result of chemical irritation, infection, and inadequate hygiene. Diabetes is a risk factor for developing balanitis. Symptoms of balanitis may include erythema or ulceration at the penile tip, penile discharge, pain, difficulty or inability to retract the penile foreskin, rash/itching, and penile edema. Treatment for balanitis depends upon the cause. Antibiotics are indicated for infectious causes, instruction on proper hygiene with an uncircumcised penis, topical steroids, and circumcision.

Gynecomastia

Gynecomastia is the increase of **glandular breast tissue** (not fat) in males; this is not related to normal changes during puberty. It may be idiopathic or caused by meds (e.g., spironolactone, verapamil, cimetidine, finasteride, anabolic steroids) or certain conditions like hypogonadism and hyperthyroidism. This is usually physiologic and self-limited; *treat* cause or discontinue the causative agent.

Male Infertility

Medical causes of **male infertility** include tumors, cryptorchidism, hormonal imbalances, antisperm antibodies, retrograde ejaculation, infections (mumps, sexually transmitted disease, prostatitis, urinary tract), inability to ejaculate, defects of the sperm ducts, celiac sprue, conditions resulting from chromosomal defects, medications (e.g., chemotherapy, anabolic steroids, testosterone replacement therapy, certain antibiotics), and erectile dysfunction. Environmental causes of male infertility include exposure to pesticides, exposure to heavy metals, radiation exposure, increased testicular temperature from sauna/hot tub use, prolonged bicycling, illegal drug use, excessive alcohol use, age, tobacco product use, mental stress, and vitamin deficiency (C, selenium, zinc, folate).

Endocrine System

Parathyroid Glands

Parathyroid Hormone and Causes of Hyperparathyroidism and Hypoparathyroidism

Parathyroid hormone (**PTH**) is secreted by the 4 parathyroid glands which sit posterior to the thyroid gland. Release of PTH is controlled by the pituitary gland's secretion of **parathyroid stimulating hormone**. The function of PTH is to control the body's **calcium (Ca^{++}) and phosphorus balance**. When the calcium levels are low, PTH secretion is increased; when calcium levels rise, PTH secretion is suppressed. PTH causes Ca^{++} to be released from bones into the circulating blood stream, renal reabsorption of Ca^{++}, renal excretion of phosphorus, and conversion of vitamin D to its active form (1, 25-dihydroxy vitamin D). **Hyperparathyroidism** can be from primary or secondary causes. **Primary hyperparathyroidism** is most commonly caused by a parathyroid adenoma which causes increased amounts of PTH to be released. With some types of cancer, there can be ectopic sources of parathyroid tissue that will secrete excess PTH. Multiple endocrine neoplasia (MEN) syndromes can affect multiple endocrine glands, including the parathyroids, and lead to hyperparathyroidism. **Secondary causes** include chronic kidney disease and vitamin D deficiency. Accidental removal of the parathyroid glands during thyroid surgery can cause **hypoparathyroidism**. Hypomagnesemia can cause there to be a decreased amount of PTH secreted by the glands. Rarely, there can be genetic causes of deficiencies in PTH secretion (e.g., DiGeorge syndrome).

Hyperparathyroidism

Hyperparathyroidism occurs when there is **overproduction of parathyroid hormone (PTH)**. Normal range is 10-55 pg/mL. This occurs more often in women and those over 50 years old. Hypercalcemia (total Ca^{++} >10.4 mg/dL) is the most common finding in hyperparathyroidism. Patients may complain about signs of hypercalcemia which can be easily remembered with bones, stones, groans, and moans. This includes **bone pain** due to demineralization, **kidney stones**, **abdominal groans** (nausea, vomiting, constipation, loss of appetite), and **psychiatric moans** (nervous system issues: muscle weakness, fatigue, lethargy, depression, confusion). Polyuria can occur with renal failure. Cardiac arrhythmias, hypertension, and even coma can occur. Ca^{++} levels >12 mg/dL may be due to cancer and therefore, cancer must be ruled out especially if Ca^{++} levels rise rapidly. *Treat* with parathyroidectomy of affected glands.

Hypoparathyroidism

Hypoparathyroidism is the **deficiency of PTH**. This is more common in women and is usually due to accidental damage during thyroid/neck surgery, radioactive iodine treatment for hyperthyroidism, radiation, or due to autoimmune causes. As Ca^{++} levels drop, patients may complain of paresthesias of the fingers, toes, and perioral area. Patients will show other signs of neuromuscular irritability with muscle aches, hyperreflexia, carpopedal spasm (tetany), laryngospasm, and facial grimacing. A positive Chvostek sign (unilateral spasm of the facial muscles when the facial nerve is tapped) and a positive Trousseau sign (carpal spasm when upper arm is compressed with a blood pressure cuff) may be present. Irritability, confusion, fatigue, seizures, brittle hair and nails, and personality changes may occur. *Diagnose* with an ionized Ca^{++} level (<4.7 mg/dL), reduced PTH, and elevated phosphate. *Treat* with Ca^{++} and vitamin D supplements. Patients with renal failure must also reduce the amount of phosphate in their diet. Patients with tetany are treated with IV calcium gluconate.

Thyroid Gland

Hyperthyroidism and Graves' Disease

Hyperthyroidism (**thyrotoxicosis**) is a disease of **excess thyroid hormone production and secretion**. It can have many causes including Graves' disease, thyroiditis, toxic multinodular goiter (Plummer disease), and toxic adenoma. **Graves' disease** is an **autoimmune disease** and is the most common cause of hyperthyroidism in the U.S. Exophthalmos and pretibial myxedema are usually present with Graves' disease whereas these two symptoms are not seen with regular hyperthyroidism. Common *signs and symptoms* of thyrotoxicosis include irritability, nervousness, tremors, muscle weakness, palpitations, HTN, atrial fibrillation (especially in the elderly), frequent bowel movements, heat intolerance, increased sweating, and weight loss with an increase in appetite. Hyperreflexia, fine or brittle hair, warm, moist skin, menstrual irregularity, and a goiter may be present. *Diagnose* clinically and with thyroid function tests. Low TSH, with high total T3 and high free T4 confirms hyperthyroidism. With Graves' disease thyroid stimulating immunoglobulins (TSIs) are positive as well as other antibodies. Radioactive iodine scanning can help differentiate between the causes of hyperthyroidism. Thyrotoxicosis can be *treated* with antithyroid drugs (e.g., methimazole, propylthiouracil (PTU)), β-blockers (e.g., atenolol) for hyperadrenergic symptoms, iodine, and thyroidectomy. Graves' disease is usually treated with radioactive iodine. Toxic multinodular goiter and toxic adenoma are treated with either radioactive iodine or surgery. *Complications* include dysrhythmias, HTN, CHF, osteoporosis, thyroid storm, and pregnancy issues including miscarriage.

Thyroid Storm

Thyroid storm (**thyrotoxic crisis**) is very rare, but life-threatening condition in which the thyroid secretes massive amounts of **thyroid hormones** at one time, causing an acute state of **thyrotoxicosis**. This can be due to a tumor, excessive manipulation during surgery, infection, trauma, or a complication of Graves' disease. Those who take excessive doses of thyroid hormones or suddenly discontinue antithyroid medications may also experience a thyroid storm. *Signs and symptoms* include high fever, extreme irritability, nausea, vomiting, diarrhea, dehydration, CHF, arrhythmias, disorientation, and delirium. This can progress to the point of seizures, coma, or death. *Diagnosis* is clinical. Since this is a medical emergency, *treatment* should not be delayed while waiting for the thyroid panel results. A patient presenting with symptoms of thyroid storm should have immediate treatment. Supportive measures, β-blockers to treat increased adrenergic tone, thioamides (e.g., methimazole, PTU) to stop new thyroid hormone synthesis, iodine to stop the release of thyroid hormones, bile acid sequestrants to slow liver recycling of hormones, and glucocorticoids to decrease T4 to T3 conversion (this also assists with adrenal insufficiency). Note that thioamides (anti-thyroids) can cause agranulocytosis in 0.2-0.5% of patients. PTU helps inhibit peripheral T4 to T3 conversion, but has been linked to severe liver injury/acute liver failure (black box warnings); therefore, use with caution. Once the crisis has passed, radioactive iodine or thyroidectomy may be used in patients with contraindications to antithyroid drugs. *Complications* include hypotension, shock, coma, and death.

Subacute Thyroiditis

Subacute thyroiditis is a self-limited disease that causes **inflammation of the thyroid gland**. Most commonly, subacute thyroiditis is caused by a viral infection (e.g., coxsackie, mumps, influenza, adenovirus). Also, it can occasionally occur with certain medications (e.g., lithium, amiodarone) or is possibly due to an autoimmune cause (e.g., subacute lymphocytic thyroiditis, subacute postpartum thyroiditis). Patients will usually have a fever with a painful, tender, asymmetrically or symmetrically enlarged thyroid gland. They may remember having symptoms of an upper respiratory infection before the thyroid symptoms began. In addition to the localized tenderness, patients may describe symptoms of either hyper- or hypothyroidism. Usually, patients are initially in a hyperthyroid state, followed by a period of hypothyroidism, and then returning to a euthyroid state. *Diagnosis* is clinical, using thyroid function tests (TSH, free T4, serum thyroglobulin), and other labs. Lab tests will show an elevated WBC and ESR. Thyroid antibodies may be positive; however, will not be as high as with Graves' disease. A fine-needle biopsy may be done, especially if a solitary nodule is found. Patients are *treated* with high-dose NSAIDs (usually ibuprofen or naproxen; *avoid* aspirin) and sometimes steroids to decrease the inflammation within the thyroid gland. Antibiotics do not have a role here because of the condition's viral etiology. The TSH and T4 levels should be monitored every 4 weeks for resolution as this can take several months. Around 95% of cases will resolve on their own in 18 months without *complications*. In the other cases, hypothyroidism will be permanent.

Hypothyroidism

Hypothyroidism, a **deficiency of thyroid hormones**, is more common in women and is most commonly due to autoimmune factors (e.g., Hashimoto thyroiditis) in the U.S. However worldwide, **iodine deficiency** is the most common cause of hypothyroidism. Hypothyroidism may be **primary** (due to diseased thyroid) or **secondary** (diseased hypothalamus or pituitary). For example, pituitary tumors can also cause a decrease in TSH secretion, which will lead to secondary hypothyroidism. *Symptoms* are often nonspecific. Patients may complain of fatigue, weakness, loss of concentration/memory, cold intolerance, constipation, weight gain, and a decreased appetite. Patients may have myxedema (a nonpitting edema of the face, periorbital area, hands, and feet), a hoarse voice, dry and coarse skin, and dry, brittle hair with hair loss. Hypertension and bradycardia may be present as well as paresthesias in the hands along the median nerve. Lab results with hypothyroidism will show an elevated TSH as the pituitary gland tries to stimulate more production of the thyroid hormones. Triiodothyronine (T3) and thyroxine (T4) are the primary thyroid hormones. Test for free T4 which will be decreased (T3 is not sensitive for hypothyroidism). With *Hashimoto thyroiditis*, thyroid peroxidase antibodies will be present. *Treatment* includes thyroid replacement hormone (levothyroxine) and careful monitoring of the thyroid hormone levels to reach therapeutic dosage. *Complications* include goiter, depression, weight gain, peripheral neuropathy, myxedema coma, infertility, miscarriage, high cholesterol, and heart failure.

Hashimoto Thyroiditis

Hashimoto thyroiditis is a **chronic autoimmune-mediated form of hypothyroidism** and the most common cause of hypothyroidism in the U.S. The body's immune system attacks the **thyroid tissue**, preventing the normal secretion of thyroid hormones. Patients may complain of the usual *symptoms* of hypothyroidism, including fatigue, cold intolerance, weight gain with a decreased appetite, forgetfulness, dry skin, a puffy face, as well as a goiter. Female patients may also have menorrhagia. Thyroid hormone levels may be normal early in the disease. The TSH level will be elevated, though, and the thyroid hormone levels will begin to decrease as the disease progresses. Anti-thyroid peroxidase (anti-TPO) antibodies can also be tested to determine an autoimmune etiology, but the autoantibodies may be negative 10-15% of the time. In this case, a biopsy will confirm the *diagnosis*. *Treatment* involves typically lifelong thyroid hormone replacement therapy and possibly surgery. TSH and free T4 levels are regularly performed, measured every 6-8 weeks after initiation and medicine adjustments, until normal levels are achieved. After that, follow-up patients every 6-12 months. To avoid maternal and fetal sequelae, treatment and careful monitoring must be continued through pregnancy. *Complications* of this disease include goiter, heart failure, depression, decreased libido, pregnancy and fetal issues, and myxedema coma.

Adrenal Gland

Adrenal Insufficiency

Adrenal insufficiency can be primary or secondary, and chronic or acute. **Primary adrenal insufficiency (Addison's disease)** is chronic, has an insidious onset, and is due to autoimmune factors, infections (e.g., TB), or disease within the adrenal gland causing a decrease in cortisol secretion from the gland. **Secondary adrenal insufficiency**, which is more common, involves a decrease in adrenocorticotropin (ACTH) production from the pituitary; therefore, aldosterone levels are not affected. Causes include a pituitary adenoma, steroid use, or discontinuation of steroids. **Adrenal crisis** is a life-threatening emergency of **acute adrenal insufficiency** usually due to rapid corticosteroid withdrawal or a stressful event (e.g., illness, accident). With adrenal insufficiency, patients may complain of fatigue, weakness, dizziness, and may have orthostatic hypotension, weight loss, nausea, and vomiting. The skin may become hyperpigmented in primary disease. With acute adrenal crisis, patients can present with signs of shock, N/V, hypotension, and abdominal pain. *Diagnose* with a high-dose ACTH stimulation test. Autoantibodies against 21-hydroxylase can help diagnose the cause. Addison disease is *treated* with cortisol replacement therapy (e.g., hydrocortisone). If the patient is aldosterone deficient, replace with the mineralocorticoid fludrocortisone. With secondary adrenal insufficiency, the cause is the focus of treatment (e.g., resection of a pituitary adenoma). When adrenal crisis is suspected, treat with immediate IV hydrocortisone. It is important that patients are slowly weaned off steroids to prevent adrenal insufficiency/adrenal crisis. *Complications* include adrenal crisis, shock, coma, and death.

Cushing Syndrome

Cushing syndrome results when **cortisol levels** are increased. Most commonly, this is due to steroid treatment with **prednisone**. Endogenous causes include a pituitary adenoma producing excess amounts of adrenocorticotropic hormone (ACTH) which leads to elevated cortisol (termed **Cushing's disease**) or a primary tumor of the adrenal gland causing increased cortisol secretion. Forms of cancer (e.g., lung, carcinoid) can present with ectopic sources of ACTH secretion. Patients will develop proximal muscle weakness, muscular atrophy, truncal obesity with thin arms and legs, round facies, buffalo hump, and purple striae usually across the abdomen. Patients may bruise easily, have non-healing sores, and women may be affected with hirsutism and oligomenorrhea/amenorrhea. Osteoporosis can occur as can glucose intolerance. For *diagnosis* a patient should be screened with one of the following: 24-hour urine free cortisol x3, low dose (1 mg) dexamethasone suppression test, midnight serum or salivary cortisol. Once Cushing syndrome is established, determine the cause using an ACTH and simultaneous cortisol measurement (elevated = adrenal adenoma or carcinoma) or a high-dose (8 mg overnight, or 2-day) dexamethasone suppression test (differentiates between pituitary cause and ectopic ACTH cause). Patients should be weaned off prednisone if possible. Removal of a pituitary adenoma can decrease ACTH production. Removal of an adrenal adenoma or other ectopic source of hormone secretion can decrease cortisol levels. *Complications* include hypertension, CV disease, DM, osteoporosis, risk of adrenal crisis, and psychosis.

Pituitary Gland

Hormones Produced by the Pituitary Gland

The **anterior pituitary gland** secretes the following hormones:

- Growth hormone – promotes growth
- Thyroid-stimulation hormone (TSH) – stimulates secretion of thyroid hormones
- Adrenocorticotropic hormone (ACTH) – stimulates secretion or glucocorticoids
- Prolactin - stimulates milk production in post-partum women
- Luteinizing hormone (LH) – stimulates secretion of sex steroids
- Follicle stimulation hormone (FSH) – stimulates follicle development

The **posterior pituitary** secretes:

- Antidiuretic hormone – water reabsorption in the kidney
- Oxytocin – stimulates uterine contraction during labor and milk let-down post-delivery

Gigantism and Acromegaly

Gigantism and acromegaly both occur from **excessive production of growth hormone (GH)**, usually due to a pituitary adenoma. **Gigantism**, which is very rare, occurs in children, before the epiphyseal plates close, while **acromegaly** occurs in adults after epiphyseal fusion. In children, GH helps with bone growth and development. Therefore, gigantism results in **excessive long bone growth**. In adulthood, the epiphyseal plates are fused and the bones are no longer able to grow. With excess GH, more calcium is laid down on the bone, causing **bony enlargement**. *Signs and symptoms* include prominent forehead and jawbones (prognathism), large hands, feet, nose, and lower lip, a deep voice, arthritis, and possible headaches. Patients may develop left ventricular hypertrophy, CHF, hypertension, and cardiac arrhythmias. IGF-I (insulin-like growth factor I), which is more consistent throughout the day than GH, and an oral glucose tolerance test checking for GH non-suppression are helpful in making the *diagnosis*. MRI is used to check for pituitary tumors. *Treatment* is aimed at treating the cause. Removal of a pituitary adenoma will decrease or stop the production of GH. However, if this does not occur, pituitary radiation and medication may help (e.g., somatostatin analogs, dopamine analogs, or GH receptor antagonists). *Complications* include diabetes, HTN, cardiomyopathy, osteoarthritis, sleep apnea, carpal tunnel syndrome, spinal cord compression, uterine fibroids, and colon polyps.

Hypopituitary Dwarfism

Hypopituitary dwarfism occurs in children who suffer from **decreased production of growth hormone (GH)** due to congenital or acquired causes (e.g., pituitary adenoma, brain injury), or it may be idiopathic. GH secretion can be decreased in adults, resulting in increased fat and decreased muscle mass, but this will not affect bone growth since the epiphyseal plates have fused. Children who have decreased secretion of GH will be very short in stature because of inadequate bone development. **Dwarfism** is categorized by the Little People of America (LPA) as a person less than 4'10" tall due to a medical or genetic condition. Patients with hypopituitary dwarfism fall below the 3rd percentile in height, but will have normal body proportions, and usually have delayed tooth development. There are no intellectual deficits associated with this. *Diagnosis* is multifactorial including history, physical, labs (e.g., low levels of insulin-like growth factor-1 [IGF-1] and IGF-binding protein-3), and imaging studies (e.g., bone age, MRI). Rule out other causes (e.g., Turner syndrome, familial short stature, malnutrition). If due to decreased GH, and not a primary skeletal disorder, the child can be *treated* with human growth hormone to try to stimulate growth. Surgery may be necessary to remove a pituitary adenoma if that is the cause. *Complications* include panhypopituitarism, delayed puberty, and complications associated with GH replacement (e.g., fluid retention, pseudotumor cerebri, slipped capital femoral epiphysis, myalgia, and arthralgia).

Disorders of Calcium Metabolism and Bone

Hypophosphatemia and Hyperphosphatemia

Phosphorus, or phosphate, (PO_4) is necessary for neuromuscular and red blood cell function and the maintenance of acid-base balance, and provides structure for teeth and bones. About 85% is in the bones, 14% in soft tissue, and <1% in ECF.

- Normal values: 2.4 – 4.5 mEq/L

Hypophosphatemia <2.4mEq/L.	Occurs with severe protein-calorie malnutrition, excess antacids with magnesium, calcium or albumin, hyperventilation, severe burns, and diabetic ketoacidosis. Symptoms include: Irritability, tremors, seizures to coma. Hemolytic anemia. Decreased myocardial function. Respiratory failure. Treatment*:* Identify and treat underlying cause and replace phosphorus.
Hyperphosphatemia > 4.5 mEq/L.	Occurs with renal failure, hypoparathyroidism, excessive intake, and neoplastic disease, diabetic ketoacidosis, muscle necrosis, and chemotherapy. Symptoms include: Tachycardia. Muscle cramping, hyperreflexia, and tetany. Nausea and diarrhea. Treatment*:* Identify and treat underlying cause, correct hypocalcemia, and provide antacids and dialysis.

Renal Osteodystrophy

Renal osteodystrophy is bone disease associated with chronic kidney disease and abnormal levels of calcium and phosphorus. In kidney failure, the kidneys can no longer make calcitriol (form of vitamin D), which is necessary for calcium absorption. Renal osteodystrophy is common in those adults who have received renal dialysis for a number of years but is more serious with children, whose bones are still developing, often resulting in short stature. Renal osteodystrophy increases the risk of fractures. Diagnosis is only by bone biopsy, but this is rarely done as it is assumed patients are at risk. Types include:

- **Osteomalacia**: Inadequate bone mineralization, resulting from hypovitaminosis D.
- **Osteitis fibrosa cystica**: Resulting from secondary hyperparathyroidism. The increased PTH stimulates osteoclasts to form bone.
- **Adynamic bone disease**: Resulting from low PTH levels, which cause a slow turnover of bone.

Treatment includes cinacalcet hydrochloride to lower PTH levels, dietary modification (reducing intake of phosphorus, increasing calcium), vitamin D/Calcitriol (to treat secondary hyperparathyroidism), and phosphorus binders, such as calcium carbonate, calcium acetate, sevelamer, and/or lanthanum. Serum phosphorus should be maintained at <4.6 mg/dL in stage 3 and 4 and 4.7 to 5.5 mg/dL in end-stage renal disease.

Endocrine Tumors

Endocrine tumors	Characteristics	Diagnosis and treatment
Insulinoma	Benign (90%) tumor of beta cells in pancreas, resulting in excess production of insulin and hypoglycemia. Neurologic symptoms include diplopia and blurred vision, confusion, amnesia, seizures, and coma. Adrenergic symptoms include diaphoresis, weakness, hunger, tremors, anxiety, tachycardia, and palpitations.	Diagnosis is per symptoms, blood glucose levels (<50 mg/dL), with relief with glucose, supervised fasting with testing of insulin and C-peptide levels, and imaging (ultrasound, CT). Treatment is by surgical excision of tumor.
Vasoactive intestinal-peptide (VIP)-secreting tumors (VIPoma)	Pancreatic tumor of non-beta islet cells, secreting VIP, which causes severe watery diarrhea (to >3000 mL/d), dehydration, nausea, vomiting, abdominal pain, dehydration, hypokalemia, and metabolic diarrhea.	Diagnosis is per symptoms, secretory diarrhea found in stool specimens, serum VIP, and imaging (PET, scintigraphy, Endoscopic US). Treatment includes managing fluid and electrolyte balance and octreotide to decrease diarrhea along with pancreatic enzymes. Chemotherapy (streptozocin and doxorubicin, temozolomide regimens, sunitinib, or everolimus) may control symptoms but does not cure. Surgical resection is curative for those with localized tumors and may decrease symptoms for metastatic lesions.
Glucagon-secreting tumors (Glucagonoma)	Tumor (usually malignant) of the pancreatic islet cells. Characterized by weight loss and 4 Ds: diabetes (hyperglycemia), dermatitis (necrolytic migratory erythema), DVT, and depression.	Diagnosis is per RIA for level of glucagonemia, GTT, FBS, CBC, nutritional assessment, liver function tests, CT and/or MRI. Treatment includes surgical excision (if possible) or chemotherapy (streptozotocin and doxorubicin or 5-FUO).
Ectopic adreno-cortico-tropic hormone (ACTH) (due to tumor)	AKA ectopic Cushing syndrome because the ACTH is produced by a tumor rather than the pituitary gland, and symptoms are consistent with those of Cushing disease (moon face, weight gain, acne, osteoporosis, hirsutism, skin infections, bruising, bone pain, weakness, hypertension, type 2 diabetes, impotence, depression).	Diagnosis is per 24-hour urine cortisol and potassium levels, laboratory tests for ACTH, cortisol, and potassium, FBS, dexamethasone suppression tests, and MRI and/or CT to locate tumor. Treatment includes surgical excision of tumor if possible, radiation, or administration of medications (aminoglutethimide, ketoconazole, metyrapone, mitotane) to block production of cortisol.

Hypothalamic Disorders

Hypothalamic disorders most often involve traumatic brain injury resulting in impaired function but can also be caused by tumors, radiation, surgery, malnutrition (anorexia, bulimia), hemochromatosis, bleeding, and some genetic disorders, such as Prader-Willi syndrome. The hypothalamus produces hormones that stimulate or inhibit the production of hormones by other organs and controls the release of hormones from the pituitary gland.

Hormone	Increase	Decrease
Antidiuretic hormone (controls kidneys' conservation of water)	SIADH (headache, nausea, vomiting, seizures)	Diabetes insipidus (polyuria, polydipsia)
Corticotropin-releasing hormone (stimulates release of ACTH)	Cushing's syndrome	Adrenocortical deficiency (Addison's disease)
Gonadotropin-releasing hormone (stimulates production of FSH and LH)	Overproduction of sex hormones (testosterone, estrogen)	Children: Stunted growth and failure to go through puberty. Adults: amenorrhea, infertility, menopause
Growth hormone releasing hormone (stimulates secretion of growth hormone)	Acromegaly, gigantism	Children: Growth failure
		Adults: Decreased muscle and bone and increased fat deposits.
Oxytocin (stimulates uterine contractions and lactation)	Benign prostatic hypertrophy, increased lactation	Inability to breastfeed, may increase risk of depression
Somatostatin (inhibits production of growth hormone and TSH)	Diabetes mellitus, cholelithiasis, dietary fat intolerance, diarrhea	Unclear, may result in excess growth hormone and acromegaly, gigantism
Thyrotropin-releasing hormone	Hyperthyroidism	Hypothyroidism

Diabetes Insipidus

Diabetes insipidus (**DI**) is a disease due to an impairment in the secretion or response to **vasopressin**, resulting in excessive thirst and urination. There are 2 main types: **central** (decreased production/secretion of antidiuretic hormone [ADH] from the hypothalamus/pituitary) or **nephrogenic** (resistance to the effects of ADH by the kidney; which may be caused by lithium use). DI can occur because of decreased levels of ADH (aka vasopressin), damage to the hypothalamus gland where ADH is produced, damage to the pituitary gland where ADH is stored, or primary kidney damage that prevents the kidneys from functioning properly. *Signs and symptoms* include polyuria, polydipsia, along with extreme thirst, and nocturia. The patient may present with dehydration, hypernatremia, and low levels of ADH. Labs show an increased urinary output (>3 L/24 hours), poorly concentrated urine (<200 mOsm/kg), and a urinary specific gravity of ≤1.005. Water deprivation testing can be used to differentiate central DI (osmolality rises after ADH is given) from nephrogenic DI (osmolality stays the same after ADH is given). An MRI is used to rule out a pituitary tumor/adenoma. A low sodium diet and desmopressin (intranasally or orally) are *treatments* of choice for central DI. Hypothalamic/pituitary tumors can be surgically removed or debulked, if possible. With nephrogenic DI, correct the cause, treat with sodium and protein restriction along with adequate water intake. Sometimes thiazide diuretics (e.g., HCTZ), amiloride, and NSAIDS are used in both central and nephrogenic DI. Electrolyte imbalances and dehydration may cause many symptoms including hypotension, tachycardia, and dysrhythmias.

Diabetes Mellitus

Type 1 Diabetes Mellitus

Type 1 diabetes mellitus (**Type I DM**), previously termed juvenile or insulin-dependent DM, is autoimmune in nature which destroys **pancreatic islet cells** causing greatly **decreased insulin production**. Type I is often diagnosed early in life before age 30, but may develop after age 30, and symptoms may appear fairly suddenly. There is ≤6% risk in those with a positive family history with 1 parent with type I DM, an almost 30% risk in those with 2 parents, and a ≤50% concordance rate in twins. Patients with type 1 DM classically have *symptoms* of polyuria, polydipsia, and polyphagia. There can be weight loss even though patients are eating more, and patients may complain of weakness and fatigue. *Diagnosis* is made when fasting plasma glucose (FPG) levels are ≥126 mg/dL, when a 2-hour PG is ≥200 mg/dL during an OGTT (75 g), or when HbA1c is ≥6.5%. These 3 tests require a second positive result to confirm the diagnosis. However, diagnosis is automatically established if the patient has classic hyperglycemic or hyperglycemic crisis (e.g., ketoacidosis) symptoms along with a random PG ≥200 mg/dL. Lifelong insulin *treatment* is required for type I DM. *Complications* include diabetic retinopathy, diabetic neuropathy, micro and macrovascular conditions (e.g., atherosclerosis, MI), and infection.

Review Video: Diabetes Mellitus: Diet, Exercise, & Medication
Visit mometrix.com/academy and enter code: 774388

Insulin Types for Controlling Glucose Levels

The different types of **insulin** available for controlling glucose levels with type 1 diabetes mellitus are explained below:

- **Rapid-acting** (Lispro®/Aspart®)
  - Onset of Action: 12-30 minutes
  - Peak Action: 30 minutes-3 hours
  - Duration of Action: 3-5 hours
- **Short-acting** (Regular insulin)
  - Onset of Action: 30 minutes
  - Peak Action: 2.5-5 hours
  - Duration of Action: 4-24 hours
- **Intermediate-acting** (NPH insulin)
  - Onset of Action: 1-1.5 hours
  - Peak Action: 6-10 hours
  - Duration of Action: 14-24 hours
- **Long-acting** (Glargine®)
  - Onset of Action: 3-4 hours
  - Peak Action: No peak
  - Duration of Action: Approx. ≥24 hours (range 11-32 hours)

Rapid-acting: Typically taken right before meals and combined with longer-acting insulin. **Short-acting**: Typically taken 30 minutes before meals and used with longer-acting insulin.

Intermediate-acting: Combined with rapid or short-acting insulin to continue coverage; given bid.
Long-acting: Can be combined with rapid or short-acting insulin, as necessary; given qd or bid.

Diabetic Ketoacidosis

Diabetic ketoacidosis (DKA) is more likely to develop in patients with type 1 diabetes. Insufficient or absent insulin results in increased gluconeogenesis and ketogenesis, leading to very elevated levels of plasma glucose and ketones. This causes an osmotic diuresis that may result in severe dehydration. Risk factors for development of DKA include infection, not taking prescribed insulin, or newly diagnosed diabetes. Classic symptoms include: abdominal pain, vomiting, dehydration, altered mental status, Kussmaul respirations, and 'ketone breath' (a fruity odor due to high ketone levels). The *diagnosis* is made by laboratory findings, including an extremely elevated glucose and a high ion gap metabolic acidosis. Immediate therapy includes IV fluids (normal saline followed by 1/2NS; glucose should be added when serum glucose is below 250 mg/dL), insulin drip, and electrolyte replacement.

Type 2 Diabetes Mellitus

Type 2 diabetes mellitus (**Type 2 DM**) is an endocrine/metabolic disorder that results in **impaired secretion and peripheral response to insulin**. There is a strong genetic predisposition towards developing type 2 DM and a 90% twin concordance. Risk factors include age ≥40, positive family history, overweight/obese, history of gestational diabetes, HTN, and African/American, American Indian, Hispanic/Latino, or Asian American descent. Many patients are asymptomatic. Patients may present with classic *symptoms* of polyuria, polydipsia, polyphagia, weight loss and signs of hyperglycemia (e.g., blurred vision, paresthesias, yeast infections). *Diagnosis* can be made in a patient presenting with classic symptoms of hyperglycemia and a random blood glucose ≥200 mg/dL. In an asymptomatic patient, diagnosis is made with a fasting blood glucose ≥126 mg/dL, a 2-hour PG ≥200 mg/dL during an OGTT (75 g), or when HbA1c is ≥6.5%. *Treatment* includes a comprehensive medical evaluation and preventive monitoring: annual fundoscopic and foot exams, and annual screening for atherosclerotic CV disease, peripheral neuropathy, and albuminuria. Dietary modification, weight reduction, and exercise are steps to slow the progression and improve glycemic control. At diagnosis, metformin therapy should be initiated with previously mentioned lifestyle changes. HbA1c should be rechecked every 6 months and every 3 months if not meeting treatment goals (e.g., HbA1c <7.0%, preprandial PG 80-130 mg/dL, postprandial <180 mg/dL). If treatment regimen is unsuccessful, add another oral or injectable medication or change to insulin. Consult endocrinologist. *Complications* include cardiovascular disease, neuropathy, diabetic retinopathy, nephropathy, and infections (especially of the foot).

Oral Medications for Controlling Glucose Levels

Oral medications available for controlling glucose levels with type 2 diabetes mellitus are discussed below:

- **Biguanide (insulin sensitizer; e.g., Metformin)**: Is the initial medication of choice for type 2 DM. It decreases hepatic gluconeogenesis, decreases intestinal absorption of glucose, and increases peripheral glucose uptake/use. It can decrease the HbA1c and decrease LDL cholesterol. It should be avoided in liver or renal disease, in those with CHF, and before receiving IV contrast. Side effects include nausea, vomiting, diarrhea, and *lactic acidosis*.

- **Sulfonylureas (insulin secretagogues; e.g., 1st gen.-glipizide, glimepiride; 2nd gen.-glyburide)**: This class stimulates insulin release from pancreatic β cells and has a great glycemic-lowering effect. Dosed once a day. They should be avoided in severe renal or hepatic impairment and are contraindicated in those with a sulfa allergy. It has been associated with an increased risk of CV death. Side effects include weight gain and hypoglycemia, but there are fewer side effects with 2nd generation meds.
- **Meglitinide (short-acting insulin secretagogues; e.g., repaglinide, nateglinide)**: Works similarly to sulfonylureas and can be used if allergic to sulfonylureas. Preprandial dosing.
- **α-glucosidase inhibitors (intestinal enzyme inhibitors; e.g., acarbose, miglitol)**: This class of drugs is best given with the 1st bite at meals and works by delaying intestinal glucose absorption and so helps decrease postprandial glucose surges. It should be avoided in intestinal, liver, or renal disease. Side effect is flatulence.
- **Thiazolidinediones (insulin sensitizers; e.g., pioglitazone, rosiglitazone)**: This class has been shown to slow the progression of DM, decrease triglycerides, and increase HDL cholesterol. Maximum effect in 12-16 weeks. Side effects include edema, macular edema, weight gain, anemia, CHF, and hepatotoxicity (rare). It should be avoided in liver disease and CHF. Access to rosiglitazone is limited due to an elevated risk of MI.
- **Dipeptidyl peptidase IV inhibitors (e.g., alogliptin, linagliptin, saxagliptin, sitagliptin)**: DPP-4 inhibitors work by prolonging the effects of incretin hormones (hormones that stimulate insulin secretion due to meals). Side effects include arthralgias, hypersensitivity reactions.
- **Na^+-glucose transporter 2 inhibitors (e.g., canagliflozin, dapagliflozin)**: SGLT-2 inhibitors work by increasing urinary glucose excretion. Side effects include genital mycotic infections, UTIs, and hypotension. Contraindicated in severe renal impairment; has been associated with lower limb amputation.

Hyperosmolar Coma and Hypoglycemia

In **hyperosmolar coma**, patients present with extremely elevated serum glucose, often >800 mg/dL, and altered mental status. This condition is a complication of type 2 diabetes mellitus. Acidosis is not present and serum pH >7.3. *Treatment* includes fluid and electrolyte replacement and insulin drip. Prognosis is guarded with mortality as high as 50%.

Hypoglycemia and hypoglycemic coma are common complications of diabetes and should be considered in any patient in a comatose state of unknown etiology. Presenting symptoms include change in mental status ranging from confusion to coma, palpitations, trembling, and tachycardia. If the patient is awake, treatment includes oral administration of glucose. Comatose patients are treated with intramuscular (IM) glucagon (1 mg) or an IV infusion of 50% glucose.

Chronic Complications of Diabetes

The **chronic complications of diabetes** can be divided into three groups: macrovascular complications, microvascular complications, and neuropathies.

- **Macrovascular** complications include coronary artery disease, which results in increased risk of myocardial infarction, stroke, and congestive heart failure. Coronary artery disease is responsible for 70% of the mortality associated with diabetes.
- **Microvascular** complications include retinopathy and nephropathy, which can result in blindness and kidney failure.
- **Neuropathies** usually affect the distal extremities and increase the patient's risk for traumatic lesions.

The diabetic patient must be followed closely for the onset of complications. Yearly eye exams, kidney functions screening, and careful foot exams are critical. Chronic complications generally start to appear five or more years following diagnosis. The onset of complications can be delayed or prevented with tight control of blood glucose levels.

Multisystem Processes and Disorders

Acidosis and Alkalosis

Metabolic Acidosis

Metabolic acidosis is a condition in which there are excess **hydrogen ions** (H^+) within the system (due to elevated H^+ or reduced HCO_3^-), resulting in a **decreased serum pH level (arterial pH <7.35)**. The body will try to **compensate** by increasing the respiratory rate and depth of respirations in an effort to "blow off" some of the excess H^+ through carbon dioxide. The excess H^+ in the system can be due to excessive intake or production of acidic substances, decreased acid excretion by the kidneys, or by GI or renal loss of bicarbonate (HCO_3^-). These can result in a high anion gap metabolic acidosis or a normal anion gap acidosis. These can be remembered by the mnemonics: (increased anion gap)=GOLD MARK (Glycols, Oxyproline, L-lactate/lactic acidosis, D-lactate, Methanol, Aspirin, Renal failure/ uremia, Ketoacidosis/DKA); (normal anion gap or hyperchloremic acidosis) = USED CARP (Ureteroenterostomy, Small bowel fistula, Extra chloride, Diarrhea, Carbonic anhydrase inhibitors, Adrenal insufficiency, Renal tubular acidosis, Pancreatic fistula. Substances that increase acid include aspirin products, methanol, ethanol, and antifreeze. *Symptoms* usually reflect the cause of the acidosis (e.g., diarrhea, h/o DM, lactic acidosis). Long, deep breaths (hyperpnea) is usually the first sign that is noted. With worsening acidosis, patients may experience N/V, headache, malaise; and stupor, Kussmaul breathing, coma, or death may result without treatment. If chronic acidosis, bone demineralization can occur. *Diagnose* with serum electrolytes and ABG which reveal a reduced pH, reduced $PaCO_2$, and reduced HCO_3^-. Determine the anion gap and amount of respiratory compensation [Winter formula = expected $PaCO_2 = (1.5 \times HCO_3^-) + 8 \pm 2$]. *Treat* the underlying cause and correct acidosis through bicarbonate (use with caution). *Complications* include coma and death.

Metabolic Alkalosis

Metabolic alkalosis occurs when the **pH of the blood** becomes elevated (pH >7.45) due to too much **bicarbonate** (HCO_3^-) in the system. This can occur due to a decrease in hydrogen ions (H^+) or a direct increase in HCO_3^-. The means by which these two actions occur is usually through the **GI tract** or through the **renal tubule system**. With the loss of hydrochloric acid (HCl) in the stomach (e.g., vomiting or NG tube suctioning), an alkalotic state can develop. Renal dysfunction or diuretic use can cause decreased secretion of HCO_3^-, which raises bicarbonate levels. Metabolic alkalosis can be divided into (1) *chloride-responsive metabolic alkalosis* (e.g., GI loss, diuretic use; Urine Cl^- <20 mEq/L) or (2) *chloride-resistant metabolic alkalosis* (e.g., increased aldosterone effect/mineralocorticoid excess, hypokalemia, edema, HTN; Urine Cl^- >20 mEq/L). *Signs and symptoms* can include hypoventilation (a compensatory mechanism), signs of hypocalcemia (+ Chvostek's sign, neuromuscular excitability, HA, changes in mental status), signs of hypokalemia (weakness, myalgias, arrhythmias), hypervolemia or hypovolemia, and hypertension. *Diagnose* through serum electrolytes and ABGs. Urine Cl^- and aldosterone levels may be helpful. Lab studies show an elevated serum pH (7.45), elevated HCO_3^- levels, and possibly elevated aldosterone levels. Expected $PCO_2 = 0.7\,[HCO_3] + 20, +/- 5$. *Treatment* consists of correction of the underlying cause, and IV sodium chloride (isotonic saline solution, 0.9%) for chloride-responsive met. alkalosis, Chloride-resistant met. alkalosis involves treating the specific cause (e.g., removal of adrenal or pituitary tumors, K^+-sparing diuretics, dexamethasone). If edema is present, potassium chloride (KCl) should be used instead to balance electrolytes and reduce the edema. *Complications* include arrhythmias, tetany, seizures, and coma.

Respiratory Acidosis

Respiratory acidosis is due to a **depressed respiratory system** that prevents carbon dioxide (CO_2) from being "blown off," leading to **elevated acid levels** in the blood (pH <7.35). This can be acute or chronic. Blood pH is affected by the amount of CO_2 or carbonic acid (H_2CO_3) in the blood; the pH is controlled thorough the bicarbonate buffering system: $CO_2 + H_2O \leftrightarrow H_2CO_3 \leftrightarrow H^+ + HCO_3^-$. With chronic respiratory acidosis, the body will compensate by renal retention of bicarbonate (HCO_3^-) over a few days. Respiratory acidosis can be due to alveolar hypoventilation (most common), overproduction of CO_2 by the body, or by an increased intake of CO_2. Some causes include COPD, asthma, sleep apnea, pneumonia, pulmonary edema, pleural effusion, pneumothorax, neuromuscular diseases (myasthenia gravis, Guillain-Barré), sedative drugs, and CNS depression. Patients may exhibit CO_2 narcosis: HA, confusion, somnolence, or stupor; but *symptoms* largely follow the underlying cause. If chronic, patients may appear asymptomatic or have subtle changes. *Diagnose* with serum electrolytes and ABGs which reveal a pH <7.35 and $PaCO_2$ >45 mmHg.

If chronic, the pH can be normal or near normal due to renal compensation. *Treat* the underlying cause and give proper respiratory support. If severe, intubation and mechanical ventilation may be necessary. If chronic, corrections need to be made slowly to avoid overcorrecting. *Complications* include confusion, seizures, coma, and respiratory failure.

Respiratory Alkalosis

Respiratory alkalosis occurs due to an excessive **loss of carbon dioxide** (CO_2) through increased depth or rate of respirations (**hyperventilation**). This can occur with chronic respiratory illnesses or may be acute in nature. It can be caused by hyperventilation from anxiety, pain, fever, pneumonia, sepsis, anemia, hyperthyroidism, hepatic failure, pneumonia, mechanical ventilation, or salicylate toxicity. Initially, the excess bicarbonate is buffered by extracellular H^+, but this is minimal. When chronic, the body will compensate by increasing the excretion of bicarbonate ions (HCO_3^-) through the urine, thus lowering the pH after a few days. **Chronic respiratory alkalosis** usually does not cause patients to experience symptoms. When **acute**, patients may experience light-headedness, dizziness, paresthesias, and syncope due to hyperventilation. On exam, patients may have a fever, be visibly hyperventilating, short of breath, and may have a positive Chvostek or Trousseau sign. *Diagnose* with serum electrolytes and ABGs which show a pH >7.45 and $PaCO_2$ <35 mmHg. *Treat* the underlying cause. With symptomatic respiratory alkalosis, effort should be made to correct the acid-base imbalance by slowing down the respiratory rate and administering oxygen (as needed). If fever is the cause, antipyretics should be given and the underlying cause of the fever should be treated. *Complications* include tetany and seizures.

Sepsis and Shock

Sepsis

Sepsis is the body's systemic response to **infection** which can cause tissue damage, organ failure, and death. Mortality rates increase as the start time of treatment is delayed; and patient survival improves if treatment is started within 3 hours. Those at risk of sepsis include children <1 year old, elderly (≥65 years old), those with chronic medical conditions, and the immunocompromised. *Symptoms* include fever (≥102° F) or hypothermia, diaphoresis, SOB, tachycardia, altered mental status, pain/discomfort, and hypotension. A quick SOFA score (Sequential Organ Failure Assessment) can help identify those with sepsis. Patients with 2 out of the 3 criteria are likely to have sepsis and include: RR ≥22/min., systolic BP ≤100 mmHg, and altered mental status. Labs to help with *diagnosis* include a CBC with differential, BUN, Cr, LFT's, and blood cultures/cultures from potential infection sites (e.g., wound or surgery site, CSF, urine) should be taken before antibiotics are started. If signs of septic shock, admit to the ICU and monitor ABG's, O_2 levels, renal function (urine output), blood glucose, lactate, and electrolytes. *Treatment* includes empiric antibiotics started immediately (follow local trends and antimicrobial resistance patterns when choosing antibiotics), reperfusion with IV fluids and vasopressors (if needed), oxygen, and other supportive measures. *Complications* include organ failure, septic shock, and death.

SIRS

Systemic inflammatory response syndrome (SIRS) suggests that there is inflammation in the body and is a way to assess for possible sepsis (assess risk of increased mortality due to sepsis).

SIRS is defined as meeting **2 or more** of the following:

- Fever >100.4 °F or <96.8 °F
- HR >90 bpm
- RR >20/min. or $PaCO_2$ <32 mmHg
- abnormal WBC count (i.e. >12,000/μL or <4,000/μL or >10% immature bands).

However, SIRS is nonspecific. Processes other than sepsis (or infection) that can meet the SIRS criteria include trauma, surgery, burns, ischemia, MI, medications, malignancies, and pancreatitis. Workup includes CBC with differential, metabolic panel, and other studies based on the patient's history and PE (i.e. various cultures: blood, sputum, urine, CSF; cardiac enzymes; blood gases, lactate, etc.). *Treatment* varies greatly and is directed toward the cause. Since infection is the most common cause of SIRS, empiric antibiotic treatment should be directed at the source of infection and follow local resistance patterns. *Complications* of SIRS may include ARDS, renal failure, DVT, hyperglycemia, DIC, and death.

Shock

Shock is defined as an emergency medical condition in which the circulatory system is unable to meet the oxygen delivery needs of the body. Shock is a medical emergency that if left untreated, can lead to irreversible organ damage and death. Shock is divided into three categories based on the etiology: hypovolemic, cardiogenic, and distributive (septic). Some of the more common causes of shock include trauma, ruptured aneurysm, cardiac failure, and sepsis. The presenting signs of shock include tachycardia, tachypnea, cool clammy skin, altered mental status, and hypotension. First attention must be given to evaluating and managing the ABCs (airway, breathing, and circulation). Intravenous access must be established. It is generally recommended that two large bore IV catheters be placed. Administer oxygen, evaluate respiratory status, and consider intubation. The cause of shock should be investigated. Work up should include CBC, metabolic panel, toxicology screen, arterial blood gas, and chest x-ray. Once the etiology is established, it should be treated. Use of pressers such as epinephrine, dopamine, and dobutamine should be considered.

Other Multisystem Complications

Toxic Ingestions

There are many **toxic substances** that can potentially be ingested. Signs and symptoms, as well as a treatment regimen, depend on identifying the substance. *General management* principles can be applied to most ingestions. The use of ipecac to induce vomiting is ineffective for treatment of ingestions and is no longer recommended. Gastric lavage is generally considered useful if it can be done within 1.5 hours of the ingestion. The airway must be protected during lavage. Patients with depressed mental status require intubation. Activated charcoal should be given as soon as possible. Some specific antidotes for ingestions include: N-acetylcysteine for acetaminophen, physostigmine for anticholinergics, hyperbaric oxygen for carbon monoxide, deferoxamine for iron, and ethylenediamine tetraacetic acid (EDTA) for lead.

Hypothermia

Hypothermia is defined as the core body temperature <35°C. It occurs when the body is unable to produce sufficient heat to make up for losses. The risk of hypothermia is increased at both ends of the age spectrum. Alcohol, drug use, and conditions that cause mental impairment, such as Alzheimer's disease or psychiatric illness, also increase the risk of hypothermia. Patients usually present with shivering, confusion, slurred speech, and clumsiness. The diagnosis is confirmed by the presence of a low core body temperature. *Treatment* involves rewarming the patient. Heat blankets, heat packs, warmed IV saline, and warmed humidified oxygen are all used. Patients may appear dead, but should not be considered dead until their core body temperature has been returned to normal.

Hyperthermia

Hyperthermia is defined as a condition in which the body produces or absorbs more heat than it can eliminate. Heat exhaustion is the milder form of hyperthermia and it is characterized by a mild increase in body temperature and dehydration. Heat stroke is a severe condition in which the body temperature rises above 41.1°C. Heat stroke is associated with a high mortality rate. The symptoms of hyperthermia include fatigue, nausea, vomiting, and an altered mental status. Physical exam is significant for tachycardia, tachypnea, and an elevated body temperature. It is a medical emergency. *Treatment* includes rapid cooling measures with ice pack and water immersion and IV hydration.

Nutrition

Thiamine (Vitamin B_1)

Thiamin or thiamine (vitamin B_1) is a water-soluble vitamin that, like all B vitamins, is used in the **metabolism** of food into usable energy. Thiamine is especially important in carbohydrate metabolism, proper nerve function, and is essential to pyruvate metabolism. **Beriberi** is the condition caused by thiamine deficiency which causes wasting, peripheral neuropathy, and rarely heart issues like CHF. Beriberi can be divided into *dry beriberi*, which refers to the nervous system effects, or *wet beriberi*, which refers to the cardiovascular effects ot thiamine deficiency. **Wernicke-Korsakoff syndrome** is another disease caused by thiamine deficiency that is characterized by a classic presentation of confusion, ataxia, and horizontal nystagmus. It is usually seen in chronic alcoholics, but may also appear in extreme malnutrition and after bariatric surgery. With proper treatment, most conditions due to thiamine deficiency are reversible until the late findings of Korsakoff syndrome (e.g., memory loss). *Treat* with parenteral thiamine until symptoms are gone. Maintaining proper levels of thiamine involves eating thiamin-rich foods including sunflower seeds, beans, oats, meat (e.g., pork), green peas, and potatoes, Thiamine is metabolized in the liver, excreted in the urine, and there are no known cases of thiamine toxicity.

Riboflavin (Vitamin B_2)

Riboflavin, or vitamin B_2, is a water-soluble vitamin that acts as a **coenzyme** which is necessary for normal **cell growth, development, and energy production**. Riboflavin also helps in red blood cell production and maintaining healthy mucous membranes. A primary deficiency in riboflavin may be due to malnutrition, though this is rare in industrialized countries. It can also be due to a secondary deficiency caused by chronic diarrhea or a malabsorption syndrome that prevents riboflavin from being absorbed. Riboflavin and thiamine deficiencies are usually seen together. *Symptoms* of riboflavin deficiency include swelling of the mucous membranes, sore throat, and cracks on the lips or corners of the mouth (angular stomatitis or cheilosis). Seborrheic dermatitis may develop without adequate levels of riboflavin, as can certain types of anemia. *Treat* with riboflavin replacement through supplements and eating beef (esp. high in beef liver), fortified cereals and breads, yogurt, cheese, eggs, spinach, and drinking milk. If there is an underlying malabsorption disorder causing the deficiency, this should be treated. Riboflavin is metabolized in the liver, excreted in the urine, and there are no known cases of riboflavin toxicity.

Niacin (Vitamin B_3)

Niacin, or vitamin B_3, is a water-soluble vitamin which is essential for **cell function and cell metabolism**. Dietary tryptophan can be metabolized to niacin. A niacin deficiency can lead to a condition called **pellagra**. This can occur with malnutrition, due to a lack of niacin in the diet (e.g., diet high in maize), because of a malabsorption syndrome, or due to certain meds (e.g., some TB meds). The "4 D's" can occur with advanced pellagra and usually appear in this order:

- Diarrhea
- Dermatitis
- Dementia
- Death

Patients may experience weakness, have a typically symmetric, erythematous rash in sun-exposed areas, and may be irritable or short-tempered before dementia becomes evident. *Treatment* involves replacing the niacin orally and eating niacin and tryptophan-rich foods (e.g., turkey, tuna, chicken, beef, peanuts, brewer's yeast). Correct malabsorption issues (e.g., alcoholism). Carcinoid tumors or gastric tumors may cause obstruction that prevents absorption of niacin, and should be surgically removed, if possible. Niacin is metabolized and stored in the liver, excreted in the urine, and niacin toxicity can occur (e.g., flushing, pruritus, N/V, hepatotoxicity).

Vitamin B_6

Vitamin B_6 is a water-soluble vitamin that is important in **protein metabolism, hemoglobin synthesis, antibody synthesis, and proper nerve function**. A deficiency can be caused by a primary deficiency (inadequate intake) or a secondary deficiency (malabsorption, alcoholism, drugs that inactivate pyridoxine). A B_6 deficiency results in peripheral neuropathy, anemia, seborrheic dermatitis, cheilosis, glossitis, a pellagra-like syndrome (characterized by diarrhea, dermatitis, and dementia), and possibly seizures. *Treatment* involves supplements and eating B_6-rich foods including liver, meat, fish, seeds, chickpeas, and bananas. Correct malabsorption issues and give patients on isoniazid concomitant pyridoxine. Vitamin B_6 is metabolized and mostly stored in the liver (also stored in muscle and brain), excreted in the urine, and megadoses can lead to B_6 toxicity which manifests as peripheral neuropathy, impaired vibratory sensation, impaired proprioception (sense of your body's position), and ataxia.

Folate (Vitamin B_9)

Folate, or vitamin B_9, is a water-soluble vitamin that is needed for **DNA synthesis, mitosis, RBC production, and proper fetal development**. This vitamin cannot be synthesized by the body so it must be ingested through foods and supplements. Folate supplements are especially important in pregnancy for prevention of neural tube defects. It is recommended to take folic acid 600-800 µg/day while pregnant and 500-800 µg/day while breastfeeding. Folate supplements must be accompanied by vitamin B_{12} supplements. This is due to the fact that both folate and B_{12} deficiencies result in a megaloblastic anemia. Therefore, if a patient is treated with folate, the anemia will appear to be correcting while the nerve damage caused by a concomitant vitamin B_{12} deficiency continues. This can result in permanent nerve damage. Folate deficiency can be due to inadequate intake, increased age, malabsorption (e.g., chronic alcohol use, IBD), and certain meds (e.g., antacids, methotrexate). Folate deficiency can result in megaloblastic anemia, glossitis, diarrhea, confusion, and neural tube defects in pregnancy. *Diagnose* with a CBC with blood smear, with serum folate or RBC folate levels, and serum vitamin B_{12} levels. *Treat* with oral folate and concomitant vit B_{12} if deficient. Foods rich in folate include dark green leafy vegetables, fruit, organ meats, and dairy products. Unlike vit B_{12}, folate is not stored in large amounts in the body. Folate is metabolized in the liver, excreted in the urine, and there appears to be no risk of toxicity.

VITAMIN B_{12}

Vitamin B_{12} or cobalamin is a water-soluble vitamin which is important for **DNA synthesis, RBC production, proper nerve function, and cell metabolism**. Vitamin B_{12} works with folate in several chemical processes including RBC production and maturation. Vitamin B_{12}, like folate, must be ingested since it cannot be produced by the body. It is only found in animal products; therefore, strict vegans are at an increased risk of a primary B_{12} deficiency. Vitamin B_{12} deficiency may also be caused by impaired absorption due to age, decreased gastric acid production, lack of intrinsic factor (i.e. pernicious anemia; often seen in the elderly), or intestinal disorders. Vitamin B_{12} deficiency can result in megaloblastic anemia, peripheral neuropathy, weight loss, glossitis, ataxia, and confusion or dementia. *Diagnose* with CBC with blood smear (hypersegmented neutrophils) and serum vitamin B_{12} and folate levels; the Schilling test (tests for intrinsic factor) is not used as often as it once was. *Treat* with oral or IM vitamin B_{12}, depending on the severity of the deficiency. Foods rich in vitamin B_{12} include clams, fish, meat, eggs, milk, and fortified cereals. Vitamin B_{12} is stored in the liver in large quantities, excreted in the urine, and there appears to be no risk of toxicity.

VITAMIN A

Vitamin A is a fat-soluble vitamin that is an **antioxidant**, is helpful in **boosting the immune system, maintains epithelial and bone/teeth integrity, keeps the eyes healthy, and is required for night/low light vision**. The antioxidant effects of vitamin A (beta-carotene) may help prevent some forms of cancer. Vitamin A comes from animal sources (retinol; preformed vit A, the body converts all forms to retinol) and vegetable sources (carotenoids; provitamin A). A primary vitamin A deficiency can be due to malnutrition but is rare in developed countries. Secondary vitamin A deficiency can be due to malabsorption, including malabsorption of fats which decreases the absorption of vitamin A, impaired vit. A transport, or liver disease. Deficiency can lead to diarrhea, increased infections, respiratory disorders, dry/brittle hair and nails, decreased growth rate, night blindness and eventually complete blindness. **Xerophthalmia**, or pathologic dry eyes, leads to keratinization, Bitot spots, and eventually corneal ulcerations and blindness. Although rare in the U.S., this blindness is especially seen in malnourished children in developing countries. Deficiency is diagnosed clinically and serum retinol levels can be measured. *Treat* by giving supplements and eating foods rich in vit A (e.g., liver, fish oils, egg yolk, sweet potatoes, dark leafy greens like spinach, and carrots). Treat malabsorption disorders if possible. Vitamin A is stored in the liver (typical reserves last ~1 year), metabolized in the cell, and toxicity can develop. Toxicity causes birth defects, N/V, headache, increased ICP, dry/rough skin, and liver damage. **Carotenemia**, or **carotenoderma**, is harmless and causes yellowing of the skin due to increased ingestion of beta-carotene.

VITAMIN C

Vitamin C or ascorbic acid is a water-soluble vitamin that acts as an **antioxidant** and is vital for **immune health, wound healing, collagen formation, proper function of blood vessels, and aids in the absorption of iron in the intestines**. Vitamin C must be ingested since the body cannot manufacture it. Those at an increased risk of a vit C deficiency include alcoholics, smokers, and the elderly/those with poor nutrition. A deficiency in vitamin C causes an illness known as **scurvy**.

Historically, this was seen in those who were at sea for extended periods of time and did not have access to foods rich in vitamin C. Scurvy causes weakness, bruising, bleeding gums/gingivitis, hemorrhages, hair and tooth loss, arthralgias, rash (e.g., perifollicular hyperkeratosis/perifollicular hemorrhage), and poor wound healing. In children, this can appear as impaired bone growth and growth delay. *Treatment* of a vitamin C deficiency requires supplementation and dietary changes that increases the consumption of foods rich in vitamin C, such as citrus fruit, strawberries, potatoes, broccoli, and red/green peppers. Vitamin C is metabolized in the liver, excreted in the urine, and is not thought to be toxic, but may cause diarrhea if taken in high doses.

Vitamin D

Vitamin D is a fat-soluble vitamin that plays a vital role in **calcium absorption** into bones to provide healthy, strong **teeth and bones**. Vitamin D is known as the "sunshine vitamin," is produced within the skin after exposure to sunlight, and 5-30 mins/day (depending on skin type, location, and time of the year) of sun exposure can help increase a person's vitamin D level. It then undergoes 2 hydroxylations in the liver and kidney to become the hormone, 1α,25-dihydroxyvitamin D (calcitriol), which is the biologically active form of vit D. A deficiency of vitamin D leads to a condition called rickets in children and osteomalacia in adults. **Rickets** will produce a bowing of the legs of children because of bone softening due to decreased bone mineralization. Bone growth will also be stifled without vitamin D. **Osteomalacia** in adults causes periosteal bone pain, muscle aches, weakness, and decreased bone mineralization or "soft bones" which places these individuals at higher risk of compression fractures. *Diagnose* with serum 25(OH)D levels, which will be low (while PTH levels may be elevated), and radiographs. *Treat* with vitamin D supplements (e.g., ergocalciferol), and by increasing intake of dairy products, fortified foods, and saltwater fish. Correct any concurrent calcium or phosphate deficiencies. Vitamin D is stored in the liver and adipose tissue, metabolized in the liver and kidney, and toxicity can occur from megadoses of supplements. Toxicity results in hypercalcemia causing bone pain, N/V, poor appetite, constipation or diarrhea, kidney stones, and kidney failure.

Vitamin E

Vitamin E is a fat-soluble vitamin that acts as a vital **antioxidant** which is important for protecting **lipids**, in the cell membrane and throughout the body, from **free radicals**. It is also important for immune function, nerve function, metabolic processes, RBC formation, and blood vessel health. There are 8 isoforms, but only **α-tocopherol**, which is the body's preference, can correct vit E deficiency. A deficiency can be due to a primary lack in the diet or a secondary cause (e.g., fat malabsorption). Vitamin E deficiency results in hemolytic anemia, muscle weakness/pain, ataxia, and nystagmus. The late effects of severe deficiency can result in cardiac arrhythmias, blindness, and dementia. *Diagnose* with a serum α-tocopherol level. *Treat* with vitamin E supplements (tocopherol) and eating foods high in vitamin E like vegetable oils, seeds, nuts, spinach, broccoli, and fortified foods. Vitamin E is stored in adipose tissue, metabolized in the liver, and toxicity can develop. Toxicity results in weakness, headache, nausea, abdominal cramps, diarrhea, and cause blood clotting issues (easy bruising/bleeding). Vitamin E interacts with anticoagulate/antiplatelet medications, interferes with the action of vitamin K, and therefore can increase the risk of bleeding.

Vitamin K

Vitamin K is a fat-soluble vitamin that acts as a coenzyme and plays a vital role in the **clotting cascade** to prevent excessive bleeding. It is involved in the formation of factors II (prothrombin), VII, IX, and X. It also helps maintain bone and tissue health. Vit K comes in 3 forms: **Vitamin K1** (from plants), **Vitamin K2** (produced by bacteria in the intestines), and **Vitamin K3** (synthetic). A deficiency in vitamin K is very rare, but it can be seen in those individuals with a malabsorption syndrome that prevents that absorption of fats from the GI tract leading to a decreased amount of vit K absorbed from foods. The blood thinning drug warfarin (Coumadin®) blocks the function of vitamin K in the clotting cascade, which promotes bleeding and a decreased clotting time. *Treatment* of a vitamin K deficiency can be reversed with injectable vitamin K1 (preferred method is SC or IM; oral also available). Also, this is given to infants IM shortly after birth (within 6 hours) to help prevent excessive bleeding. Diet is the main source of vit K and it is found in abundant supply in green, leafy vegetables. Malabsorption issues that prevent absorption of fats from the GI tract should be treated, if possible. Vitamin K has low stores in the body, is metabolized in the liver, excreted in the feces and urine, and toxicity can occur with vit K3. This causes jaundice in newborns and hemolytic anemia, and therefore is no longer used to treat vit K deficiencies.

Obesity

Obesity is a condition in which the person has too much body fat. Diagnosis may include lipid levels, liver function tests, blood glucose, and thyroid function tests. The Body Mass Index (BMI) formula is a measurement that uses height and weight as an indicator of obesity/malnutrition:

Calculating BMI	Resulting scores
For adults ≥age 20: BMI formula using pounds and inches: $BMI = (weight\ in\ pounds \times \frac{703}{Height\ in\ inches^2}$ BMI formula using kilograms and meters: $BMI = \frac{weight\ in\ kilograms}{Height\ in\ meters^2}$	Below 18.5: Underweight 18.5-24.9: Normal weight 25.0-29.9: Overweight 30 and above: Obese
For children and those <age 20: Uses age-gender specific charts provided by the CDC, containing a curved line that indicates percentiles.	<5th percentile: Underweight 85th-<95 percentile: At risk for overweight >95th percentile: Overweight

Risk factors include genetics, unhealthy eating habits/diet, lack of activity, medical conditions (Cushing's syndrome, hypothyroidism, arthritis), older age, pregnancy, smoking cessation, inadequate sleep, and socioeconomic issues. Treatment options include dietary modification (low fat, low carbohydrate, low calorie), increased exercises, behavioral changes, weight loss medications (orlistat, lorcaserin, phentermine-topiramate, naltrexone-bupropion, liraglutide), and/or bariatric surgery.

TPN

Total parenteral nutrition (TPN) is an intravenous hypertonic solution containing glucose, fat emulsion, protein, minerals, and vitamins, delivering nutrients to maintain body mass, energy, and strength. Long (24 inch) PICCs may be inserted in the basilic or cephalic veins and advanced into central circulation for short-term TPN. Central venous catheters are usually inserted into the subclavian or jugular vein and advanced to the tip of the superior vena cava for long-term TPN. Central solutions are more hypertonic than peripheral. Commercially-prepared TPN solutions contain dextrose and protein (amino acids), but electrolytes, vitamins, and trace elements are individualized. A total nutrient admixture that contains fat emulsion, dextrose, and amino acids is widely used although fat emulsion may be administered separately. Generally, fat emulsions should not provide >30% of total energy, with maximum dose of 2.5/g/kg per day. Protein levels of 1.5 to 2 g/kg/ per day are common. Complications include hypoglycemia, hyperglycemia, electrolyte imbalance, fluid imbalance, phlebitis, infection, air embolus, phlebitis, thrombosis, and nutritional deficiencies. Because hyperglycemia is a common complication, blood glucose levels should be monitored every 4 to 6 hours at bedside. Insulin may be ordered (sliding scale) to maintain glucose level <150 mg/dL, or insulin is included in the TPN and blood sugar levels are monitored.

Biostatistics and Epidemiology/Population Health and Interpretation of Medical Literature/Social Science

Population Health

Importance of Disease Prevention and Education in Family Medicine

Disease and injury prevention and education are the foundations for effective family medicine, with the healthcare provider focusing on providing anticipatory guidance to patients and family members based on evidence-based guidelines that are appropriate for the patient's age and gender. The healthcare provider should be prepared to collaborate with the patient and family in a culturally-sensitive manner and should have tools ready to help patients make lifestyle changes to improve health when they engage in unhealthy practices, such as drug use, alcohol abuse, unhealthy eating habits, inactivity, multiple sex partners, and smoking. The healthcare provider must have a clear understand of behavioral change and the importance of independence to patients and family. Additionally, the healthcare provider must provide information about periodic health screening guidelines recommended by organizations such as the U.S. Preventive Task Force (USPSTF) and the American Academy of Pediatrics and must share information about local, regional, and national resources that are available to assist the patient and family members.

Primary, Secondary, and Tertiary Prevention

Primary prevention describes measures undertaken to avoid the development of disease. There are many examples of primary prevention, including: immunizations, counseling high-risk behavior, and prophylactic medicines.

Secondary prevention is action taken to prevent the progression of a disease. This includes early detection, as in cancer screening, HIV screening, and blood pressure monitoring.

Tertiary prevention is aimed at minimizing damage and complications from a particular disease. Examples of tertiary prevention include cancer chemotherapy, antihypertensive medication, insulin for blood glucose control in diabetics, and renal dialysis.

Key Health Policies Relevant to Family Medicine

Key health policies relevant to family medicine include:

- **Health is Primary**: Advocates for the values and practices of family medicine to be incorporated into the provision of primary care with a focus on the needs of the patient.
- **American Academy of Family Physicians:** Clinical policies include:
    - Support for regulation of alcohol advertising aimed at adolescents and the need to recognize problems associated with underage drinking.
    - Recognition of inappropriate antibiotic use and the importance of utilizing evidence-based research when prescribing antibiotics.
    - Healthcare providers should utilize clinical practice guidelines that are evidence-based and patient centered.

- **Health Insurance Portability and Accountability Act (HIPAA):** Protects the privacy of individuals and provides regulation concerning security of electronic records.
- **Healthy People 2030:** Sets leading health indications and goals for many aspects of patient care, including promotion of breastfeeding, screening recommendations, initiatives to reduce infant deaths, exercise and weight recommendations, and tobacco use.
- **CDC:** Provides policies and guidelines regarding infectious diseases and reporting requirement.

Cancer Screening Guidelines for Cervical, Breast, and Colon Cancer

The following are recommended **cancer screening procedures**:

- **Cervical cancer** – Annual PAP tests for all women within 3 years onset of sexual activity and not later than age 21 years. Women over the age of 70 years who have had 3 consecutive normal PAP tests no longer require screening. Women who have had a total hysterectomy do not require screening.
- **Breast cancer** – Yearly mammograms should be performed beginning at the age of 40 years. Breast self-exam should be taught to women beginning in their twenties.
- **Colon cancer** – Patients over the age of 50 years should have annual screening for occult blood in the stool and sigmoidoscopy every 3 to 5 years or colonoscopy every 10 years. Patients with a family history of colon cancer should begin screening at the age of 40 years.

Cancer Screening Guidelines for Prostate, Skin, Testicular, and Ovarian Cancer

The following are **recommended screening procedures**:

- **Prostate cancer** – Digital rectal exam and prostate-specific antigen (PSA) annually beginning at age 50 years. High-risk men (African-American or positive family history) should be screened beginning at age 40 years.
- **Skin cancer** – Patients should be counseled regarding suspicious skin lesions and receive a skin exam every 3 years. Patients should also be advised about the importance of using sunscreen.
- **Testicular cancer** – All men should receive an annual testicular exam by a physician. Patients should be taught and encouraged to do testicular self-exam.
- **Ovarian cancer** – There is no recommended screening procedure for ovarian cancer.

Recommendations for Adult Immunization

The following **vaccines are recommended for adults**:

- **Tetanus and diphtheria** –Give primary series if not performed in childhood, followed by boosters every 10 years.
- **Measles, mumps, rubella** – Patients born after 1957 and not previously immunized should be given two doses a minimum of 1 month apart.
- **Influenza** – Yearly vaccine is recommended for patients over the age of 50 years or patients at risk for severe disease. This includes immunocompromised patients and patients with chronic disease.
- **Pneumococcal** – All patients over the age of 65 years, or high-risk patients over the age of 50 years.
- **Varicella** – Should be given to all adults without evidence of immunity. Two doses should be administered 4 to 8 weeks apart.
- **Human papilloma virus (HPV)** – Three dose series should be given to all women <26 years of age who have not been previously immunized.

- **Meningococcal** -- All asplenic adults and first-year college students who will be living in a dormitory.
- **Herpes zoster** – All adults over the age of 60 years.
- **Hepatitis A and B** – Recommended for patients at risk due to lifestyle, occupation, or travel plans.

Diseases That Must Be Reported to the Health Department

The requirement for **reporting diseases** to the state health department varies by state, but most states require reporting of the following:

- Animal bites requiring rabies prophylaxis
- Anthrax
- Botulism
- Brucellosis
- Cholera
- Diphtheria
- Encephalitis
- Glanders
- Hantavirus
- Hepatitis A in a food handler
- Measles, mumps or rubella
- Severe acute respiratory syndrome (SARS)
- Meningococcemia
- Smallpox
- Syphilis
- Tuberculosis
- Typhoid

Other diseases may mandate reporting and a physician should be aware of the requirements of the state in which they are practicing.

Smoking Cessation Methods

Smoking is the leading cause of preventable death in the United States today. The benefits of quitting are well-established. Nicotine is addictive and smoking cessation leads to symptoms of withdrawal. This issue should be addressed by the primary care physician. The Public Health Service recommends the 4-A's approach to aid patients with **smoking cessation**:

- **Asking** about smoking.
- **Advise** an approach to quitting and setting a date to quit.
- **Assistance** – Provide counseling as well as pharmacologic aids. Counseling options include smoking cessation groups and hypnosis. It should include the possibility of weight gain and advice about diet and exercise. Drugs available to help include nicotine replacement products available as patches, gum, nasal spray, and inhalers. Bupropion is an antidepressant used to aid in smoking cessation. It is contraindicated in patients with a history of seizures.
- **Arrange** a follow-up appointment 2 to 4 weeks after the date set for quitting.

The combination of counseling and support groups with drug therapy has a smoking cessation success rate of about 50%.

Obesity and BMI

Obesity is defined as being greater than 20% above one's ideal body weight. It is estimated that approximately one third of Americans are obese. Family history, increased age, and female gender all increase the risk of obesity. Obesity is most often caused by a poor diet and sedentary lifestyle. Occasionally, obesity can be due to a medical condition such as hypothyroidism or Cushing's disease, or as it can be a side effect of a medication. Obesity increases an individual's risk of cardiovascular disease, stroke, diabetes, hypertension, and certain cancers. Treatment options include dietary changes, exercise, and other lifestyle changes. Drug therapy can sometimes be helpful. Medications such as sibutramine, which decreases appetite, and orlistat, which reduces fat absorption, have been shown to be helpful. In severe cases, weight-loss surgery may be considered.

Body mass index (BMI) is an approximation of body fat based on height and weight. It is calculated by dividing weight (kilograms) by height (in meters squared): BMI = weight (kg) / height (m^2).

Domestic Violence/Partner Abuse

Domestic abuse often begins subtly and progresses over time. Initial signs include a partner that is overly controlling and jealous. The abuser is often extremely controlling of finances, social activities, and even everyday issues such as clothing. This can progress to threats, physical and sexual violence. Signs that should lead to suspicion of domestic partner abuse include inconsistent or implausible explanation of injuries, frequent emergency room visits, or delay in seeking medical care. Women are far more likely to be abused by their male partners. Same sex couples are estimated to have about the same incidence of abuse as heterosexual couples. An abused partner is most likely to be killed when attempting to leave the relationship. Mandatory reporting of domestic violence is not required in most states.

Child Abuse

Child abuse includes the physical, psychological, or sexual mistreatment of a child. Neglect is also a form of child abuse. Child abuse can occur in any socioeconomic or ethnic group. Physicians are mandated to report cases of suspected child abuse. Signs exhibited by children that should arouse suspicion of abuse include a sudden change in behavior, missing school, social withdrawal, and inappropriate sexual behavior. Unexplained cuts, bruises, or burns are also indications there may be abuse. A parental explanation that is vague, changes, or inconsistent with the injuries seen is also a reason to suspect abuse. If abuse is suspected, appropriate authorities must be notified. Careful documentation of the history and injuries is important. Photographs of injuries should be taken.

Elder Abuse

The different types of **elder abuse** include physical, sexual, emotional, financial, and neglect. The most likely perpetrator is a family member. Institutional caregivers are also potential abusers of the elderly. Women and individuals over the age of 80 years are more likely to be abused. The more dependent an elderly individual, the greater the chances of abuse. Signs of abuse include unexplained cuts, bruises, burns, or other injuries. Weight loss, poor hygiene, and other unmet needs are also signs that there may be abuse. Improper management of valuables and finances should also lead to suspicion of abuse. Physicians should routinely question elderly patients about the possibility of abuse and take appropriate action if abuse is suspected.

Herbal Medicines

There are numerous **herbal medicines** are readily available over the counter for patients. Most are safe, but some can have toxic effects or unwanted drug interactions. Some of the more commonly used herbal remedies include aloe vera gel for burn relief, Echinacea for colds and flu, ginseng for numerous disorders, and green tea extract as an antioxidative medication. Some common herbal remedies with potentially toxic effects include kava (which is toxic to the liver and may alter the effect of other medications), ephedra (which can cause palpitations and other autonomic hyperactivity), and ginseng (which may be linked to some unwanted health effects). Patients should routinely be asked about their use of herbal remedies and advised accordingly.

Medicare and Medicaid

An individual is eligible for **Medicare** if they are age 65 years or older and are either receiving or are eligible to receive social security benefits. They are also eligible when not yet 65 years old if they are receiving social security disability benefits or have end-stage renal disease. Part A of Medicare is free and covers inpatient costs, nursing facilities, home health care, and hospice care. Part B requires a premium payment and covers outpatient care, x-rays, and lab work. Part C (Medicare Advantage) covers enrollment in HMOs or PPOs if they are approved. Part D is the Medicare prescription drug benefit.

Persons eligible for **Medicaid** include pregnant women and children under the age of 6 years whose family income is <133% of the poverty level. All children <18 years are eligible if their family income is <100% of the poverty level. Elderly and disabled individuals who are below the poverty level are also eligible.

AMA Code of Medical Ethics

The **AMA code of medical ethics** is a set of standards developed by the American Medical Association that physicians are expected to adhere. The code of medical ethics was first developed and published in 1847. It is revised on a regular basis. There are nine basic principles that make up the code. In summary, the nine principles state that a physician should: be dedicated and competent and uphold standards of professionalism at all times. Physicians should abide by the law and respect the rights and privacy of patients. A physician should commit to continuing medical education and to improving the health of the community. The principles also state that physicians are free to choose where and to whom they will provide medical care, except in cases of an emergency.

Biostatistics and Epidemiology

Impact of Biostatistics and Epidemiology on Preventative Medicine

Preventive medicine draws from knowledge and skills of all branches of medicine and depends on evidence-based research to develop the most cost-effective and efficient models of prevention. Two critical elements include:

- **Biostatistics:** This is the application of statistical methods to research in the field of medicine. Data are collected and analyzed in order to reach conclusions (such as which type of treatment is most effective) or to make predictions (such as regarding health challenges in the future). In preventive medicine, it's critical that the most effective model be promoted in order to see results, and accurate predictions can help to determine future needs.
- **Epidemiology:** This is the study and analysis of incidence, distribution, and patterns in health, treatment, and disease. Epidemiologists try to find where and to whom diseases occur and the causes of disease and health outcomes. Preventive medicine must be able to identify needs and target populations and develop programs that meet those needs.

Incidence and Prevalence

Incidence is defined as the number of new cases of a disease that develop over a certain period of time in a population that is at risk for developing the disease. Incidence is a measure of risk. It is calculated as follows:

Incidence per 1,000 = [(Number of new cases during time period) / (total number of persons at risk)] x 1,000

Prevalence is defined as the number of cases that currently exist at a specified time. Prevalence is not a measure of risk. Prevalence is influenced by the duration of a disease. Therapies that prolong the survival of patients with a particular disease will increase the prevalence of that disease. It is calculated as follows:

Prevalence per 1,000 = [(Number of cases) / (Number of persons in population at the current time)] x 1,000

Cross-Sectional Studies

A **cross-sectional study** is a study in which exposure to a particular risk factor and development of a disease are assessed simultaneously. This type of study measures prevalent cases of the disease of interest and is also known as a prevalence study. A cross-sectional study cannot assess risk because the chronology of the risk factor and disease development are not known. Cross-sectional studies can only identify an association between a certain factor and disease development and suggest possible risk. The advantages of cross-sectional studies are that they are generally quicker to complete and the cost is lower.

Case-Control Studies and Cohort Studies

In a **case-control study**, the researcher begins with a group of individuals with the disease of interest (cases) and a comparable disease-free group (controls). The groups are then examined for the history of exposure to the factor of interest. The goal is to determine if a particular factor increases the risk of developing a particular disease.

In a **cohort study**, the investigator begins with a group of individuals with a history of exposure to the factor of interest and a comparable group of non-exposed individuals. The groups can then be followed for a period of time to identify the development of a disease (prospective cohort study). An investigator can also begin with a group of individuals whose exposure was documented at a certain time in the past as well as a comparable group of non-exposed people. Records can then be examined to determine the number who developed the disease of interest (retrospective cohort study).

Sensitivity, Specificity, Positive Predictive Value, and Negative Predictive Value

Sensitivity (Sn), specificity (Sp), positive predictive value (PPV), and negative predictive value (NPV) are ways of assessing the **validity** of diagnostic tests.

- **Sensitivity** is defined as the proportion of individuals correctly identified as positive by a particular test. It is expressed as a percent.
- **Specificity** is defined as the proportion of disease-free individuals identified as negative by a particular diagnostic test. It is also expressed as a percent.

- **Positive predictive value** is defined as the proportion of individuals who test positive that actually have the disease. It is expressed as a percent.
- **Negative predictive value** is defined as the proportion of individuals who test negative that are disease-free. It is also expressed as a percent.

P-Value, Type I Error (Alpha), and Type II Error (Beta)

A **type I error**, or alpha, is the probability that the study will conclude that there is a difference between the intervention group and the control when in fact no difference exists. This is also known as the **P-value.** The P-value identifies whether or not a result is statistically significant. A $P<0.05$ is considered significant. This means there is less than a five percent chance that no real difference between the two groups exists.

A **type II error**, or beta- the study will conclude there is no difference between the groups, when in fact a difference does exist.

Confounding, Recall Bias, and Selection Bias

Confounding occurs when a variable that is a known risk factor for a disease is associated with the factor being studied. An example is a study looking at the relationship between drinking coffee and pancreatic cancer. Smoking is associated with drinking coffee and is known to be a risk factor for pancreatic cancer. Therefore, an observed association between coffee drinking and pancreatic cancer may not be causal, but it may be due to the confounding factor of smoking.

Recall bias occurs in case-control studies when the cases studied recall issues differently based on their situation. It is also known as rumination bias.

Selection bias is an error in the selection of the study groups that changes the study outcome. An example of a selection bias occurs when a particular segment of a group being studied is less likely to complete a survey or follow through with the entire study.

Quality Improvement

Quality improvement is a systematic method of analyzing performance and improving the quality of performance, usually across an entire organization although more localized quality improvement methods may be employed. Methods of quality improvement include:

- **Continuous Quality Improvement** (CQI): Emphasizes the organization and systems and processes within that organization rather than individuals. It recognizes internal customers (staff) and external customers (patients) and utilizes data to improve processes.
- **Total Quality Management** (TQM): Espouses a commitment to meeting the needs of the customers at all levels within an organization, promoting not only continuous improvement but also a dedication to quality in all aspects of an organization. Outcomes should include increased customer satisfaction, productivity, and increased profits through efficiency and reduction in costs.
- **Six Sigma®**: A data-driven performance model that aims to eliminate "defects" in processes that involve products or services. The first model for Six Sigma® is DMAIC (define, measure, analyze, improve, control) and is used when existing processes or products need improvement and is utilized in healthcare quality.

SPEX Practice Test

Want to take this practice test in an online interactive format?
Check out the online resources page, which includes interactive practice questions and much more: **mometrix.com/resources719/spex**

1. A 57-year-old man goes to see his physician because of intermittent chest pain. It sometimes occurs with effort, and sometimes at rest, and usually lasts 5 to 10 minutes. It is midsternal with some radiation to the throat. He has a history of high blood pressure. He discontinued smoking at about age 50. His only medication is amlodipine 10 mg daily. He has a family history of hypertension and diabetes type 2. He denies other significant medical problems. On examination his blood pressure is 135/85, pulse 76 and regular, height 70 inches and weight 210 lb. His chest is clear and no cardiac murmurs or rubs are heard. The balance of the examination is negative. His electrocardiogram (ECG) is normal.

What is the next logical procedure most likely to provide a diagnosis?

a. Lipid profile
b. Hemoglobin A_{1c}
c. Technetium Tc-99m sestamibi stress test
d. Coronary angiography
e. Esophagogastroduodenoscopy (EGD)

2. Two days later the above patient awakens with severe, persistent chest pain. There is mild diaphoresis but no nausea or vomiting. He is given 2 chewable aspirin tablets and nitroglycerin spray by the paramedics and taken to the emergency room. His blood pressure is now 160/90 and electrocardiogram shows a sinus tachycardia with ST depressions and some inverted T waves in the lateral precordial leads. His chest pain has diminished somewhat.

What would be the next most reasonable course of action?

a. Send the patient to the catheterization laboratory immediately
b. Draw blood for a troponin level
c. Obtain a high-resolution CT scan of the chest
d. Request a cardiac ultrasound
e. Start clopidogrel

3. The above patient has angiography that shows a 90% obstruction in a major branch of the left anterior descending artery (LAD). The other arteries appear less than 30% obstructed. A drug-eluting stent is placed in the severely obstructed vessel after balloon angioplasty and the patient then reports he is pain free at rest and with exercise. The resting electrocardiogram is now normal and an isotopic stress test fails to show evidence of myocardial ischemia.

The patient may be discharged on all the following drugs EXCEPT:

a. clopidogrel.
b. warfarin.
c. an angiotensin-converting enzyme (ACE) inhibitor.
d. a statin.
e. aspirin.

4. A 67-year-old woman consults her physician because of several episodes of weakness in the right arm and hand, accompanied by slightly garbled speech. There is no loss of conscience. The events last 5 to 15 minutes, after which she returns to her normal state. She is a widow, living alone, and right-handed. She has been treated for high blood pressure and diabetes for the past 5 years and is taking a diuretic and an angiotensin receptor blocker (ARB) and metformin. She denies blurred vision, seizures, vertigo, or other neurologic disease, or heart disease. Her last hemoglobin A_{1c} was 6.6%. On examination her blood pressure is 150/80, pulse regular. A bruit is heard over the left carotid artery. There is a grade 2/6 midsystolic murmur at the cardiac base but no other abnormalities. Neurologic exam does not reveal extremity weakness, abnormal reflexes, or motor or sensory abnormalities. Her cranial nerves are intact.

What is the most likely diagnosis that accounts for her symptoms?

a. Transient ischemic attacks (TIA)
b. Left hemispheric stroke
c. Seizure disorder
d. Vertebrobasilar insufficiency
e. Aortic stenosis

5. Routine blood tests for the above patient show a normal CBC and platelet count, a fasting glucose of 150 mg/dL, and mild transaminase elevations. A chest x-ray indicates a borderline enlarged cardiac silhouette and clear lung fields. An electrocardiogram is read as normal sinus rhythm with a left anterior hemiblock but without ST changes or Q waves.

The next diagnostic procedure should be:

a. echocardiogram.
b. referral to a vascular surgeon.
c. cerebral angiography.
d. duplex carotid scan.
e. MR angiography.

6. This patient was found to have a 95% stenosis of the left carotid artery on cerebral angiography and underwent a successful endarterectomy. No evidence of prior stroke was found on brain MRI and her cardiac ultrasound confirmed mild left ventricular hypertrophy but no abnormalities of wall motion or possible sources of emboli.

Appropriate discharge medication(s) should include:

a. low molecular weight heparin.
b. aspirin and clopidogrel.
c. warfarin.
d. aspirin alone.
e. aspirin and a statin.

7. A 25-year-old single man is seen for a routine preemployment physical. His medical history reveals an appendectomy at age 16 but no serious medical illness. He had a febrile illness with swollen glands, fatigue, and fever to 101 °F several months ago, but it resolved by itself and he did not see a doctor. Further questioning reveals that he is bisexual and has had sexual encounters with men and women but has a steady girlfriend at this time. He is vague about condom use. He denies sexually transmitted disease or intravenous drug use but occasionally snorts a little cocaine. Physical examination is essentially negative except for the appendectomy scar. No oropharyngeal abnormalities are noted and there is no evidence of lymphadenopathy or hepatosplenomegaly. A chest x-ray is negative. CBC, liver function tests, VDRL, and hepatitis panel are all negative. An HIV screening test is positive and confirmed by Western blot. A purified protein derivative (PPD) test is negative.

What is an appropriate next course of action with this patient?

a. Observation only with repeat examination and blood tests in 6 months
b. Observation only with HIV testing of his girlfriend
c. Begin highly active antiretroviral therapy (HAART)
d. Obtain a CD4 T-lymphocyte count
e. Obtain a CD4 T-lymphocyte count and a plasma HIV RNA determination

8. Results of the above patient's follow-up testing are a CD4 T-cell count of 400/mL and a plasma HIV RNA value of 75,000. HIV screening of his girlfriend was negative but 1 male sexual contact was found to be positive. He was warned to practice safe sex with latex condoms and avoid homosexual contacts if possible. Follow-up testing in 6 months showed a CD4 T-cell decline to 340/mL and a rise in the viral load to 110,000. He remains asymptomatic.

How should he be treated now?

a. Continued observation and repeat testing
b. A nonnucleoside reverse transcriptase inhibitor (NNRTI) only
c. A protease inhibitor (PI) only
d. A protease inhibitor and a nucleoside reverse transcriptase inhibitor (NRTI)
e. An NNRTI and a PI

9. The young man begins treatment with a protease inhibitor and NRTI. Six months later his girlfriend is found to be HIV positive. They admit to having unprotected sex several times. She is also 5 weeks pregnant and referred by her obstetrician for possible treatment. She feels well except for some morning sickness and has an essentially clean medical history. Her CD4 T-cell level is 500/mL and the HIV RNA is 20,000 copies/mL.

What is the most prudent treatment option for her to prevent transmission to the fetus?

a. Zidovudine monotherapy
b. No therapy until her HIV RNA is above 50,000
c. Combination ART immediately
d. Combination ART after her first trimester is completed
e. Defer treatment until just before delivery

10. A 74-year-old white man is in for an annual physical examination. His major complaint is joint pain and stiffness, especially in the knees, for which he takes naproxen regularly and an occasional hydrocodone. He has a history of angina in his mid-60s and underwent an angioplasty. He is also taking atorvastatin, low-dose aspirin, and an angiotensin receptor blocker. He is not diabetic and has no history of gastrointestinal or genitourinary disorders. He denies chest pain or dyspnea as well as abdominal pain or changes in bowel habits. His weight has been stable at 170 lb. On exam his blood pressure is 140/85, regular pulse at 70. Head, neck, chest, and cardiac examination are negative. The abdomen is slightly tender but there is no rebound or guarding, palpable mass, or hepatosplenomegaly. The prostate is enlarged but benign. Rectal exam is otherwise negative. Typical osteoarthritic changes of the hands are noted. Fecal occult blood testing is positive. A CBC shows hypochromic anemia with a hemoglobin of 10 g/dL and serum iron of 10 mcg/mL and a ferritin level of 5 ng/mL. He denies hematemesis, obvious rectal bleeding, or maroon-colored feces.

What is the most likely cause of the occult blood loss in this patient?

a. Diverticular bleeding
b. Angiodysplasia
c. Colon cancer
d. Gastric ulceration
e. Hemorrhoids

11. The above patient is advised to stop the aspirin and naproxen and to report any obvious rectal bleeding. He is then referred to a gastroenterologist for further workup.

What should be the next diagnostic procedure?

a. Upper gastrointestinal endoscopy (EGD)
b. Colonoscopy
c. Both EGD and colonoscopy
d. Angiography
e. Air contrast barium enema

12. The patient undergoes both upper and lower endoscopy but no bleeding lesion or clot is noted. No gastric or duodenal ulcer is seen and the esophageal mucosa appears intact. He has scattered diverticula and a few small colonic polyps that are removed and reported as benign by pathology. A repeat EGD remains negative but occult blood in the stool tests remain positive.

What should be the next diagnostic step?

a. Isotopic red blood cell scan
b. Surgical intraoperative enteroscopy
c. Angiography
d. Capsule endoscopy
e. Push enteroscopy

13. A 45-year-old man goes to see his physician because his wife insists that he gets a physical. He feels well but has gained some weight over the past 10 to 15 years and gets little exercise. He is an attorney and is usually too busy to worry about his diet. He had a melanoma removed from his arm about 8 years ago. His mother has high blood pressure and diabetes and his father died of an apparent heart attack in his late 50s. His blood pressure is 140/88, regular pulse, afebrile, and BMR of 30.2 kg/m^2. A surgical scar from the melanoma excision is present on his left forearm but no suspect lesions are noted on skin exam. His physical examination is fairly unremarkable except for abdominal obesity with a waist/hip ratio of 1.3. An electrocardiogram is normal. Blood tests and urinalysis are unremarkable except for a fasting glucose of 180 mg/dL and a hemoglobin A_{1c} of 7.8%

What is the most appropriate treatment for this patient now?

a. Referral to a dietitian for a low-carbohydrate diet and an exercise program
b. Answer A and start metformin
c. Answer A and start a sulfonylurea
d. Answer A and start a thiazolidinedione
e. Answer A and start insulin

14. The above patient is seen 3 months after his initial visit. He has lost only 2 lb. He says he is too busy with a big case to follow a diet or get much exercise. His blood pressure is now 150/90, the total cholesterol 280 mg/dL with an LDL-C of 140 mg/dL and an HDL-C of 35 mg/dL. The triglycerides are 400 mg/dL. His hemoglobin A_{1c} is 7.6%

What treatment is most appropriate now?

a. Increase metformin
b. Begin a statin and maintain metformin
c. Begin a sulfonylurea and a statin
d. Begin a diuretic or beta-blocker
e. Begin insulin

15. Six months later, the patient is taking a statin, metformin, and losartan. His blood pressure is now 130/80, his LDL-C is 100 mg/dL, and the hemoglobin A_{1c} is 6.8%. He has lost about 5 lb. The following year, on the same therapy, his numbers are as follows: blood pressure 135/85, LDL-C 90 mg/dL, HDL-C 40 mg/dL, and hemoglobin A_{1c} 8.5%. He now complains of fatigue and occasional thirst and polyuria.

What action should be taken now?

a. Add a sulfonylurea
b. Add a non-sulfonylurea secretagogue
c. Add a thiazolidinedione
d. Add an alpha-glucosidase inhibitor
e. Any of the above and consider adding long-acting niacin

16. A 24-year-old man presents with a persistent productive cough and fever of 101°. He states he has had a "cold" for about a week with cough and fever in the 100° to 101° range. He is otherwise healthy, on no medications, and denies smoking, illicit drug use, and homosexual activity. He has never had a "pneumonia shot." He is slightly short of breath with exertion and has mild left-sided pleuritic pain on deep inspiration. He has some crackles and percussion dullness over the left lower lobe. There is no leg swelling or calf tenderness. Oxygen saturation is 93%.

What is the most likely diagnosis?

a. Legionnaire disease
b. Streptococcus pneumoniae pneumonia
c. Pulmonary embolus
d. Mycoplasma pneumonia
e. Pneumocystis pneumonia

17. All of the following would be appropriate in the management of this case EXCEPT:

a. chest x-ray.
b. CBC with differential.
c. hospitalization for intravenous cephalosporin.
d. azithromycin 500 mg as a single dose on the first day followed by 250 mg daily.
e. doxycycline 100 mg orally twice daily.

18. A 45-year-old female school teacher complains of pain and tenderness in both hands and wrists for the past 3 to 4 weeks. She also has some diffuse muscle tenderness and notes that she gets extremely fatigued while jogging, her major activity. No other joints are painful and she denies fever, back pain, and ocular, cardiopulmonary, or gastrointestinal symptoms. She has no family history of rheumatic disease. On examination there is warmth and tenderness over the wrist and metacarpal joints with some swelling and limited range of motion. Other joints appear intact and the rest of the exam is negative.

At this point, what is the most likely diagnosis?

a. Systemic lupus erythematosus (SLE)
b. Rheumatoid arthritis (RA)
c. Polymyalgia rheumatica (PR)
d. Fibromyalgia (FM)
e. Osteoarthritis (OA)

19. The above patient is sent for blood tests and imaging studies.

Which of the following would be most useful in establishing a diagnosis?

a. Joint aspiration and analysis
b. C-reactive protein (CRP)
c. Rheumatoid factor (RF)
d. Plain x-rays of the hands and wrists
e. Anti-cyclic citrullinated protein (anti-CCP)

20. A 50-year-old retired firefighter presents with weight loss, frequent palpitations, and a blood pressure of 170/70. He states his appetite has been good but he sweats a lot and his bowel movement frequency has increased but there has been no diarrhea. On examination he has a lid lag and brisk deep tendon reflexes. His thyroid is diffusely enlarged with an audible bruit but is nontender and no nodules are present. Blood testing reveals the presence of antithyroid antibodies. An ECG shows sinus tachycardia with occasional runs of atrial fibrillation.

Which of these lab results (TSH = thyroid-stimulating hormone and T4= free serum thyroxine) are most consistent with the clinical diagnosis (normal ranges: TSH 0.5 to 5 mcIU/mL and free T4 5 to 15 mcg/dL)?

a. TSH 0.1 mcIU/mL, free T4 20.5 mcg/dL
b. TSH 0.2 mcIU/mL, free T4 15 mcg/dL
c. TSH 7.5 mcIU/mL, free T4 14 mcg/dL
d. TSH 3 mcIU/mL, free T4 7.4 mcg/dL
e. TSH 14.5 mcIU/mL, free T4 2 mcg/dL

21. The above patient has typical symptoms and signs of thyrotoxicosis.

Any of the following may be employed in his immediate treatment EXCEPT:

a. propranolol.
b. radioactive iodine (RAI).
c. methimazole.
d. subtotal thyroidectomy.
e. saturated solution of potassium iodide (SSKI or Lugol's solution).

22. A 24-year-old medical student has noted a change in the size and color of a mole on his back. He is in good health with no family history of skin cancer. He is light-skinned and worked as a lifeguard for 2 summers while in college but does not remember a severe sunburn as a child. He has had occasional itching in the mole recently that called his attention to it. The lesion is on the left upper back just below the shoulder and measures 0.8 cm with a somewhat irregular border. No nodule is palpable but the color is somewhat variegated. No ulceration is noted on magnifying lens inspection. The balance of his physical examination is unremarkable except for a few benign-appearing skin nevi. There is no evidence of lymphadenopathy in the cervical, supraclavicular, or axillary regions. A wide excisional biopsy of the mole is performed.

Which of the following clinical and pathologic findings is most important in estimating prognosis?

a. Tumor thickness
b. Depth of penetration
c. Age of patient
d. Location of the melanoma
e. Sex of the patient

23. The pathology report for the above patient indicates a superficial spreading melanoma with a thickness of 1.2 mm, a slight ulceration, and a normal mitotic rate. Imaging studies for metastatic disease are negative.

What is the next step in managing this patient?

a. Axillary lymph node dissection
b. Observation only
c. Sentinel node biopsy
d. Radiation therapy to the regional lymph nodes
e. Adjuvant chemotherapy

24. A 61-year-old woman comes to the emergency room complaining of increasing shortness of breath for the past few days, especially while walking her dog. There is also a component of chest pain that subsides when she is at rest. She has a history of hypertension, hyperlipidemia, hypothyroidism, and thrombocythemia, the latter well controlled on hydroxyurea. There is no history of myocardial infarction or thromboembolic disease but she has 2 male siblings with premature heart disease. She is taking atenolol, ezetimibe, simvastatin, hydrochlorothiazide, L-thyroxine, and estrogen. She is diaphoretic and nauseated. Her blood pressure is 150/90, oxygen saturation 96% on room air, otherwise normal physical with clear lungs, no murmurs, rubs, or gallop sounds. Her legs are not tender nor is there swelling or ankle edema. A portable chest shows a slightly prominent left hilum but clear lung fields. Her EKG shows sinus rhythm with no Q waves, ST, or T-wave changes. She is sent to the CCU.

Which set of lab and imaging studies would be ordered next?

a. CBC, follow troponin levels and EKGs, chest PA and lateral when stable
b. Answer A plus coagulation panel (including PT, PTT, and D-dimer assay)
c. Answer B plus isotopic stress test
d. Answer B plus spiral CT of the chest
e. Answer B plus immediate cardiac catheterization

25. The above patient's stress test showed some evidence of septal reversibility. She was then taken to the catheterization laboratory; results showed a 50% obstruction in the LAD with collaterals from the right coronary artery (RCA) and a 30% obstruction in a dominant RCa. Ventricular ejection fraction was 70%. Shortly after returning to the CCU she developed severe dyspnea and hypoxemia, hypotension, and chest discomfort. There was no evidence of bleeding at the catheterization site. Review of her laboratory results showed a platelet count of 550,000/mm^3, a normal INR and PTT, but a D-dimer of 6 mcg/mL (normal is less than 0.5). She had been receiving enoxaparin, aspirin, and sublingual nitroglycerin for presumed coronary artery syndrome. Nasal oxygen was begun.

What treatment option is most appropriate now?

a. Switch to unfractionated heparin intravenously
b. Vascular surgery consult to install vena cava filter
c. Intravenous morphine and diuretic
d. Thrombolytic therapy with recombinant tissue plasminogen activator (TPA)
e. Cardiovascular surgical consult for emergency coronary bypass

26. A 26-year-old man complains of vague abdominal discomfort and intermittent diarrhea for several years. Recently, it has become worse with more bouts of diarrhea and intense pain, especially in the right lower abdomen. These episodes are often accompanied by low-grade fever, nausea, and vomiting. He has lost about 10 lb over the past 6 months. His medical history is unremarkable and both parents and 2 sisters are alive and well. He is referred for colonoscopy and a follow-up small bowel barium study. Multiple aphthous ulcers are found at the ileocecal junction and scattered throughout the colon with areas of normal mucosa and sparing of the rectum. The small bowel study indicates some luminal narrowing and mucosal ulceration.

What is the most likely diagnosis?

a. Ulcerative colitis (UC)
b. Diverticulitis
c. Irritable bowel syndrome
d. Ulcerating carcinoma of the colon
e. Crohn's disease (CD)

27. The above patient was started on prednisone 40 mg/day and had considerable improvement in his symptoms over the next 2 weeks. However, tapering the dosage to 20 mg/day results in a flare-up of the disease.

What is the next step in managing this patient?

a. Increase the steroid and maintain him on this indefinitely
b. Temporarily increase the steroid, and then add an immunosuppressant such as 6-mercaptopurine (6-MP) or azathioprine
c. Segmental resection of the terminal ileum
d. Begin a 5-aminosalicylic acid-containing drug
e. Add powdered opium and belladonna along with a nonsteroidal anti-inflammatory drug (NSAID)

28. A 30-year-old man presents with fatigue, nausea, and dark urine for about a week and is evaluated in the clinic. He denies sex with men or sexually transmitted disease but admits to some alcohol abuse and heroin use with needle sharing. He had mononucleosis as a teenager but has no history of hepatobiliary disease or blood transfusion. Laboratory values include markedly elevated aminotransferases with mild LDH, direct/total bilirubin, and alkaline phosphatase elevations. HIV and VDRL tests are negative. Antibody tests for hepatitis A, B, and C are negative. IgG levels are normal and ANA and anti-liver cytosol type 1 antibody tests are also negative and a gamma-glutamyl transferase (GGT) level is also normal.

What is the most likely diagnosis?

a. Acute viral hepatitis A
b. Acute viral hepatitis B
c. Acute viral hepatitis C
d. Cholestatic jaundice
e. Autoimmune hepatitis

29. The above patient's HCV RNA was found to be quite elevated and an HCV antibody test was positive 3 months later. His jaundice and symptoms resolved, but follow-up aminotransferases were persistently elevated, though fluctuating in value.

What treatment should now be started?

a. None, follow-up only
b. Prednisone
c. Acyclovir
d. Peginterferon and ribavirin
e. Ribavirin only

30. A 26-year-old woman who is 30 weeks pregnant consults her PCP at the suggestion of her obstetrician. This is her first pregnancy and it has been normal thus far. There is no family history of high blood pressure or cardiovascular disease. Her pre-pregnancy blood pressures were 115 to 120/70 to 75 and her blood glucose levels were normal. She has gained about 15 lb. There is no history of seizures. Her exam today reveals a blood pressure of 150/90, and normal heart and lungs with an obvious pregnancy. Her CBC and serum chemistries are normal but there is trace proteinuria. She is given a 24-hour urine collection bottle and 1 week later her blood pressure is 160/100 and the 24-hour urine shows 500 mg of protein.

What is the most likely diagnosis?

a. Preeclampsia
b. Eclampsia
c. Gestational hypertension
d. Chronic essential hypertension
e. None of the above

31. The above patient is treated with bed rest and close monitoring but her blood pressure remains elevated and the urinalysis continues to show 1+ to 2+ proteinuria at 32 weeks.

What should be recommended now?

a. Immediate delivery
b. Magnesium sulfate intravenously
c. Calcium supplements and low-dose aspirin
d. Antihypertensive treatment with an angiotensin-converting enzyme (ACE) inhibitor
e. Antihypertensive treatment with methyldopa.

32. A 65-year-old man with type 2 diabetes sees his physician for an annual exam. The onset of the diabetes was about 10 years ago and after treatment with several oral hypoglycemic drugs, he has been on insulin for the past 2 years. He is also taking amlodipine for moderate hypertension. He denies visual changes or genitourinary problems. His blood pressure is 140/85 and his prostate is somewhat enlarged without nodules. There is trace ankle edema. A hemoglobin A_{1c} is 6.9% and a urine dipstick is 2+ positive for protein, otherwise negative. A 24-hour excretion of total protein is 800 mg. A GFR is 35 mL/min/m^2.

What changes in his therapy are now appropriate?

a. No changes are needed
b. Increase his insulin dose
c. Start a diuretic
d. Stop amlodipine and start an angiotensin receptor blocker (ARB)
e. Continue amlodipine and begin dietary protein restriction

33. Five years later, the above patient's proteinuria has increased to 4 g per 24 hours and his GFR is now less than 15 mL/min/m^2. He has symptoms of mild uremia.

What should be the best step in managing his case?

a. Refer for peritoneal dialysis
b. Refer for hemodialysis
c. Kidney transplant using compatible cadaver kidney
d. Kidney transplant if live compatible donor kidney is available
e. Medical therapy only

34. A 33-year-old married woman consults her PCP because her mother died of breast cancer in her 40s and her older sister has just been diagnosed with it. She is Jewish and her grandparents emigrated from Poland. She wants to know her risk of getting the disease and what she can do about it. She is in good health, and has a 5-year-old child and is thinking about having one or two more. Breast examination is normal. Genetic testing shows she is positive for the *BRCA2* gene. Bilateral mastectomy is discussed but she refuses to consider it.

What would be the best approach to managing her case?

a. Schedule a mammogram and if negative, order an annual mammogram
b. Schedule an MRI of the breasts and if negative, annual examination only
c. Schedule an MRI of the breasts and if negative, start tamoxifen
d. Refer to an oncologist for adjuvant chemotherapy
e. Refer to a radiation therapist for prophylactic radiation treatment to both breasts

35. The above patient begins tamoxifen but discontinues it after several months because of adverse effects. She returns 3 years later with a 2 to 3 cm nodule in her left breast that is diagnosed as a carcinoma on follow-up imaging and needle aspiration biopsy. She undergoes a lumpectomy and a sentinel node biopsy, which is positive for cancer. Axillary node dissection is negative for other nodes. Her tumor is 3 cm in diameter and estrogen and progesterone receptor–positive but human epidermal growth factor receptor type 2 (HER2)–negative. A metastatic screen is negative.

What is the most appropriate treatment?

a. No further treatment, observation only
b. Trastuzumab (Herceptin)
c. Adjuvant chemotherapy
d. Aromatase inhibitor
e. Hormonal and adjuvant chemotherapy

36. An 18-year-old woman consults her physician for easy bruising and menorrhagia. Her gynecologist reports a normal pelvic exam. Further history reveals bruising after minor trauma from childhood, occasional spontaneous epistaxis, and heavy periods since menarche at age 13. She has had no surgery but she did experience persistent bleeding after a dental extraction and the dentist recommended a workup for a bleeding disorder. She has had no deep intramuscular or joint bleeding. She is not taking aspirin or other drugs that disturb platelet function. She was adopted so family history is absent. Her physical exam is normal except for some bruises on the extremities. A mild iron deficiency anemia is present.

Which of the following laboratory tests is most likely to confirm the clinical diagnosis?

a. Prothrombin time (PT)
b. Activated partial thromboplastin time (aPTT)
c. Ristocetin-induced platelet aggregation (RIPA)
d. Platelet count
e. Factor VIII assay

37. A 68-year-old man states that he had urinary frequency and nocturia for the past 6 months. He had acute prostatitis in his 20s but no other history of genitourinary disease, diabetes, or sexually transmitted disease. His international prostate symptom score (IPSS) is 12 (0 to 8 mild, 9 to 18 moderate, 19 to 35 severe), and he is bothered by the symptoms (4 out of a possible 6). There is no organ enlargement or bladder distension and digital rectal examination (DRE) reveals a firm, nontender prostate 2+ to 3+ enlarged without nodules and normal male genitalia consistent with his age.

All of the following diagnostic tests should be done at this point EXCEPT:

a. urinalysis.
b. prostate-specific antigen (PSA).
c. serum calcium level.
d. ultrasound-guided biopsy of the prostate.
e. urine culture.

38. A 35-year-old auto mechanic presents with the sudden onset of severe upper abdominal pain with vomiting shortly after his evening meal, about 3 hours ago. No blood was regurgitated. He describes the pain as intense, mostly in the left upper quadrant with radiation to the epigastrium and mid-back. There is no definite history of gastrointestinal disease but he does state he occasionally has some vague abdominal discomfort after fast food ingestion. He drinks 3 to 4 beers most days. He lies very still, holding his upper abdomen. There is diffuse tenderness and guarding over much of the abdomen and bowel sounds are diminished to absent. There is no fever but his WBC count is elevated at 16,000/mm^3.

What is the most likely diagnosis and the best lab or imaging study to diagnose it?

a. Acute pancreatitis; serum amylase
b. Acute pancreatitis; CT of the abdomen
c. Acute pancreatitis; ultrasound of the abdomen
d. Acute cholecystitis; CT of the abdomen
e. Acute cholecystitis; ultrasound of the abdomen

39. A 16-year-old high school basketball player develops an erythematous painful swelling on his calf several days after a fall during a game. It is warm to the touch and slightly fluctuant. He has had no fever or other complaints but leg pain is keeping him from practice and a big game is coming up. Medical history is unremarkable except for an appendectomy at age 13. His pre-athletics high school physical was normal. The lesion is drained of obviously purulent fluid and sent for culture and sensitivities. A plain x-ray of the leg is normal.

What antibiotic treatment should be begun?

a. None, wait for culture and sensitivity report
b. Methicillin
c. A cephalosporin
d. Vancomycin
e. A fluoroquinolone

40. A healthy 24-year-old man who plans a trip to southeast Asia consults his PCP for travel prophylaxis. He is a member of and will be traveling with a wilderness group that plans hiking in countryside and jungle areas of Thailand, Cambodia, Vietnam, and Laos.

All of the following immunizations and medications are appropriate EXCEPT:

a. hepatitis A vaccine.
b. meningococcal vaccine.
c. malaria prophylaxis with doxycycline.
d. malaria prophylaxis with mefloquine.
e. azithromycin.

41. A 65-year-old man consults his physician because of trembling and shakiness in his right arm and hand at rest, and he also notes that it occurs while he is walking. He complains of some dizziness and weakness on arising from bed but has not fainted. On examination he speaks slowly without inflections and there is a reduced arm swing and some imbalance in his slow gait. There is a mild right-hand tremor with a cycle of 4 to 5 cycles per second which disappears with movement of the arm to a new position. There is some rigidity on passive movement of his right arm, exacerbated when the left arm is moved. Cranial nerves, deep tendon reflexes, and sensory function are intact on the rest of the neurologic exam and cognitive and memory screening are normal for his age.

What are the probable diagnosis and an important next step in confirming it?

a. Parkinson disease and an MRI of the brain
b. Parkinson disease and a careful drug history
c. Wilson disease and serum ceruloplasmin and slit lamp exam
d. Alzheimer disease and MRI of the brain
e. Normal pressure hydrocephalus and trial of levodopa

42. A 74-year-old woman is seen in the emergency room complaining of shortness of breath and palpitations for the past 24 hours. She is found to be in atrial fibrillation (AF) with a ventricular rate of 100 and a blood pressure of 100/70 mm Hg. She is anticoagulated with heparin and converted to normal sinus rhythm with intravenous diltiazem. There is no clinical, imaging, or laboratory indication of heart failure, left atrial thrombi, or significant coronary artery disease.

Which of the following would be reasonable discharge medications?

a. Sotalol
b. Amiodarone
c. Warfarin
d. Digoxin
e. Any of the above

43. A 50-year-old man has had increasing dyspnea for several months, especially with effort. He has a chronic nonproductive cough that has become worse but no blood has been seen. There is a smoking history of 30 pack-years, although he recently quit. He was once told he had asthma and treated with a beta-adrenergic inhaler, which resulted in some relief but has not helped his current symptoms. He has hypertension but no history of chest pain or cardiovascular disease. On exam he is afebrile, blood pressure 190/100 but there is no cyanosis or neck vein distension, the chest is slightly increased in AP diameter with diffuse wheezing and some dullness at the lung bases. There is a short midsystolic murmur at the base but a gallop sound cannot be heard. There is no ascites, hepatosplenomegaly, or pedal edema. An ABG shows P02 of 55, pCO_2 of 48 and pH of 7.37. A chest x-ray shows a borderline enlarged cardiac silhouette, some hyperinflation of the lungs, and streaky densities in the lower lung fields. An ECG shows a sinus tachycardia with a left bundle branch block but no acute ST-T changes. Beta-natriuretic peptide (BNP) is 700 pg/mL.

What is the most likely diagnosis?

a. Asthma
b. Pneumonia
c. Heart failure (HF)
d. COPD with exacerbation
e. COPD and HF

44. A 69-year-old man consults his PCP because of low energy and sleep problems. He has had difficulty falling asleep and often awakens very early in the morning. He is a widower and he states that he has had a sad mood and poor concentration since his wife died of cancer 2 years ago. He thinks about her all the time. He has lost interest in things he used to enjoy: swimming, hiking, and socializing with friends. He has had brief suicidal thoughts but no attempts and has not experienced delusions, hallucinations, or episodic mood swings. He lives alone and has 2 or 3 alcoholic drinks daily but avoids other drugs of abuse. He has 2 adult children but they live out of state and he does not see them often. He has mild hypertension and benign prostatic hypertrophy and takes the alpha-adrenergic blocker tamsulosin (*Flomax*).

What is the most likely diagnosis and what treatment should be begun?

a. Major depression; refer to a psychiatrist
b. Major depression; start sertraline (Zoloft)
c. Drug-induced depression; stop Flomax
d. Dysthymia; start trazodone
e. Bipolar disorder; start lithium

45. A 33-year-old woman complains of fatigue and intermittent pain in the left upper abdomen. She had no fever, swollen glands, or bruising. She is married with 2 children and her medical history is confined to minor, self-limited ailments. Her examination is negative except for slight conjunctival pallor and a spleen tip felt 3 cm below the left costal margin. A CBC result is: hemoglobin 10 g/dL; WBC count 45,000/mm^3 with a marked shift to the left including myelocytes and promyelocytes and increased basophils; platelet count of 500,000/mm^3. Serum levels of uric acid and LDH are elevated but bilirubin and alkaline phosphates are normal. A bone marrow exam with cytogenetic analysis shows marked hypercellularity with a myeloid/erythroid ratio of 15:1. A t-(9;22)(q34;q11.2) chromosome abnormality is present on cytogenetic analysis.

What treatment should be recommended for this patient?

a. Cytosine arabinoside
b. Busulfan (Myleran)
c. Imatinib mesylate (Gleevec)
d. Allogenic bone marrow transplant
e. Interferon (IFN-alpha)

46. A 30-year-old married man is brought to the emergency room with severe head trauma sustained in a motor vehicle accident. He is in a coma and is on life support, including a ventilator, intravenous hydration, and nutrition. Neurologic examination, brain imaging studies, and electroencephalogram (EEG) are all consistent with a diagnosis of brain death. He left no living will or other instructions regarding terminal care but according to his driver's license he wished to be an organ donor. His wife wishes to terminate all his support and proceed with organ donation but his parents and brother object; their wish is to give him more time on life support, hoping for a "miracle" and not allowing organ donation.

What is the responsible physician to do in these circumstances?

a. Continue life support and call in clergy or a bioethics specialist to make the decision
b. Stop artificial ventilation but maintain hydration and nutrition
c. Call a transplant surgeon to manage the case
d. Stop all life support per the wife's wishes and proceed with the organ donation
e. Add morphine or potassium chloride to his intravenous line to try to hasten cardiorespiratory death

47. A previously healthy 15-year-old boy has had a gastroenteritis syndrome for about 3 days characterized by low-grade fever, nausea, and vomiting. He complains of constantly being thirsty and having to urinate frequently. On day 4 he is less alert than usual and breathing heavily. He is brought to the emergency room where his pulse is 110 and regular, blood pressure 90/60, and deep rapid respirations are noted. His skin is dry and there is tenting. Oxygen saturation is 98% while blood pH is 7.2. A fingerstick glucose is 650 mg/dL and serum is positive for ketones. A corrected serum sodium is 150 mEq/L and potassium is 5.3 mEq/L. Urinalysis, chest and abdominal x-rays, and 12-lead ECG are ordered, and he is placed on a cardiac monitor.

All of the following treatment measures are appropriate EXCEPT:

a. infusion of 0.45% saline at 1,000 mL/hr.
b. add 20 mEq of potassium chloride per liter of saline.
c. add 1 ampule (44 mEq) of bicarbonate per liter of saline.
d. give a regular insulin bolus intravenously at 0.15 U/kg.
e. add 0.1 U/kg regular insulin to the saline infusion at 1,000 mL/hr.

48. A 60-year-old white woman consults her PCP because of nagging back pain for about 3 months. She has no history of prior back pain, sciatica, or fractures. Heating pads and nonprescription medications have been of little help and the pain is interfering with her daily activities. She took estrogen and progesterone orally for about 3 years for menopausal symptoms but stopped when she was 50 because of the Women's Health Initiative study indicating that hormone replacement therapy increased the risk of breast cancer. She currently is not taking any medications regularly. On examination she is a small and somewhat thin woman. There is some localized tenderness over the upper lumbar and lower thoracic vertebrae but full range of motion of the extremities and no neurologic abnormalities are noted.

Which of the following laboratory and imaging tests would best confirm the diagnosis?

a. Vitamin D level
b. TSH and thyroxine levels
c. Bone mineral density by dual-energy x-ray absorptiometry (DXA)
d. Urine hydroxyproline excretion
e. Quantitative CT scanning of the vertebrae

49. A 30-year-old mother of two complains of frequent nasal congestion, headaches with facial and dental pain, and a cloudy nasal discharge. She denies fever and cough but has some ear pressure. She believes she is allergic to animal dander from experience with a childhood cat and to some trees and grasses but the latter occurs only in the spring and it is now winter. She has no pets. She has tried a variety of nonprescription medications, including antihistamines, mucolytics, and decongestants, with only minor and temporary relief of her symptoms. She had a typical cold several weeks ago and she believes her current symptom began shortly afterwards.. Nasal speculum exam reveals a reddish mucosa, some purulent discharge in the middle meatus, but no polyps or masses. Ear examination is normal as is hearing.

On the basis of the above history and physical findings, what is the diagnosis and treatment?

a. Acute sinusitis, treat with intranasal steroid spray
b. Acute sinusitis, treat with a macrolide antibiotic
c. Chronic sinusitis, treat with oral steroids and a beta-lactamase–resistant antibiotic
d. Viral rhinitis, treat with nasal decongestants and steam inhalation
e. Allergic rhinitis, treat with antihistamines

50. A reserve soldier returns from his 1-year tour of duty in Iraq in the late spring and resumes his favorite leisure outdoor activities: hiking and fishing. He consults his physician complaining of myalgias, fatigue, headaches, and intermittent fever for several weeks. He had a reddish, circular rash on his back but it has now faded. He also notes some joint pain but there is no swelling or erythema. He cannot recall insect bites while in the woods but does remember being bitten by desert sand flies while in Iraq. He did not travel to other parts of the Middle East or Africa during his tour and he had the usual series of immunizations for soldiers departing for service abroad. He denies any sexual encounters while he was there and has had no genital lesions or inguinal swelling. A VDRL is negative.

What organism is the most likely cause of this man's symptoms?

a. *Borrelia burgdorferi*
b. *Ixodes scapularis*
c. *Treponema pallidum*
d. *Plasmodium falciparum*
e. *Treponema pertenue*

Answer Key and Explanations

1. C: The most important objective is to determine if this man has coronary artery disease (CAD). A lipid profile may indicate his risk for the condition but he already has elevated risk due to his history of smoking, high blood pressure, and possibly diabetes. The hemoglobin A_{1c} will offer information about the latter but not about CAD. EGD may be useful to rule out an upper gastrointestinal cause of his symptoms, such as gastroesophageal reflux or esophageal spasm. Most important is to detect the presence of coronary disease. Since he is stable and pain free, an isotopic stress test is preferred to immediate angiography.

2. B: From the clinical presentation, this man has an acute coronary syndrome (ACS), most likely a non–ST-segment elevation myocardial infarction (NSTEMI). Recent evidence has shown that ST depression confers a worse prognosis than T-wave inversion alone. An elevated troponin level will indicate myocardial damage and results are now available quickly. Thirty-day mortality has been shown to be proportional to the degree of troponin I elevation. Since he is in the high-risk category, he should then be sent to the catheterization laboratory for coronary angiography as soon as possible with balloon angioplasty and stenting if needed. High-resolution CT scanning may detect coronary calcifications but angiography remains the "gold standard" for the detection of CAD. Clopidogrel is indicated for ACS patients whose catheterization is delayed more than 24 hours. Cardiac ultrasound may show some abnormalities of wall motion but will only delay the necessary heart catheterization.

3. B: Warfarin is not usually indicated for CAD patients unless complicated by atrial fibrillation or venous thromboembolism. Clopidogrel, a platelet inhibitor, is generally prescribed to diminish the chance of stent thrombosis, although some patients (15% to 48%) are resistant and higher doses or a new drug, prasugrel, may be required. A statin is definitely indicated even if the LDL cholesterol is in the normal range. Many cardiologists believe that the LDL cholesterol should be reduced to less than 70 mg/dL in patients such as this one. Low-dose aspirin is often added unless there is a history of gastrointestinal or other bleeding risk. ACE inhibitors have also been shown to have a beneficial effect in these patients in addition to their antihypertensive action.

4. A: This woman has been experiencing transient ischemic attacks, presumably arising from vascular disease of the left carotid artery. These attacks may last up to an hour or two before resolution but persistence of these symptoms beyond 24 hours suggests a completed stroke. Her diabetes and hypertension are risk factors for cerebrovascular disease and the bruit suggests narrowing of the vessel. Her symptoms do not suggest a seizure disorder. The absence of vertigo, visual symptoms, or drop attacks rules against vertebrobasilar disease. She may well have a degree of aortic stenosis but this alone should not explain her constellation of symptoms.

5. D: Since the presumptive diagnosis is carotid stenosis leading to transient ischemic attacks, duplex scanning of the carotids is a reasonable initial and noninvasive test. It combines B-mode ultrasonography and range-gated pulsed Doppler. It will usually disclose the luminal diameter and blood velocity, although only that portion of the carotid circulation between the clavicles and mandible may be visualized. This study is probably best done before referral to a vascular or neurosurgeon so that the results will be available if the consultation is required. Cerebral angiography is usually performed prior to endarterectomy to determine if the patient is likely to benefit from the surgical procedure. It exposes the patient to ionizing radiation and contrast material. MR angiography is useful for large lesions but less useful for smaller ones and tends to exaggerate the degree of stenosis. This patient should also have a cardiac ultrasound because there is a suggestion of left ventricular prominence and to rule out a possible cardiac source of emboli. A CT or MRI of the brain should also be done to exclude a previous stroke or other brain lesion.

6. E: All patients who have had a stroke or TIA should undergo secondary prophylaxis. Aspirin and other antiplatelet drugs may reduce the incidence of another stroke by 30%. The daily dose of aspirin has not been established with certainty. Clopidogrel may also be used at a 75 mg/day dosage but the combination of aspirin and clopidogrel is not found to be superior to aspirin alone, it costs considerably more, and probably increases the bleeding risk. All patients with cerebrovascular disease should be treated aggressively with statins, which have been found to reduce the stroke rate by 25%. Warfarin and low molecular weight heparin have not been found to be effective in stroke prevention and are quite inconvenient since one requires frequent laboratory testing and the other subcutaneous injection.

7. E: Since this patient is asymptomatic and free of obvious opportunistic infection, there is no rush to treat him based only on the positive HIV test. His history of a febrile illness with lymphadenopathy may or may not be related to the initial phase of HIV viremia. Decisions regarding treatment in an asymptomatic patient such as this are largely based on the CD4 count and the plasma viral load. Therefore, both values should be obtained for a decision regarding immediate treatment and as a baseline for follow-up. There is some controversy about the indications for treatment based on these values; some doctors begin therapy with CD4 T-cell levels as high as 500/mL. Standard guidelines to initiate treatment are if CD4 T-cell levels are below 200/mL; strongly consider if the count is between 200/mL and 350/mL. Many AIDS experts will treat if the count is over 350/mL and the viral load exceeds 100,000 copies. Therapy may be deferred if the count is greater than 350/mL and the viral load is less than 100,000, although some experts believe that viral counts above 55,000 should be treated regardless of the CD4 T-cell count. The girlfriend and any other named sexual contacts should be screened. There is some very recent evidence that sexual transmission of the virus to an HIV-negative partner may be blocked by early ART.

8. D: HAART therapy in a new HIV-positive patient should be initiated with combination drug therapy to discourage the emergence of resistant strains. There are numerous drugs on the market in each major category and several combinations of 2 and 3 drugs that make taking them easier. Lists of possible adverse effects from each drug must be gone over carefully with the patient before initiating therapy. Authorities recommend the combination of a PI and an NNRTI with a NRTI. Therefore, reasonable combinations might be atazanavir and ritonavir (PI) with zidovudine/lamivudine (NRTI) or efavirenz (NNRTI) with zidovudine/lamivudine. Three drug treatments appear as satisfactory as four in new patients. Treatment should reduce the HIV viral load 0.5 to 0.75 log by week 4 and 1 log at week 8. There should be no detection of the virus by 4 to 6 months. A rising CD4 T-cell level usually accompanies a diminution in the viral RNA.

9. D: Treatment of HIV-infected pregnant women has evolved over the past few years. Instead of zidovudine or nevirapine monotherapy, combination ART including zidovudine is recommended for those who have HIV RNA levels above 1,000 copies/mL. Women with levels lower than this have a small risk of transmission to the newborn. While most ART drugs are not teratogenic, many have not been studied adequately and some may contribute to the adverse effects of pregnancy. Waiting until the second trimester is probably safest.

10. D: All the answers are possible causes of occult gastrointestinal bleeding in this age group but an upper gastrointestinal source is 5 times more likely than a lower one. Gastric ulceration is common in patients taking NSAIDs and/or aspirin, often without abdominal pain. Hemorrhoidal bleeding may be the most common cause of lower gastrointestinal bleeding but most often the blood is fresh and mixed with stool. The negative rectal exam tends to make this source less likely. Angiodysplasia (telangiectasia), a small vascular malformation of the gut, sometimes multiple, is increasingly reported as a cause of gastrointestinal bleeding, frequently intermittent. Diverticular bleeding, often maroon in color, is another possibility. Finally, colon cancer is the cause of lower gastrointestinal bleeding in about 3% to 5% of cases and may be present without other symptoms, especially if it is in the ascending or transverse colon.

11. C: Both the upper and lower gastrointestinal tract should be examined in patients with occult blood loss since there may be more than 1 lesion. This is often done one after another for patient convenience and to avoid giving anesthesia twice. Barium enema is now rarely used since colonoscopy can identify a bleeding lesion or clot and take a biopsy and/or coagulate it. Angiography is useful for brisk bleeding lesions (at least 1 mL/min) when endoscopy has failed to detect the source or is obscured by blood.

12. D: Capsule endoscopy (patient swallows a small camera within an ingestible capsule and images are transmitted to a receiver on the patient's abdomen for review) has a good diagnostic yield (60% to 90%) in occult bleeding cases in which traditional endoscopy has failed to detect a lesion. Angiography is mostly useful for rapid bleeding. Isotope tagged red blood cell scintigraphy may identify the site of gastrointestinal bleeding at lower blood flows (0.1 mL/min) but cannot determine the cause. Push enteroscopy of the small bowel has a yield of 38% to 75% and may be tried if the bleeding is not rapid. If all of the above fail to disclose the source and bleeding continues, surgical intervention with intraoperative enteroscopy may be tried. In all cases, iron therapy and follow-up hemoglobin values should be carried out with transfusion if necessary.

13. A: Asymptomatic but overweight diabetic patients with a hemoglobin A_{1c} less than 8% should probably be given a short trial of diet and exercise before beginning hypoglycemic therapy. The current guidelines from the American Diabetes Association require reduction to less than 7%. Some other authorities demand a reduction to less than 6.5%, although a recent clinical trial indicates that too aggressive treatment may be counterproductive. The patient should be seen at 3- to 4-month intervals with follow-up blood testing. Monitoring of blood pressure, lipid levels, and abdominal girth is also recommended. If glycemic control is not achieved, metformin or one of the others may be started.

14. B: It is clear that this patient is unlikely to be controlled on diet and exercise, so hypoglycemic therapy is indicated. His weight, abdominal girth, elevated blood pressure, high triglycerides, and low HDL-C suggest he has metabolic syndrome, although this designation is somewhat controversial. He needs reduction of his LDL-C and hemoglobin A1c, as well as his blood pressure. The best approach would be to maintain the previously started metformin and introduce a statin immediately, saving the introduction of an antihypertensive at a follow-up visit as starting three drugs at once may obscure adverse effects or cause noncompliance. Most doctors would prefer metformin for this patient since it does not cause weight gain and has been shown to reduce macrovascular complications of diabetes mellitus. Using a sulfonylurea is a second choice since it tends to increase weight and it is an insulin secretagogue, and the likelihood of hypoglycemic episodes is greater than with metformin. Insulin may ultimately be required in type 2 diabetic patients but a trial of oral therapy is preferred for a patient such as this. When antihypertensive therapy is started, an ACE inhibitor or an ARB would be preferable to a beta-blocker or diuretic since the latter drugs have a tendency to raise the blood sugar, though modestly. A reduction to less than 140 mm Hg systolic is advisable.

15. E: This patient now has mild symptoms and his glycohemoglobin has risen to greater than 8%. Some doctors would begin insulin at this point but most authorities suggest a trial of a second daytime oral drug. The exact type depends on the patient's compliance, cost of the medication, and adverse effects. Sooner or later most patients fail on oral therapy but many doctors would try a third agent from a different class before submitting the patient to the nuisance and hazards of insulin. Use of a daytime sulfonylurea and bedtime insulin is a popular regimen instead of adding a third oral drug. Adding long-acting niacin may be considered to try to raise the HDL-C and lower triglycerides but liver function tests must be followed.

16. B: This man appears to have community-acquired pneumonia. Sometimes the pathogen may be suspected by the clinical presentation but there is considerable overlap. The most likely cause is *Streptococcus pneumoniae*, which still is the most common cause of a community-acquired bacterial pneumonia. The crackles, dullness, and pleuritic pain with slightly low oxygen saturation favor this diagnosis. A mycoplasma etiology cannot be ruled out without further diagnostic testing but this is frequently skipped unless the patient does not respond to empiric antibiotic therapy. Legionella pneumonia is most common in those older than 40 who smoke or are receiving chemotherapy or immunosuppressant drugs. Pneumocystis pneumonia is usually seen in HIV-positive patients or those on prolonged steroid therapy. Pulmonary embolus can sometimes mimic pneumonia but would be very unusual in this young man without predisposing conditions.

17. C: Decisions regarding the management of pneumonia patients are largely based on certain risk factors, such as age, presence of complicating conditions, and extent of disease. This patient is young and otherwise healthy and only mildly impaired physically. A chest x-ray and CBC are always indicated in pneumonia patients to further indicate the extent and severity of the disease and possibly discover additional risk factors. A macrolide antibiotic is usually the first choice for empiric treatment since it covers most of the common community-acquired pathogens. Doxycycline may also be used if the patient is allergic to or does not tolerate macrolides. Intravenous antibiotic therapy is usually not required for this type of patient unless he fails to respond to initial therapy or a complication develops.

18. B: This patient's age, sex, history, and physical findings of joint inflammation are typical of RA. Symmetric synovitis of the wrist and metacarpal joints with morning stiffness and limited range of motion is a common presentation. SLE cannot be ruled out at this point as it often presents with joint pain and swelling, although usually in younger women along with constitutional symptoms. Polymyalgia rheumatica tends to occur in older patients and chiefly presents with head and neck pain and sometimes tenderness over the temporal artery. Fibromyalgia does not show signs of acute inflammation but tenderness over numerous joint and soft tissue spots is present along with constitutional symptoms such as poor sleep, mental "fogginess," and prominent fatigue. Osteoarthritis is a degenerative disorder of joint cartilage, tends to occur in older people, is often asymmetric, and may affect distal joints of the hands or larger joints, such as knees and hips.

19. E: Joint aspiration, if possible, is most useful for distinguishing inflammatory (greater than 2,000 cells/mm^3, mostly polys) from noninflammatory (less than 2,000 cells/mm^3, mostly mononuclear) arthritis, septic joints (gram stain and culture), and crystal-induced arthritis (gout). CRP is an acute-phase reactant, usually elevated in inflammatory arthritis but not specific for a particular disease though useful for following the degree of inflammation and prognosis. RF is a family of antibodies, usually immunoglobulin M (IgM), that bind to IgG. It is elevated in about 80% of patients with RA but may also be elevated in other immune and inflammatory disorders and in healthy, usually older individuals. Perhaps the immune test most specific for RA is the anti-CCP test, which is positive in 60% to 70% of patients with RA and uncommon in those with other inflammatory disorders. It may even be positive before the onset of symptoms and may be useful for screening those at high risk for the disease. Plain radiographs are an important part of evaluation and progress of all arthritic disorders. While joint space narrowing, erosions, and subluxation of the MCP and PIP joints are common in RA, they may not be seen at the onset of the disease; however, the films are inexpensive, easily obtained, and very useful for following the course of the disease.

20. B: This patient most likely has Graves' disease with the presence of thyroid antibodies, which causes predominantly T3 (triiodothyronine) thyrotoxicosis. The TSH will be suppressed, the T3 level increased (greater than 35% resin uptake), and the T4 high normal or borderline elevated. Answer A is more typical of a T4 thyrotoxicosis as seen in subacute thyroiditis. Answer C is most consistent with a TSH-secreting pituitary adenoma where the TSH and the T4 are both elevated. Answer D shows normal values while E is consistent with hypothyroidism.

21. D: Propranolol or other long-acting beta-blockers may offer rapid symptomatic relief to hyperthyroid patients, especially for palpitations, tremor, or anxiety. They may be started while more definitive treatment is planned. Thioamides, such as methimazole or propylthiouracil, inhibit organification of iodine and iodotyrosine coupling but do not prevent the secretion of preformed thyroid hormone from the gland. Thus, they may take from 3 to 8 weeks to become effective in patients with Graves' disease. RAI with I131 is the most commonly used treatment to destroy thyroid tissue and is often effective after a single dose. RAI treatment, however, usually results in persistent hypothyroidism so that thyroid hormone supplementation and thyroid monitoring is usually necessary. SSKI inhibits synthesis and release of thyroid hormone from the gland and may be used in conjunction with other treatments for severe hypothyroidism or prior to thyroid surgery. Surgical resection of thyroid tissue is usually not recommended in Graves' disease unless other therapies are ineffective or contraindicated or a nodule suspicious for malignancy is present.

22. A: Melanoma thickness is the strongest predictor of survival, as well local, regional, or distant metastatic disease. Ulceration and mitotic rate of the tumor cells are also strong predictors of outcome. Ulceration and increased mitotic rate imply a more aggressive tumor with higher incidence of lymph node involvement and a decreased survival. Although depth of penetration has been used as a prognostic factor for many years, it is less reliable than the actual thickness of the melanoma and/or the presence of ulceration. Men in general have a worse prognosis than women and head, neck, and trunk primaries have an inferior survival to those on the extremities. There is also a diminution in survival with advancing age.

23. C: Appropriate staging of the tumor by American Joint Committee on Cancer (AJCC) criteria include thickness and presence or absence of ulceration of the primary lesion, the number of positive regional lymph nodes and whether they are macroscopically or microscopically involved, and the presence or absence of distant metastases. For patients such as this with a lesion depth greater than 1 mm and clinically negative lymph nodes, a sentinel node biopsy is usually performed. If positive, then a regional lymphadenectomy may be done. Some clinical trials of radiation and adjuvant chemotherapy for stage III patients have shown some improvement in disease-free survival but not overall survival. Overall, 15-year survival is 80% for stage I patients, 50% for stage II, 30% to 40% for stage III, and less than 10% for stage IV.

24. C: This is a complex case and the differential diagnosis includes coronary artery syndrome, pulmonary embolus (PE), heart failure, pneumothorax, pneumonia or exacerbation of COPD, and several others. Most likely are coronary artery syndrome and PE. A good screening test for the latter is the D-dimer assay, which if elevated suggests possible PE. A spiral CT of the chest (if available) would then be appropriate; if not available, then a V/Q lung scan, venous ultrasound of the lower extremities, and even pulmonary angiography would be appropriate. She should have a stress test if no signs of myocardial infarction develop. If they do or if the stress test is positive or nondiagnostic, then cardiac catheterization would likely be appropriate.

25. D: This patient has a life-threatening situation with a presumptive clinical diagnosis of massive pulmonary embolus. This occurred while she was receiving low molecular weight heparin, which actually has several advantages over unfractionated heparin. Heparin can prevent further clot formation and allow the thrombolytic system to work more efficiently, but it may not be effective in dissolving a large thrombus. A vena cava filter is indicated for those patients with recurrent thromboemboli on adequate anticoagulant therapy but is not useful for a pulmonary embolus that has already occurred. Since this patient is hypotensive and hypoxic, morphine and a diuretic are contraindicated, especially since her cardiac ejection fraction was normal and there is no other indication of heart failure. Pressor support with dopamine or norepinephrine is indicated. Since there was evidence of only mild to moderate coronary obstruction and good collaterals, bypass surgery is not indicated. The situation is dire, so thrombolytic therapy with streptokinase (SK) or TPA should be started even without imaging confirmation of the embolus.

26. E: The clinical presentation of this patient is fairly typical of young patients with Crohn's disease. Vague pain with intermittent diarrhea, occasionally bloody, is common. With progression, especially if ileal disease is prominent, right lower quadrant pain and tenderness becomes more intense. The pattern of diarrhea to some extent depends on the anatomic location of the disease: rectal involvement leads to urgency and tenesmus while in disease confined to the small bowel these symptoms are absent and stools are larger. The colonoscopic and small bowel contrast study findings described are typical of Crohn's disease; abscess, stricture, and perianal disease are common complications. Ulcerative colitis is characterized on colonoscopy with diffuse erythema and loss of the fine vascular pattern and extreme friability of the mucosa, occasionally with a yellowish exudate. There may be small ulceration and spontaneous bleeding. In a small percent of cases, UC cannot be differentiated from CD, even with biopsy. While both diseases have an increased risk of colon cancer, UC more than CD, the endoscopic findings in this case do not suggest that diagnosis. Diverticulitis can be excluded by the colonoscopic findings and a CT scan with contrast is usually done. Irritable bowel syndrome is a functional disorder and no anatomic lesions of the bowel should be present.

27. B: While corticosteroids orally or intravenously are the main remission-inducing agents for Crohn's disease, they cannot be continued indefinitely because of their considerable adverse effects. Antibiotics, such as metronidazole and/or ciprofloxacin, may also be used as initial therapy. If a flare-up of the disease occurs while tapering steroids, the best approach is to temporarily increase the steroid dose and then add an immunosuppressant. Steroid tapering may then be tried again after several weeks on the immunosuppressant drug. Surgery early in the disease is usually necessary only for patients who are refractory to medical therapy or who develop a fistula, abscess, or intestinal obstruction. Drugs containing 5-aminosalicylic acid (sulfasalazine, olsalazine) may be used for maintenance therapy in Crohn's patients in remission but are more useful in ulcerative colitis. Powdered opium and belladonna are antidiarrheal and antispasmodic medications that may relieve symptoms but have no effect on the disease itself. NSAIDs may sometimes exacerbate inflammatory bowel disease and should be avoided if possible.

28. C: The clinical picture of an acute onset illness with jaundice and high aminotransferases and modest elevations in the other liver function tests is most suggestive of acute viral hepatitis. In cholestasis, the alkaline phosphatase elevation would predominate and the GGT is usually elevated. Autoimmune hepatitis is characterized by elevated IgG levels and a positive ANA or anti-liver cytosol type 1 antibody. Antibodies in hepatitis A (IgM anti-HAV) and B (IgM anti-HBc) appear early in the disease and are usually increased when symptoms and jaundice are present. However, in hepatitis C, the rise in anti-HCV antibody titer is usually delayed for 2 to 3 months after the onset of symptoms. For this reason, a follow-up HCV antibody level should be obtained several months after the onset of illness in cases in which A and B antibodies are negative. HCV RNA by polymerase chain reaction is usually elevated early in the illness and may be diagnostic in cases such as the one presented.

29. D: Up to 80% of acute hepatitis C cases progress to chronic hepatitis with persistence of HCV RNA. The transaminases are usually elevated to less than 10 times normal but may be normal in up to one-third of patients. Liver biopsy will show evidence of chronic hepatitis. Clinical trials have shown that treatment with peginterferon with or without ribavirin for 24 weeks results in a 90% resolution of HVC with sustained disappearance of HCV RNA. The treatment may be begun within 2 or 3 months after the onset of symptoms if viral RNA persists. As many as 50% of patients who present only with elevated transaminases may be successfully treated with this regimen. Acyclovir and prednisone have no role to play in the antiviral treatment.

30. A: Hypertension during pregnancy is fairly common and should be characterized as preeclampsia, chronic hypertension, chronic hypertension plus preeclampsia, or gestational hypertension. Preeclampsia is present if the blood pressure is elevated higher than 140/90 seated on 2 occasions and there is proteinuria greater than 300 mg per 24 hours. Pre-pregnancy blood pressures are normal. Hypertension that develops during pregnancy without proteinuria is referred to as gestational hypertension but may develop into preeclampsia during the course of the pregnancy, usually in the third trimester. Eclampsia is defined by seizures. Since this patient had normal pre-pregnancy blood pressures, chronic essential hypertension is excluded. The possibility of other less common causes of elevated blood pressure (e.g., renal artery stenosis, coarctation of the aorta, pheochromocytoma) should be considered but are rare.

31. E: Delivery is curative of both preeclampsia and gestational hypertension but must be weighed against the risk of prematurity. Most obstetricians will not deliver before 36 weeks unless the blood pressure cannot be controlled or evidence of end-organ failure develops. Magnesium sulfate is effective for eclampsia seizure control but is not indicated for preeclampsia or gestational hypertension. Calcium supplements and low-dose aspirin are most useful for prevention of preeclampsia and should be considered for any future pregnancies this woman may have. ACE inhibitors and angiotensin II receptor blockers are contraindicated for pregnant women as they may cause renal damage to the fetus or even fetal death or malformation. Methyldopa has been used extensively in pregnant hypertensive patients since it has a very good safety record and reduces vascular resistance while maintaining cardiac output and uteroplacental perfusion. Alpha- and beta-blockers may also be used.

32. D: This patient most likely has stage 3 diabetic nephropathy, which accounts for more than 80% of patients with end-stage renal disease. Many of these patients, unlike type 1 diabetes, are hypertensive and require blood pressure as well as diabetes control. His hemoglobin A_{1c} is under 7%, which conforms to the American Diabetes Association recommendation for adequate control. A diuretic may cause dehydration and possibly raise the blood glucose or cause electrolyte abnormalities. There is evidence that a dihydropyridine-type calcium channel blocker, such as amlodipine, may augment renal deterioration so this drug should be stopped and an ACE inhibitor or ARB should be started. ACE inhibitors and ARBs have shown some evidence of retarding the proteinuria and slowing kidney deterioration. While some protein restriction for this patient may be advisable (to 0.8 g/kg of ideal body weight per day), the amlodipine should be stopped.

33. D: With a GFR less than 15 $mL/min/m^2$ and proteinuria greater than 3.5 g per 24 hours, this patient now has nephrotic syndrome and end-stage renal disease. Hemodialysis is preferred to peritoneal dialysis because of greater efficiency, less discomfort for the patient, and a lower risk of infection. However, diabetic patients should be evaluated for immediate renal transplant if a live or cadaver compatible kidney is available. The 1-year allograft survival of kidneys from living donors is about 93%, somewhat better than that for a cadaver kidney transplant. Patients with type 1 diabetes should be considered for a live donor kidney transplant followed by a cadaver pancreas or islet cell transplant.

34. C: Patients who test positive for a *BRCA1* or *BRCA2* gene mutation represent less than 5% of all breast cancers, but they make up to 40% of hereditary breast cancer patients, with a frequency of 1 in 40 in Ashkenazi Jewish women. This woman has a 56% to 85% lifetime risk of breast cancer and 10% to 20% risk of ovarian cancer. In *BRCA* patients, MRI screening is considered superior to conventional mammography or ultrasound. For premenopausal women at high risk, tamoxifen 20 mg daily has been shown to reduce the risk by 50% for both invasive and noninvasive breast cancer. Raloxifene may also be used as it has a similar rate of risk reduction with fewer adverse effects than tamoxifen. A variety of other drugs are in clinical trials. Neither radiation nor chemotherapy is appropriate at this point.

35. E: This woman has a stage IIB breast cancer. This classification is based on the TNM staging system: a tumor more than 2 cm but less than 5 cm (T2); nodal involvement in 1 to 3 ipsilateral lymph nodes (N1); and no evidence of metastatic disease (M0). Thus, T2N1M0 is stage IIB. Her 10-year recurrence-free survival would be 45% to 55% without additional therapy. Since she is hormone receptor–positive and HER2-negative, her prognosis is probably somewhat better than most. Addition of adjuvant chemotherapy and hormone therapy should result in a significant improvement in her survival chances. Since she could not tolerate tamoxifen, other antiestrogen drugs may be tried. Trastuzumab is a monoclonal antibody that complexes with the HER2 protein in the tumor cells and inhibits cell proliferation in HER2-positive patients; however, this patient is HER2-negative. Aromatase inhibitors may be used for postmenopausal patients to block the conversion of androgen to estrogen but are ineffective in premenstrual women since any decrement in circulating estrogen stimulates pituitary gonadotropin release to fuel the ovaries to produce more estrogen. In this patient, hormonal therapy, if tolerated, and adjuvant chemotherapy would be advisable.

36. C: This young woman has a history typical of type 1 von Willebrand disease (vWD). This is the most common bleeding disorder affecting both sexes, 1% to 3% of the population. The vWF factor is a large multimeric glycoprotein with its gene located on chromosome 12. It is inherited as an autosomal dominant in type 1 vWD, which accounts for 75% to 80% of cases. The PTT may be elevated and factor VIII level reduced due to the absence or abnormality of the vWF protein that usually complexes with factor VIII and prevents its clearance from the circulation. The PT is usually normal or only slightly elevated. The platelet count is normal. Since the hemophilias (A and B) have an x-linked mode of inheritance they are rare in females, although a mutation may occur. The absence of deep bleeding in the muscle or joints eliminates a diagnosis of hemophilia; vWD bleeding is usual cutaneous or mucosal and menorrhagia is common in postpuberty females. The ristocetin cofactor assay (vWF:RCoF) is the most specific and sensitive diagnostic test for vWF. RIPA may only be slightly reduced in the standard assay but is markedly reduced or absent in the low ristocetin dose assay.

37. D: This man most likely has benign prostatic hypertrophy (BPH), but prostate cancer and chronic prostatitis should also be considered since the symptoms often overlap. Pelvic or genital pain may be a symptom suggesting chronic prostatitis and is often associated with urinary tract infections. A urinalysis and urine culture may be useful for diagnosing chronic prostatitis and other disorders of the kidney and urogenital tract. A calcium level should be a part of a serum chemistry screen along with diabetes screening test (hemoglobin A_{1c}) since elevations of either may be causing the urinary symptoms. PSA screening has become somewhat controversial recently because it has a poor sensitivity in this type of situation. PSA levels greater than 4 ng/mL should suggest the need for an ultrasound-guided prostate biopsy but it should be realized that about 50% of men with levels above 10 ng/mL have prostate cancer while about 25% with levels from 4.1 to 10 ng/mL have cancer. About 15% of patients with normal PSA values will have prostatic cancer. A rapidly rising PSA, especially in younger men, is an indication for prostate biopsy.

38. B: This patient is quite typical of men in the 30- to 50-year age range with acute abdominal pain who have no or only a vague history of abdominal complaints. His history suggests that the most likely differential is between acute cholecystitis and acute pancreatitis; however other entities such as perforated ulcer or intestinal obstruction must be considered. His description of the pain location and radiation are more consistent with pancreatic origin, since in cholecystitis the pain is usually in the right upper quadrant with radiation to the right scapular area. A serum amylase of greater than 3 times normal favors acute pancreatitis but may be elevated in intestinal obstruction, perforation or infarction, or even extra-gastrointestinal causes such as tubo-ovarian disease, renal failure, or macroamylasemia. CT (or MRI) of the abdomen is the best imaging test if pancreatitis is suspected since abdominal ultrasound of the pancreas is limited by intestinal gas or adipose tissue in 30% to 40% of patients. However, ultrasound is probably the best imaging study for acute cholelithiasis since it is fast, provides a good image, and does not require contrast injection.

39. D: This patient has a cutaneous abscess, almost certainly caused by *Staphylococcus aureus*. There is an increasing incidence of methicillin-resistant *Staphylococcus aureus* (MRSA) infections in the community, especially among athletes and children. These may represent 8% to 20% of community-acquired *Staph*. The community-acquired strains differ somewhat from the hospital-acquired nosocomial infections in that they almost always cause skin infections (furunculosis) versus the hospital-acquired bacteremias and wound infections. Prison inmates, native populations, and male homosexuals are most prone, in addition to children and athletes. These strains are resistant to beta-lactam and macrolide antibiotics and increasingly to fluoroquinolones. Vancomycin is the appropriate antibiotic in this setting until the culture and sensitivity report is available. Unfortunately, many of the hospital strains are multidrug resistant, including vancomycin, and treatment of these can be a major problem.

40. B: Travel prophylaxis is complex and dependent on the countries visited and whether a traveler plans to visit only urban areas or explore the countryside. Up-to-date information about appropriate chemoprophylaxis for specific countries may be obtained at the CDC website, http://www.cdc.gov. Practically all travelers should receive hepatitis A vaccine, especially those who travel to rural areas of developing countries where the risk is significant. Chloroquine malaria prophylaxis is appropriate for those areas with disease sensitive to this drug; chloroquine-resistant parasites are quite common in southeast Asia so drugs such as doxycycline (daily) or mefloquine (weekly) are preferred. Azithromycin is gradually replacing fluoroquinolones as treatment for traveler's diarrhea because of resistant strains but should not be used prophylactically. Meningococcal vaccine is only indicated for sub-Saharan Africa travel to the "meningitis belt" (Mali to Ethiopia), especially during the dry season from December through June. This is also a good time to make sure routine immunizations such as tetanus and diphtheria, influenza, pneumococcal, and varicella-zoster are up to date for appropriate patients.

41. B: This patient presents with classic signs and symptoms of early Parkinson disease: unilateral resting tremor, rigidity, and hypokinesia. While tremor is often less prominent in drug-induced parkinsonism and clinical features more symmetrical, a careful drug history is mandatory with special attention to neuroleptics, metoclopramide, certain calcium blockers, reserpine, methyldopa, and lithium. While the brain MRI is usually normal in classic Parkinson, it should be carried out to exclude other neurodegenerative diseases, as well as vascular and neoplastic disease. Wilson disease usually presents in younger patients but may be excluded by a 24-hour urine copper, serum ceruloplasmin, and slit-lamp exam for Kayser-Fleischer rings. Since cognitive function is usually normal in early Parkinson disease and impaired in Alzheimer disease, the latter is unlikely and may be excluded with an MRI. Normal-pressure hydrocephalus (NPH) may present with "lower-half" Parkinson-like features but urinary complaints are common and cognitive disturbances frequent. Response to levodopa is poor in NPH.

42. E: AF is the most common sustained arrhythmia and is especially common in elderly patients. It may be paroxysmal or continuous and may or may not result in overt symptoms. Many patients have palpitations, chest pain, or dyspnea. Cardioversion, intravenous beta-blockers, or certain calcium channel blockers may be use to restore sinus rhythm acutely. Anticoagulation is necessary to reduce the risk of stroke from embolization of thrombus, often present in the left atrial appendage. Some authorities suggest use of transesophageal echocardiography to detect a stroke and, if present, anticoagulate for 3 weeks before elective cardioversion. Long-term anticoagulation with warfarin is mandatory, although newer anticoagulants that are easier to manage are under active clinical trials. Amiodarone is the most likely drug to sustain sinus rhythm, but because of its numerous adverse effects, many doctors will initially try sotalol or propafenone for rhythm control. There is considerable evidence that rate control is just as effective in patient management as rhythm control and the former may be attempted with beta-blockers, diltiazem, or digoxin. Currently there has been considerable success with radio frequency ablation of AF focus, usually in the pulmonary veins, but this still remains secondary treatment. Finally, a catheter-placed filter over the opening of the left atrial appendage to block embolization of clots may allow discontinuation of anticoagulation.

43. E: This case illustrates a common emergency room problem, the differential diagnosis of dyspnea. History is of importance in that the man was a long-time smoker with a chronic cough that has recently changed in frequency and he has had increasing dyspnea. Asthma is doubtful since it usually begins at an earlier age and responds quickly to bronchodilators, although many patients with COPD also derive benefit from this therapy. The change in the cough and the increasing dyspnea suggest COPD with an exacerbation. This must commonly be differentiated from pneumonia or heart failure. In this case, ECG findings, the borderline enlarged heart (COPD patients often have a narrow cardiac shadow due to lung hyperinflation), and especially the BNP elevation point to heart failure. S3 gallop sounds are often hard to hear in COPD patients because of lung hyperinflation. BNP values in the 100 to 500 pg/mL range are in a so-called "gray zone," but values above this nearly always point to heart failure. Cardiac ultrasonography, ventricular scintigraphy, and cardiac catheterization usually will provide further diagnostic information. The lack of fever, sputum, or a definite pulmonary infiltrate makes pneumonia less likely.

44. A: Many depressed patients seek assistance from their primary care doctor for somatic complaints and the underlying depressive disorder is missed. In this case, the depressed mood and loss of concentration and no interest in things that he used to find pleasurable signals a major depression. Suicidal thoughts, even if brief and not acted upon, are particularly worrisome. Older people who are socially isolated and excessive users of drugs of abuse or alcohol are at a high risk of suicide and should be referred to a psychiatrist as soon as possible. Other patients may be started on a selective serotonin reuptake inhibitor (SSRI), such as fluoxetine (*Prozac*), sertraline (*Zoloft*), or paroxetine (*Paxil*), with psychotherapy added if there is an inadequate response. Several studies have indicated that combined drug and psychological therapy is most beneficial in many depressed patients. *Flomax* may cause dizziness but depressive symptoms are unusual. The suicidal thoughts take this diagnosis beyond dysthymia. While trazodone is useful for sleep disorders and may be used as a second drug, referral to a specialist is preferable. Since there is no history of mood swings or manic behavior, bipolar disorder is unlikely.

45. C: This patient has classic physical and hematologic findings of chronic myelocytic leukemia (CML). Sometimes the differential diagnosis includes polycythemia vera, thrombocythemia, myelomonocytic leukemia, and myeloid metaplasia. The diagnosis is confirmed by the finding of the cytogenetic abnormality termed a Philadelphia chromosome (Ph). If patients with apparent CML are Ph-negative, about one-third will have a hybrid BCR-ABL gene. This woman's disease is in chronic phase, which may last several years, but usually, if untreated, will transform into an accelerated phase and then a blastic phase with worsening symptoms, anemia, and increasing numbers of blasts in the peripheral blood. Imatinib has dramatically changed the prognosis for the disease. It has prolonged 5-year survival to 95% of those in chronic phase and lengthened survival significantly for those in the accelerated phases. Because of the success of imatinib, older treatments such as busulfan, IFA-alpha, or cytosine arabinoside are rarely used. Allogenic bone marrow transplant, if a donor is available, may potentially cure the disease, but subjects the recipient to potential adverse effects, including graft-versus-host disease (GVHD), infections, and second tumors. At this time, most hematologists will start the patient on imatinib and reserve allogenic bone marrow transplant for those who show disease progression.

46. D: How to manage a patient who is brain dead on life support is one of the more difficult ethical problems a physician must face, especially if the patient is young and otherwise healthy. It becomes even more complicated when the patient leaves no living will or even oral instructions to the spouse or other close family members about extraordinary measures at the end of life. It grows even more difficult when there is disagreement among family members and the possibility of organ donation is present. According to law, all interventions, including termination of artificial respiration, hydration, and nutrition, may be done ethically and legally. While members of the clergy and bioethics specialists may advise, they cannot make the final decision. The transplant surgeon is not allowed to manage the potential donor, and death is not allowed to be hastened by pharmacologic agents. This latter act by a transplant surgeon in California resulted in criminal charges, although he was acquitted. In cases in which there is dispute among the family members, the spouse's decision prevails, followed by adult children, parents, siblings, and available relatives. This situation arose in the well-known Terri Schiavo case; the husband's wishes ultimately prevailed after numerous court battles and federal intervention.

47. C: This boy has a typical onset of diabetic ketoacidosis, often preceded by an acute infection that triggers the syndrome. Dehydration is a characteristic because of polyuria exacerbated in this case by vomiting. Restoration of fluid volume is critical. Many doctors will start with normal saline, but if a corrected serum sodium is elevated, 0.45% may be preferable. Potassium should be added to the infusion if the serum level is less than 5.5 mEq/L because insulin therapy will cause a drop in the potassium level and he may already be deficient because of the vomiting. Levels should be obtained frequently. Regular insulin should be given as an intravenous bolus followed by a continuous infusion with follow-up doses based on the level of hyperglycemia, which should be checked hourly. A fall in the glucose concentration of 50 to 80 mg/dL/h is a reasonable goal. Too rapid a correction in hyperglycemia may lead to an osmotically driven cerebral edema or acute respiratory distress, especially in children. In general, addition of bicarbonate with a pH greater than 7 is not necessary since the insulin treatment should restore the acid-base abnormality. Sudden shifts in pH may further provoke hypoglycemia and impair tissue oxygen delivery by shifting the oxyhemoglobin dissociation curve to the left.

48. C: Bone mineral density declines fairly rapidly with age and menopause, although this woman may have delayed it somewhat with her short use of estrogen in her late 40s. Osteoporotic fractures of the spine, wrist, and hip may be presenting symptoms. The risk is greater among Caucasian women, especially those of slight stature. There may be a history of loss of height related to spinal compression fractures, usually in the lumbar or lower thoracic region. A plain x-ray of the spine may show the fractures with osteopenia and kyphosis. While low vitamin D levels and hyperthyroidism may be secondary causes of osteoporosis, the diagnosis is best established by DXA scanning. This technique is accurate, reproducible, and confers a relatively low radiation exposure. T scores below −2.5 SD (standard deviation) compared with age- and gender-matched controls is diagnostic of osteoporosis. Hip and spine values may differ in the same patient because of differences in the ratio of cortical to trabecular bone in these sites (higher in the hip). Urinary excretion of hydroxyproline has largely been abandoned as nonspecific with poor precision. Quantitative CT scanning is accurate and can detect early bone loss but is less reliable for follow-up with therapy and exposes the patient to considerable radiation.

49. B: This patient has acute sinusitis, most likely developing after a viral rhinitis, a common presentation. Nasal obstruction, facial pain, purulent discharge, and fever are considered major symptoms, while dental pain, cough, headache, and fever may also be present. This must be treated with antibiotics: amoxicillin or a macrolide is commonly used with amoxicillin with clavulanic acid or clindamycin as backups for beta-lactamase–resistant or anaerobic organisms. Culture is often not productive but if required should be done by a specialist via nasal endoscopy and CT guidance. This is often useful for chronic sinusitis. Persistent viral rhinitis is best treated with the usually array of oral decongestants, mucolytics, ipratropium bromide intranasal sprays, and steam inhalation. Allergic rhinitis usually presents with pale and swollen inferior turbinates; intranasal or oral steroids and antihistamines are indicated.

50. A: This man's symptoms and history of an erythematous rash are most suggestive of Lyme disease, caused by the spirochete *Borrelia burgdorferi*, and transmitted to humans by ticks, usually *Ixodes scapularis* in the Northeast and upper Midwest during the May to November period with a peak incidence in June and July. Often patients will not remember the tick bite. The characteristic rash, called erythema migrans, is a spreading, target-like lesion that often fades over a period of weeks. The organism, if untreated, may then spread and affect other anatomic sites, especially the nervous system, heart, and joints, often producing frank arthritis. *Treponema pallidum* is the cause of syphilis, which may present with similar symptoms in the secondary phase, but there is no history of a primary lesion and no positive VDRL. *Plasmodium falciparum* is the cause of falciparum malaria, which would be unlikely without travel to sub-Saharan Africa or Southeast Asia. *Treponema pertenue* infection causes yaws, which may cause skin, bone, and joint symptoms, but is usually found in children in tropical regions. Sand flies may transmit leishmaniasis but not Lyme disease.

How to Overcome Test Anxiety

Just the thought of taking a test is enough to make most people a little nervous. A test is an important event that can have a long-term impact on your future, so it's important to take it seriously and it's natural to feel anxious about performing well. But just because anxiety is normal, that doesn't mean that it's helpful in test taking, or that you should simply accept it as part of your life. Anxiety can have a variety of effects. These effects can be mild, like making you feel slightly nervous, or severe, like blocking your ability to focus or remember even a simple detail.

If you experience test anxiety—whether severe or mild—it's important to know how to beat it. To discover this, first you need to understand what causes test anxiety.

Causes of Test Anxiety

While we often think of anxiety as an uncontrollable emotional state, it can actually be caused by simple, practical things. One of the most common causes of test anxiety is that a person does not feel adequately prepared for their test. This feeling can be the result of many different issues such as poor study habits or lack of organization, but the most common culprit is time management. Starting to study too late, failing to organize your study time to cover all of the material, or being distracted while you study will mean that you're not well prepared for the test. This may lead to cramming the night before, which will cause you to be physically and mentally exhausted for the test. Poor time management also contributes to feelings of stress, fear, and hopelessness as you realize you are not well prepared but don't know what to do about it.

Other times, test anxiety is not related to your preparation for the test but comes from unresolved fear. This may be a past failure on a test, or poor performance on tests in general. It may come from comparing yourself to others who seem to be performing better or from the stress of living up to expectations. Anxiety may be driven by fears of the future—how failure on this test would affect your educational and career goals. These fears are often completely irrational, but they can still negatively impact your test performance.

Elements of Test Anxiety

As mentioned earlier, test anxiety is considered to be an emotional state, but it has physical and mental components as well. Sometimes you may not even realize that you are suffering from test anxiety until you notice the physical symptoms. These can include trembling hands, rapid heartbeat, sweating, nausea, and tense muscles. Extreme anxiety may lead to fainting or vomiting. Obviously, any of these symptoms can have a negative impact on testing. It is important to recognize them as soon as they begin to occur so that you can address the problem before it damages your performance.

The mental components of test anxiety include trouble focusing and inability to remember learned information. During a test, your mind is on high alert, which can help you recall information and stay focused for an extended period of time. However, anxiety interferes with your mind's natural processes, causing you to blank out, even on the questions you know well. The strain of testing during anxiety makes it difficult to stay focused, especially on a test that may take several hours. Extreme anxiety can take a huge mental toll, making it difficult not only to recall test information but even to understand the test questions or pull your thoughts together.

Effects of Test Anxiety

Test anxiety is like a disease—if left untreated, it will get progressively worse. Anxiety leads to poor performance, and this reinforces the feelings of fear and failure, which in turn lead to poor performances on subsequent tests. It can grow from a mild nervousness to a crippling condition. If allowed to progress, test anxiety can have a big impact on your schooling, and consequently on your future.

Test anxiety can spread to other parts of your life. Anxiety on tests can become anxiety in any stressful situation, and blanking on a test can turn into panicking in a job situation. But fortunately, you don't have to let anxiety rule your testing and determine your grades. There are a number of relatively simple steps you can take to move past anxiety and function normally on a test and in the rest of life.

Physical Steps for Beating Test Anxiety

While test anxiety is a serious problem, the good news is that it can be overcome. It doesn't have to control your ability to think and remember information. While it may take time, you can begin taking steps today to beat anxiety.

Just as your first hint that you may be struggling with anxiety comes from the physical symptoms, the first step to treating it is also physical. Rest is crucial for having a clear, strong mind. If you are tired, it is much easier to give in to anxiety. But if you establish good sleep habits, your body and mind will be ready to perform optimally, without the strain of exhaustion. Additionally, sleeping well helps you to retain information better, so you're more likely to recall the answers when you see the test questions.

Getting good sleep means more than going to bed on time. It's important to allow your brain time to relax. Take study breaks from time to time so it doesn't get overworked, and don't study right before bed. Take time to rest your mind before trying to rest your body, or you may find it difficult to fall asleep.

Along with sleep, other aspects of physical health are important in preparing for a test. Good nutrition is vital for good brain function. Sugary foods and drinks may give a burst of energy but this burst is followed by a crash, both physically and emotionally. Instead, fuel your body with protein and vitamin-rich foods.

Also, drink plenty of water. Dehydration can lead to headaches and exhaustion, especially if your brain is already under stress from the rigors of the test. Particularly if your test is a long one, drink water during the breaks. And if possible, take an energy-boosting snack to eat between sections.

Along with sleep and diet, a third important part of physical health is exercise. Maintaining a steady workout schedule is helpful, but even taking 5-minute study breaks to walk can help get your blood pumping faster and clear your head. Exercise also releases endorphins, which contribute to a positive feeling and can help combat test anxiety.

When you nurture your physical health, you are also contributing to your mental health. If your body is healthy, your mind is much more likely to be healthy as well. So take time to rest, nourish your body with healthy food and water, and get moving as much as possible. Taking these physical steps will make you stronger and more able to take the mental steps necessary to overcome test anxiety.

Mental Steps for Beating Test Anxiety

Working on the mental side of test anxiety can be more challenging, but as with the physical side, there are clear steps you can take to overcome it. As mentioned earlier, test anxiety often stems from lack of preparation, so the obvious solution is to prepare for the test. Effective studying may be the most important weapon you have for beating test anxiety, but you can and should employ several other mental tools to combat fear.

First, boost your confidence by reminding yourself of past success—tests or projects that you aced. If you're putting as much effort into preparing for this test as you did for those, there's no reason you should expect to fail here. Work hard to prepare; then trust your preparation.

Second, surround yourself with encouraging people. It can be helpful to find a study group, but be sure that the people you're around will encourage a positive attitude. If you spend time with others who are anxious or cynical, this will only contribute to your own anxiety. Look for others who are motivated to study hard from a desire to succeed, not from a fear of failure.

Third, reward yourself. A test is physically and mentally tiring, even without anxiety, and it can be helpful to have something to look forward to. Plan an activity following the test, regardless of the outcome, such as going to a movie or getting ice cream.

When you are taking the test, if you find yourself beginning to feel anxious, remind yourself that you know the material. Visualize successfully completing the test. Then take a few deep, relaxing breaths and return to it. Work through the questions carefully but with confidence, knowing that you are capable of succeeding.

Developing a healthy mental approach to test taking will also aid in other areas of life. Test anxiety affects more than just the actual test—it can be damaging to your mental health and even contribute to depression. It's important to beat test anxiety before it becomes a problem for more than testing.

Study Strategy

Being prepared for the test is necessary to combat anxiety, but what does being prepared look like? You may study for hours on end and still not feel prepared. What you need is a strategy for test prep. The next few pages outline our recommended steps to help you plan out and conquer the challenge of preparation.

Step 1: Scope Out the Test

Learn everything you can about the format (multiple choice, essay, etc.) and what will be on the test. Gather any study materials, course outlines, or sample exams that may be available. Not only will this help you to prepare, but knowing what to expect can help to alleviate test anxiety.

Step 2: Map Out the Material

Look through the textbook or study guide and make note of how many chapters or sections it has. Then divide these over the time you have. For example, if a book has 15 chapters and you have five days to study, you need to cover three chapters each day. Even better, if you have the time, leave an extra day at the end for overall review after you have gone through the material in depth.

If time is limited, you may need to prioritize the material. Look through it and make note of which sections you think you already have a good grasp on, and which need review. While you are studying, skim quickly through the familiar sections and take more time on the challenging parts.

Write out your plan so you don't get lost as you go. Having a written plan also helps you feel more in control of the study, so anxiety is less likely to arise from feeling overwhelmed at the amount to cover.

Step 3: Gather Your Tools

Decide what study method works best for you. Do you prefer to highlight in the book as you study and then go back over the highlighted portions? Or do you type out notes of the important information? Or is it helpful to make flashcards that you can carry with you? Assemble the pens, index cards, highlighters, post-it notes, and any other materials you may need so you won't be distracted by getting up to find things while you study.

If you're having a hard time retaining the information or organizing your notes, experiment with different methods. For example, try color-coding by subject with colored pens, highlighters, or post-it notes. If you learn better by hearing, try recording yourself reading your notes so you can listen while in the car, working out, or simply sitting at your desk. Ask a friend to quiz you from your flashcards, or try teaching someone the material to solidify it in your mind.

Step 4: Create Your Environment

It's important to avoid distractions while you study. This includes both the obvious distractions like visitors and the subtle distractions like an uncomfortable chair (or a too-comfortable couch that makes you want to fall asleep). Set up the best study environment possible: good lighting and a comfortable work area. If background music helps you focus, you may want to turn it on, but otherwise keep the room quiet. If you are using a computer to take notes, be sure you don't have any other windows open, especially applications like social media, games, or anything else that could distract you. Silence your phone and turn off notifications. Be sure to keep water close by so you stay hydrated while you study (but avoid unhealthy drinks and snacks).

Also, take into account the best time of day to study. Are you freshest first thing in the morning? Try to set aside some time then to work through the material. Is your mind clearer in the afternoon or evening? Schedule your study session then. Another method is to study at the same time of day that you will take the test, so that your brain gets used to working on the material at that time and will be ready to focus at test time.

Step 5: Study!

Once you have done all the study preparation, it's time to settle into the actual studying. Sit down, take a few moments to settle your mind so you can focus, and begin to follow your study plan. Don't give in to distractions or let yourself procrastinate. This is your time to prepare so you'll be ready to fearlessly approach the test. Make the most of the time and stay focused.

Of course, you don't want to burn out. If you study too long you may find that you're not retaining the information very well. Take regular study breaks. For example, taking five minutes out of every hour to walk briskly, breathing deeply and swinging your arms, can help your mind stay fresh.

As you get to the end of each chapter or section, it's a good idea to do a quick review. Remind yourself of what you learned and work on any difficult parts. When you feel that you've mastered the material, move on to the next part. At the end of your study session, briefly skim through your notes again.

But while review is helpful, cramming last minute is NOT. If at all possible, work ahead so that you won't need to fit all your study into the last day. Cramming overloads your brain with more information than it can process and retain, and your tired mind may struggle to recall even previously learned information when it is overwhelmed with last-minute study. Also, the urgent nature of cramming and the stress placed on your brain contribute to anxiety. You'll be more likely to go to the test feeling unprepared and having trouble thinking clearly.

So don't cram, and don't stay up late before the test, even just to review your notes at a leisurely pace. Your brain needs rest more than it needs to go over the information again. In fact, plan to finish your studies by noon or early afternoon the day before the test. Give your brain the rest of the day to relax or focus on other things, and get a good night's sleep. Then you will be fresh for the test and better able to recall what you've studied.

Step 6: Take a Practice Test

Many courses offer sample tests, either online or in the study materials. This is an excellent resource to check whether you have mastered the material, as well as to prepare for the test format and environment.

Check the test format ahead of time: the number of questions, the type (multiple choice, free response, etc.), and the time limit. Then create a plan for working through them. For example, if you have 30 minutes to take a 60-question test, your limit is 30 seconds per question. Spend less time on the questions you know well so that you can take more time on the difficult ones.

If you have time to take several practice tests, take the first one open book, with no time limit. Work through the questions at your own pace and make sure you fully understand them. Gradually work up to taking a test under test conditions: sit at a desk with all study materials put away and set a timer. Pace yourself to make sure you finish the test with time to spare and go back to check your answers if you have time.

After each test, check your answers. On the questions you missed, be sure you understand why you missed them. Did you misread the question (tests can use tricky wording)? Did you forget the information? Or was it something you hadn't learned? Go back and study any shaky areas that the practice tests reveal.

Taking these tests not only helps with your grade, but also aids in combating test anxiety. If you're already used to the test conditions, you're less likely to worry about it, and working through tests until you're scoring well gives you a confidence boost. Go through the practice tests until you feel comfortable, and then you can go into the test knowing that you're ready for it.

Test Tips

On test day, you should be confident, knowing that you've prepared well and are ready to answer the questions. But aside from preparation, there are several test day strategies you can employ to maximize your performance.

First, as stated before, get a good night's sleep the night before the test (and for several nights before that, if possible). Go into the test with a fresh, alert mind rather than staying up late to study.

Try not to change too much about your normal routine on the day of the test. It's important to eat a nutritious breakfast, but if you normally don't eat breakfast at all, consider eating just a protein bar. If you're a coffee drinker, go ahead and have your normal coffee. Just make sure you time it so that the caffeine doesn't wear off right in the middle of your test. Avoid sugary beverages, and drink enough water to stay hydrated but not so much that you need a restroom break 10 minutes into the test. If your test isn't first thing in the morning, consider going for a walk or doing a light workout before the test to get your blood flowing.

Allow yourself enough time to get ready, and leave for the test with plenty of time to spare so you won't have the anxiety of scrambling to arrive in time. Another reason to be early is to select a good seat. It's helpful to sit away from doors and windows, which can be distracting. Find a good seat, get out your supplies, and settle your mind before the test begins.

When the test begins, start by going over the instructions carefully, even if you already know what to expect. Make sure you avoid any careless mistakes by following the directions.

Then begin working through the questions, pacing yourself as you've practiced. If you're not sure on an answer, don't spend too much time on it, and don't let it shake your confidence. Either skip it and come back later, or eliminate as many wrong answers as possible and guess among the remaining ones. Don't dwell on these questions as you continue—put them out of your mind and focus on what lies ahead.

Be sure to read all of the answer choices, even if you're sure the first one is the right answer. Sometimes you'll find a better one if you keep reading. But don't second-guess yourself if you do immediately know the answer. Your gut instinct is usually right. Don't let test anxiety rob you of the information you know.

If you have time at the end of the test (and if the test format allows), go back and review your answers. Be cautious about changing any, since your first instinct tends to be correct, but make sure you didn't misread any of the questions or accidentally mark the wrong answer choice. Look over any you skipped and make an educated guess.

At the end, leave the test feeling confident. You've done your best, so don't waste time worrying about your performance or wishing you could change anything. Instead, celebrate the successful completion of this test. And finally, use this test to learn how to deal with anxiety even better next time.

Review Video: Test Anxiety
Visit mometrix.com/academy and enter code: 100340

Important Qualification

Not all anxiety is created equal. If your test anxiety is causing major issues in your life beyond the classroom or testing center, or if you are experiencing troubling physical symptoms related to your anxiety, it may be a sign of a serious physiological or psychological condition. If this sounds like your situation, we strongly encourage you to seek professional help.

Online Resources

Due to our efforts to try to keep this book to a manageable length, we've created a link that will give you access to all of your online resources:

mometrix.com/resources719/spex

It's Your Moment, Let's Celebrate It!

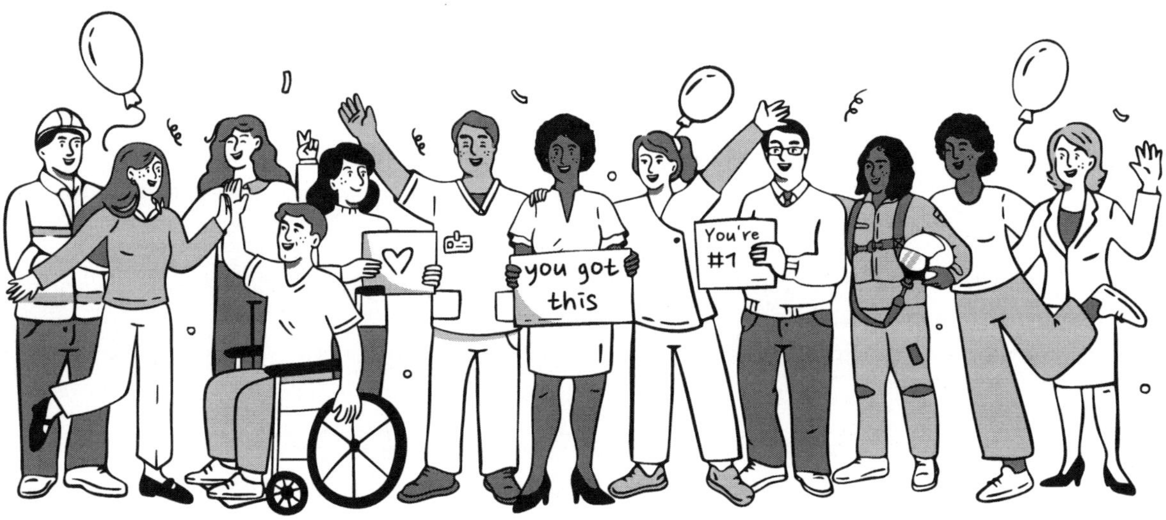

Share your story @mometrixtestpreparation

Mometrix TEST PREPARATION

SPEX®

Secrets Study Guide

Part 1 of 2

Dear Future Exam Success Story

First of all, **THANK YOU** for purchasing Mometrix study materials!

Second, congratulations! You are one of the few determined test-takers who are committed to doing whatever it takes to excel on your exam. **You have come to the right place.** We developed these study materials with one goal in mind: to deliver you the information you need in a format that's concise and easy to use.

In addition to optimizing your guide for the content of the test, we've outlined our recommended steps for breaking down the preparation process into small, attainable goals so you can make sure you stay on track.

We've also analyzed the entire test-taking process, identifying the most common pitfalls and showing how you can overcome them and be ready for any curveball the test throws you.

Standardized testing is one of the biggest obstacles on your road to success, which only increases the importance of doing well in the high-pressure, high-stakes environment of test day. Your results on this test could have a significant impact on your future, and this guide provides the information and practical advice to help you achieve your full potential on test day.

Your success is our success

We would love to hear from you! If you would like to share the story of your exam success or if you have any questions or comments in regard to our products, please contact us at **800-673-8175** or **support@mometrix.com**.

Thanks again for your business and we wish you continued success!

Sincerely,
The Mometrix Test Preparation Team

Need more help? Check out our flashcards at:
http://mometrixflashcards.com/SPEX

Written and edited by the Mometrix Exam Secrets Test Prep Team
Printed in the United States of America

TABLE OF CONTENTS

Introduction

Thank you for purchasing this resource! You have made the choice to prepare yourself for a test that could have a huge impact on your future, and this guide is designed to help you be fully ready for test day. Obviously, it's important to have a solid understanding of the test material, but you also need to be prepared for the unique environment and stressors of the test, so that you can perform to the best of your abilities.

For this purpose, the first section that appears in this guide is the **Secret Keys**. We've devoted countless hours to meticulously researching what works and what doesn't, and we've boiled down our findings to the five most impactful steps you can take to improve your performance on the test. We start at the beginning with study planning and move through the preparation process, all the way to the testing strategies that will help you get the most out of what you know when you're finally sitting in front of the test.

We recommend that you start preparing for your test as far in advance as possible. However, if you've bought this guide as a last-minute study resource and only have a few days before your test, we recommend that you skip over the first two Secret Keys since they address a long-term study plan.

If you struggle with **test anxiety**, we strongly encourage you to check out our recommendations for how you can overcome it. Test anxiety is a formidable foe, but it can be beaten, and we want to make sure you have the tools you need to defeat it.

Secret Key #1 – Plan Big, Study Small

There's a lot riding on your performance. If you want to ace this test, you're going to need to keep your skills sharp and the material fresh in your mind. You need a plan that lets you review everything you need to know while still fitting in your schedule. We'll break this strategy down into three categories.

Information Organization

Start with the information you already have: the official test outline. From this, you can make a complete list of all the concepts you need to cover before the test. Organize these concepts into groups that can be studied together, and create a list of any related vocabulary you need to learn so you can brush up on any difficult terms. You'll want to keep this vocabulary list handy once you actually start studying since you may need to add to it along the way.

Time Management

Once you have your set of study concepts, decide how to spread them out over the time you have left before the test. Break your study plan into small, clear goals so you have a manageable task for each day and know exactly what you're doing. Then just focus on one small step at a time. When you manage your time this way, you don't need to spend hours at a time studying. Studying a small block of content for a short period each day helps you retain information better and avoid stressing over how much you have left to do. You can relax knowing that you have a plan to cover everything in time. In order for this strategy to be effective though, you have to start studying early and stick to your schedule. Avoid the exhaustion and futility that comes from last-minute cramming!

Study Environment

The environment you study in has a big impact on your learning. Studying in a coffee shop, while probably more enjoyable, is not likely to be as fruitful as studying in a quiet room. It's important to keep distractions to a minimum. You're only planning to study for a short block of time, so make the most of it. Don't pause to check your phone or get up to find a snack. It's also important to **avoid multitasking**. Research has consistently shown that multitasking will make your studying dramatically less effective. Your study area should also be comfortable and well-lit so you don't have the distraction of straining your eyes or sitting on an uncomfortable chair.

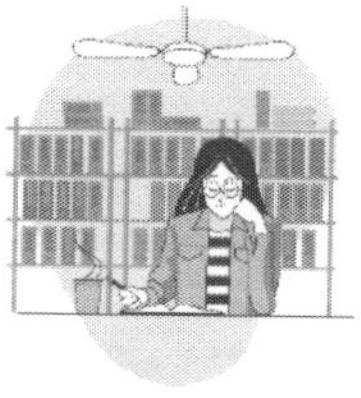

The time of day you study is also important. You want to be rested and alert. Don't wait until just before bedtime. Study when you'll be most likely to comprehend and remember. Even better, if you know what time of day your test will be, set that time aside for study. That way your brain will be used to working on that subject at that specific time and you'll have a better chance of recalling information.

Finally, it can be helpful to team up with others who are studying for the same test. Your actual studying should be done in as isolated an environment as possible, but the work of organizing the information and setting up the study plan can be divided up. In between study sessions, you can discuss with your teammates the concepts that you're all studying and quiz each other on the details. Just be sure that your teammates are as serious about the test as you are. If you find that your study time is being replaced with social time, you might need to find a new team.

Secret Key #2 – Make Your Studying Count

You're devoting a lot of time and effort to preparing for this test, so you want to be absolutely certain it will pay off. This means doing more than just reading the content and hoping you can remember it on test day. It's important to make every minute of study count. There are two main areas you can focus on to make your studying count.

Retention

It doesn't matter how much time you study if you can't remember the material. You need to make sure you are retaining the concepts. To check your retention of the information you're learning, try recalling it at later times with minimal prompting. Try carrying around flashcards and glance at one or two from time to time or ask a friend who's also studying for the test to quiz you.

To enhance your retention, look for ways to put the information into practice so that you can apply it rather than simply recalling it. If you're using the information in practical ways, it will be much easier to remember. Similarly, it helps to solidify a concept in your mind if you're not only reading it to yourself but also explaining it to someone else. Ask a friend to let you teach them about a concept you're a little shaky on (or speak aloud to an imaginary audience if necessary). As you try to summarize, define, give examples, and answer your friend's questions, you'll understand the concepts better and they will stay with you longer. Finally, step back for a big picture view and ask yourself how each piece of information fits with the whole subject. When you link the different concepts together and see them working together as a whole, it's easier to remember the individual components.

Finally, practice showing your work on any multi-step problems, even if you're just studying. Writing out each step you take to solve a problem will help solidify the process in your mind, and you'll be more likely to remember it during the test.

Modality

Modality simply refers to the means or method by which you study. Choosing a study modality that fits your own individual learning style is crucial. No two people learn best in exactly the same way, so it's important to know your strengths and use them to your advantage.

For example, if you learn best by visualization, focus on visualizing a concept in your mind and draw an image or a diagram. Try color-coding your notes, illustrating them, or creating symbols that will trigger your mind to recall a learned concept. If you learn best by hearing or discussing information, find a study partner who learns the same way or read aloud to yourself. Think about how to put the information in your own words. Imagine that you are giving a lecture on the topic and record yourself so you can listen to it later.

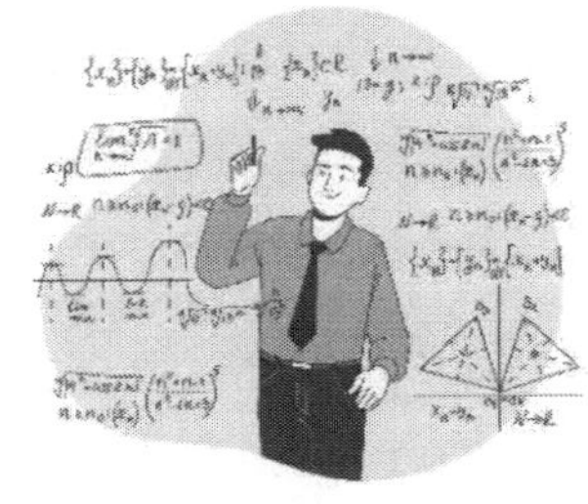

For any learning style, flashcards can be helpful. Organize the information so you can take advantage of spare moments to review. Underline key words or phrases. Use different colors for different categories. Mnemonic devices (such as creating a short list in which every item starts with the same letter) can also help with retention. Find what works best for you and use it to store the information in your mind most effectively and easily.

Secret Key #3 – Practice the Right Way

Your success on test day depends not only on how many hours you put into preparing, but also on whether you prepared the right way. It's good to check along the way to see if your studying is paying off. One of the most effective ways to do this is by taking practice tests to evaluate your progress. Practice tests are useful because they show exactly where you need to improve. Every time you take a practice test, pay special attention to these three groups of questions:

- The questions you got wrong
- The questions you had to guess on, even if you guessed right
- The questions you found difficult or slow to work through

This will show you exactly what your weak areas are, and where you need to devote more study time. Ask yourself why each of these questions gave you trouble. Was it because you didn't understand the material? Was it because you didn't remember the vocabulary? Do you need more repetitions on this type of question to build speed and confidence? Dig into those questions and figure out how you can strengthen your weak areas as you go back to review the material.

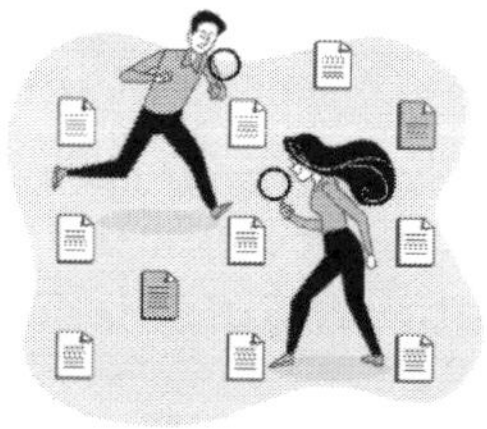

Additionally, many practice tests have a section explaining the answer choices. It can be tempting to read the explanation and think that you now have a good understanding of the concept. However, an explanation likely only covers part of the question's broader context. Even if the explanation makes perfect sense, **go back and investigate** every concept related to the question until you're positive you have a thorough understanding.

As you go along, keep in mind that the practice test is just that: practice. Memorizing these questions and answers will not be very helpful on the actual test because it is unlikely to have any of the same exact questions. If you only know the right answers to the sample questions, you won't be prepared for the real thing. **Study the concepts** until you understand them fully, and then you'll be able to answer any question that shows up on the test.

It's important to wait on the practice tests until you're ready. If you take a test on your first day of study, you may be overwhelmed by the amount of material covered and how much you need to learn. Work up to it gradually.

On test day, you'll need to be prepared for answering questions, managing your time, and using the test-taking strategies you've learned. It's a lot to balance, like a mental marathon that will have a big impact on your future. Like training for a marathon, you'll need to start slowly and work your way up. When test day arrives, you'll be ready.

Start with the strategies you've read in the first two Secret Keys—plan your course and study in the way that works best for you. If you have time, consider using multiple study resources to get different approaches to the same concepts. It can be helpful to see difficult concepts from more than one angle. Then find a good source for practice tests. Many times, the test website will suggest potential study resources or provide sample tests.

Practice Test Strategy

If you're able to find at least three practice tests, we recommend this strategy:

Untimed and Open-Book Practice

Take the first test with no time constraints and with your notes and study guide handy. Take your time and focus on applying the strategies you've learned.

Timed and Open-Book Practice

Take the second practice test open-book as well, but set a timer and practice pacing yourself to finish in time.

Timed and Closed-Book Practice

Take any other practice tests as if it were test day. Set a timer and put away your study materials. Sit at a table or desk in a quiet room, imagine yourself at the testing center, and answer questions as quickly and accurately as possible.

Keep repeating timed and closed-book tests on a regular basis until you run out of practice tests or it's time for the actual test. Your mind will be ready for the schedule and stress of test day, and you'll be able to focus on recalling the material you've learned.

Secret Key #4 – Pace Yourself

Once you're fully prepared for the material on the test, your biggest challenge on test day will be managing your time. Just knowing that the clock is ticking can make you panic even if you have plenty of time left. Work on pacing yourself so you can build confidence against the time constraints of the exam. Pacing is a difficult skill to master, especially in a high-pressure environment, so **practice is vital**.

Set time expectations for your pace based on how much time is available. For example, if a section has 60 questions and the time limit is 30 minutes, you know you have to average 30 seconds or less per question in order to answer them all. Although 30 seconds is the hard limit, set 25 seconds per question as your goal, so you reserve extra time to spend on harder questions. When you budget extra time for the harder questions, you no longer have any reason to stress when those questions take longer to answer.

Don't let this time expectation distract you from working through the test at a calm, steady pace, but keep it in mind so you don't spend too much time on any one question. Recognize that taking extra time on one question you don't understand may keep you from answering two that you do understand later in the test. If your time limit for a question is up and you're still not sure of the answer, mark it and move on, and come back to it later if the time and the test format allow. If the testing format doesn't allow you to return to earlier questions, just make an educated guess; then put it out of your mind and move on.

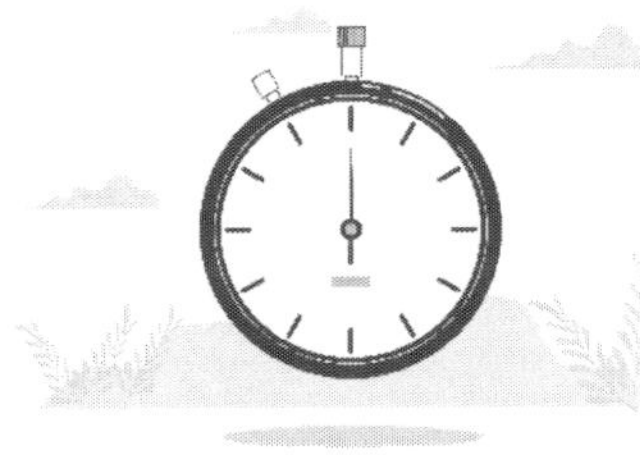

On the easier questions, be careful not to rush. It may seem wise to hurry through them so you have more time for the challenging ones, but it's not worth missing one if you know the concept and just didn't take the time to read the question fully. Work efficiently but make sure you understand the question and have looked at all of the answer choices, since more than one may seem right at first.

Even if you're paying attention to the time, you may find yourself a little behind at some point. You should speed up to get back on track, but do so wisely. Don't panic; just take a few seconds less on each question until you're caught up. Don't guess without thinking, but do look through the answer choices and eliminate any you know are wrong. If you can get down to two choices, it is often worthwhile to guess from those. Once you've chosen an answer, move on and don't dwell on any that you skipped or had to hurry through. If a question was taking too long, chances are it was one of the harder ones, so you weren't as likely to get it right anyway.

On the other hand, if you find yourself getting ahead of schedule, it may be beneficial to slow down a little. The more quickly you work, the more likely you are to make a careless mistake that will affect your score. You've budgeted time for each question, so don't be afraid to spend that time. Practice an efficient but careful pace to get the most out of the time you have.

Secret Key #5 – Have a Plan for Guessing

When you're taking the test, you may find yourself stuck on a question. Some of the answer choices seem better than others, but you don't see the one answer choice that is obviously correct. What do you do?

The scenario described above is very common, yet most test takers have not effectively prepared for it. Developing and practicing a plan for guessing may be one of the single most effective uses of your time as you get ready for the exam.

In developing your plan for guessing, there are three questions to address:

- When should you start the guessing process?
- How should you narrow down the choices?
- Which answer should you choose?

When to Start the Guessing Process

Unless your plan for guessing is to select C every time (which, despite its merits, is not what we recommend), you need to leave yourself enough time to apply your answer elimination strategies. Since you have a limited amount of time for each question, that means that if you're going to give yourself the best shot at guessing correctly, you have to decide quickly whether or not you will guess.

Of course, the best-case scenario is that you don't have to guess at all, so first, see if you can answer the question based on your knowledge of the subject and basic reasoning skills. Focus on the key words in the question and try to jog your memory of related topics. Give yourself a chance to bring the knowledge to mind, but once you realize that you don't have (or you can't access) the knowledge you need to answer the question, it's time to start the guessing process.

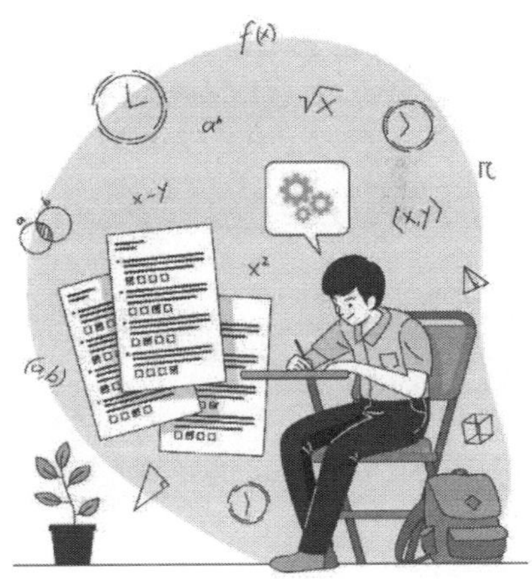

It's almost always better to start the guessing process too early than too late. It only takes a few seconds to remember something and answer the question from knowledge. Carefully eliminating wrong answer choices takes longer. Plus, going through the process of eliminating answer choices can actually help jog your memory.

Summary: Start the guessing process as soon as you decide that you can't answer the question based on your knowledge.

How to Narrow Down the Choices

The next chapter in this book (**Test-Taking Strategies**) includes a wide range of strategies for how to approach questions and how to look for answer choices to eliminate. You will definitely want to read those carefully, practice them, and figure out which ones work best for you. Here though, we're going to address a mindset rather than a particular strategy.

Your odds of guessing an answer correctly depend on how many options you are choosing from.

Number of options left	5	4	3	2	1
Odds of guessing correctly	20%	25%	33%	50%	100%

You can see from this chart just how valuable it is to be able to eliminate incorrect answers and make an educated guess, but there are two things that many test takers do that cause them to miss out on the benefits of guessing:

- Accidentally eliminating the correct answer
- Selecting an answer based on an impression

We'll look at the first one here, and the second one in the next section.

To avoid accidentally eliminating the correct answer, we recommend a thought exercise called **the $5 challenge**. In this challenge, you only eliminate an answer choice from contention if you are willing to bet $5 on it being wrong. Why $5? Five dollars is a small but not insignificant amount of money. It's an amount you could afford to lose but wouldn't want to throw away. And while losing $5 once might not hurt too much, doing it twenty times will set you back $100. In the same way, each small decision you make—eliminating a choice here, guessing on a question there—won't by itself impact your score very much, but when you put them all together, they can make a big difference. By holding each answer choice elimination decision to a higher standard, you can reduce the risk of accidentally eliminating the correct answer.

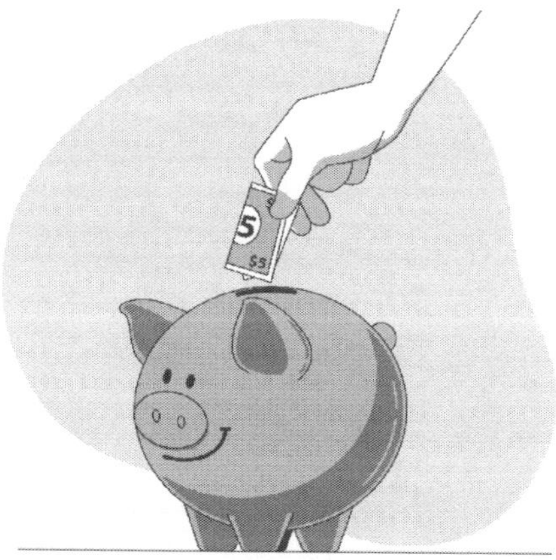

The $5 challenge can also be applied in a positive sense: If you are willing to bet $5 that an answer choice *is* correct, go ahead and mark it as correct.

Summary: Only eliminate an answer choice if you are willing to bet $5 that it is wrong.

Which Answer to Choose

You're taking the test. You've run into a hard question and decided you'll have to guess. You've eliminated all the answer choices you're willing to bet $5 on. Now you have to pick an answer. Why do we even need to talk about this? Why can't you just pick whichever one you feel like when the time comes?

The answer to these questions is that if you don't come into the test with a plan, you'll rely on your impression to select an answer choice, and if you do that, you risk falling into a trap. The test writers know that everyone who takes their test will be guessing on some of the questions, so they intentionally write wrong answer choices to seem plausible. You still have to pick an answer though, and if the wrong answer choices are designed to look right, how can you ever be sure that you're not falling for their trap? The best solution we've found to this dilemma is to take the decision out of your hands entirely. Here is the process we recommend:

Once you've eliminated any choices that you are confident (willing to bet $5) are wrong, select the first remaining choice as your answer.

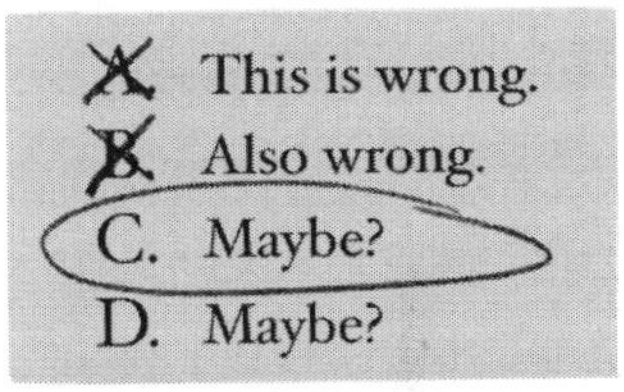

Whether you choose to select the first remaining choice, the second, or the last, the important thing is that you use some preselected standard. Using this approach guarantees that you will not be enticed into selecting an answer choice that looks right, because you are not basing your decision on how the answer choices look.

This is not meant to make you question your knowledge. Instead, it is to help you recognize the difference between your knowledge and your impressions. There's a huge difference between thinking an answer is right because of what you know, and thinking an answer is right because it looks or sounds like it should be right.

Summary: To ensure that your selection is appropriately random, make a predetermined selection from among all answer choices you have not eliminated.

Test-Taking Strategies

This section contains a list of test-taking strategies that you may find helpful as you work through the test. By taking what you know and applying logical thought, you can maximize your chances of answering any question correctly!

It is very important to realize that every question is different and every person is different: no single strategy will work on every question, and no single strategy will work for every person. That's why we've included all of them here, so you can try them out and determine which ones work best for different types of questions and which ones work best for you.

Question Strategies

✓ Read Carefully

Read the question and the answer choices carefully. Don't miss the question because you misread the terms. You have plenty of time to read each question thoroughly and make sure you understand what is being asked. Yet a happy medium must be attained, so don't waste too much time. You must read carefully and efficiently.

✓ Contextual Clues

Look for contextual clues. If the question includes a word you are not familiar with, look at the immediate context for some indication of what the word might mean. Contextual clues can often give you all the information you need to decipher the meaning of an unfamiliar word. Even if you can't determine the meaning, you may be able to narrow down the possibilities enough to make a solid guess at the answer to the question.

✓ Prefixes

If you're having trouble with a word in the question or answer choices, try dissecting it. Take advantage of every clue that the word might include. Prefixes can be a huge help. Usually, they allow you to determine a basic meaning. *Pre-* means before, *post-* means after, *pro-* is positive, *de-* is negative. From prefixes, you can get an idea of the general meaning of the word and try to put it into context.

✓ Hedge Words

Watch out for critical hedge words, such as *likely, may, can, often, almost, mostly, usually, generally, rarely,* and *sometimes*. Question writers insert these hedge phrases to cover every possibility. Often an answer choice will be wrong simply because it leaves no room for exception. Be on guard for answer choices that have definitive words such as *exactly* and *always*.

✓ Switchback Words

Stay alert for *switchbacks*. These are the words and phrases frequently used to alert you to shifts in thought. The most common switchback words are *but, although*, and *however*. Others include *nevertheless, on the other hand, even though, while, in spite of, despite*, and *regardless of*. Switchback words are important to catch because they can change the direction of the question or an answer choice.

⊘ FACE VALUE

When in doubt, use common sense. Accept the situation in the problem at face value. Don't read too much into it. These problems will not require you to make wild assumptions. If you have to go beyond creativity and warp time or space in order to have an answer choice fit the question, then you should move on and consider the other answer choices. These are normal problems rooted in reality. The applicable relationship or explanation may not be readily apparent, but it is there for you to figure out. Use your common sense to interpret anything that isn't clear.

Answer Choice Strategies

⊘ ANSWER SELECTION

The most thorough way to pick an answer choice is to identify and eliminate wrong answers until only one is left, then confirm it is the correct answer. Sometimes an answer choice may immediately seem right, but be careful. The test writers will usually put more than one reasonable answer choice on each question, so take a second to read all of them and make sure that the other choices are not equally obvious. As long as you have time left, it is better to read every answer choice than to pick the first one that looks right without checking the others.

⊘ ANSWER CHOICE FAMILIES

An answer choice family consists of two (in rare cases, three) answer choices that are very similar in construction and cannot all be true at the same time. If you see two answer choices that are direct opposites or parallels, one of them is usually the correct answer. For instance, if one answer choice says that quantity *x* increases and another either says that quantity *x* decreases (opposite) or says that quantity *y* increases (parallel), then those answer choices would fall into the same family. An answer choice that doesn't match the construction of the answer choice family is more likely to be incorrect. Most questions will not have answer choice families, but when they do appear, you should be prepared to recognize them.

⊘ ELIMINATE ANSWERS

Eliminate answer choices as soon as you realize they are wrong, but make sure you consider all possibilities. If you are eliminating answer choices and realize that the last one you are left with is also wrong, don't panic. Start over and consider each choice again. There may be something you missed the first time that you will realize on the second pass.

⊘ AVOID FACT TRAPS

Don't be distracted by an answer choice that is factually true but doesn't answer the question. You are looking for the choice that answers the question. Stay focused on what the question is asking for so you don't accidentally pick an answer that is true but incorrect. Always go back to the question and make sure the answer choice you've selected actually answers the question and is not merely a true statement.

⊘ EXTREME STATEMENTS

In general, you should avoid answers that put forth extreme actions as standard practice or proclaim controversial ideas as established fact. An answer choice that states the "process should be used in certain situations, if..." is much more likely to be correct than one that states the "process should be discontinued completely." The first is a calm rational statement and doesn't even make a definitive, uncompromising stance, using a hedge word *if* to provide wiggle room, whereas the second choice is far more extreme.

✓ Benchmark

As you read through the answer choices and you come across one that seems to answer the question well, mentally select that answer choice. This is not your final answer, but it's the one that will help you evaluate the other answer choices. The one that you selected is your benchmark or standard for judging each of the other answer choices. Every other answer choice must be compared to your benchmark. That choice is correct until proven otherwise by another answer choice beating it. If you find a better answer, then that one becomes your new benchmark. Once you've decided that no other choice answers the question as well as your benchmark, you have your final answer.

✓ Predict the Answer

Before you even start looking at the answer choices, it is often best to try to predict the answer. When you come up with the answer on your own, it is easier to avoid distractions and traps because you will know exactly what to look for. The right answer choice is unlikely to be word-for-word what you came up with, but it should be a close match. Even if you are confident that you have the right answer, you should still take the time to read each option before moving on.

General Strategies

✓ Tough Questions

If you are stumped on a problem or it appears too hard or too difficult, don't waste time. Move on! Remember though, if you can quickly check for obviously incorrect answer choices, your chances of guessing correctly are greatly improved. Before you completely give up, at least try to knock out a couple of possible answers. Eliminate what you can and then guess at the remaining answer choices before moving on.

✓ Check Your Work

Since you will probably not know every term listed and the answer to every question, it is important that you get credit for the ones that you do know. Don't miss any questions through careless mistakes. If at all possible, try to take a second to look back over your answer selection and make sure you've selected the correct answer choice and haven't made a costly careless mistake (such as marking an answer choice that you didn't mean to mark). This quick double check should more than pay for itself in caught mistakes for the time it costs.

✓ Pace Yourself

It's easy to be overwhelmed when you're looking at a page full of questions; your mind is confused and full of random thoughts, and the clock is ticking down faster than you would like. Calm down and maintain the pace that you have set for yourself. Especially as you get down to the last few minutes of the test, don't let the small numbers on the clock make you panic. As long as you are on track by monitoring your pace, you are guaranteed to have time for each question.

✓ Don't Rush

It is very easy to make errors when you are in a hurry. Maintaining a fast pace in answering questions is pointless if it makes you miss questions that you would have gotten right otherwise. Test writers like to include distracting information and wrong answers that seem right. Taking a little extra time to avoid careless mistakes can make all the difference in your test score. Find a pace that allows you to be confident in the answers that you select.

✓ KEEP MOVING

Panicking will not help you pass the test, so do your best to stay calm and keep moving. Taking deep breaths and going through the answer elimination steps you practiced can help to break through a stress barrier and keep your pace.

Final Notes

The combination of a solid foundation of content knowledge and the confidence that comes from practicing your plan for applying that knowledge is the key to maximizing your performance on test day. As your foundation of content knowledge is built up and strengthened, you'll find that the strategies included in this chapter become more and more effective in helping you quickly sift through the distractions and traps of the test to isolate the correct answer.

Now that you're preparing to move forward into the test content chapters of this book, be sure to keep your goal in mind. As you read, think about how you will be able to apply this information on the test. If you've already seen sample questions for the test and you have an idea of the question format and style, try to come up with questions of your own that you can answer based on what you're reading. This will give you valuable practice applying your knowledge in the same ways you can expect to on test day.

Good luck and good studying!

General Principles

Geriatrics

Urge Incontinence in Elderly Patients

Urinary incontinence is the involuntary loss of urine. There are several types of urinary incontinence in geriatric patients and urge incontinence is the most common type. It is characterized by a sudden intense urge to urinate followed by loss of urine. This occurs frequently and often at night. The diagnosis is made by measuring post-void residual, which will be >200 mL. Workup should include a urinalysis (U/A) and culture to rule out urinary tract infection (UTI). Urge incontinence can be caused by multiple sclerosis (MS) or Parkinson's disease. It can also be associated with Alzheimer's disease. *Treatment* options include pelvic muscle strengthening, bladder training, reducing caffeine, and scheduling frequent bathroom trips. Drug treatments include anticholinergics, oxybutynin, tolterodine, and nortriptyline.

Stress Incontinence

Stress incontinence is the involuntary loss or urine when increased pressure is placed on the bladder. This can occur with sneezing, coughing, laughing, heavy lifting, or during exercise. Stress incontinence is much more common in women and is due to weakening of the pelvic floor muscles. Risk factors include advanced age, history of multiple deliveries, and obesity. Patients present with a history of involuntary urination during sneezing, coughing, laughing, etc. The diagnosis is generally made by history. Urinary tract infection should be ruled out. A urinary stress test is sometimes performed. *Treatment* options include pelvic floor muscle exercises, limiting caffeine and fluid consumption, pads and urethral plugs, and pelvic surgery.

Overflow Incontinence

Overflow incontinence is characterized by a continuous leak of small amounts of urine. It is most often seen in men and is due to enlargement of the prostate. It can also be caused by obstruction of the bladder due to tumors or scar tissue, neurologic damage and medications such as anticholinergics, calcium channel blockers, and narcotics. The diagnosis is made by history and physical exam. Post-void residual will generally be greater than 450 mL. Urodynamic testing can be helpful in determining the cause. Acute urinary retention may require bladder catheterization. Alpha-blockers are used to relax the internal sphincter.

Pediatrics

Apgar Score

The **Apgar score** was developed in 1952 by Dr. Virginia Apgar as a way to rapidly assess the health status of a newborn. The score is given at one and five minutes after birth. The score can be repeated at ten minutes and beyond if it remains low. A newborn is given a score of 0, 1, or 2 in five different categories: heart rate, respiratory effort, muscle tone, skin color, and reflex irritability. An Apgar score of eight or greater is considered normal. An Apgar score of less than three indicates a critically ill newborn. The five-minute Apgar score is considered more indicative of long-term prognosis.

Physical Exam Findings of Down Syndrome in Newborns

Down syndrome, or trisomy 21, is one of the most common congenital abnormalities, with an incidence of approximately 1 in 700 births. The risk increases with increasing maternal age, especially after the age of 35 years. The diagnosis is suspected by the presence of certain physical features on the newborn exam. The following features are suggestive of Down syndrome: hypotonia, increased flexibility, redundant skin on the back of the neck, simian crease (single transverse palmar crease), slanted palpebral fissures, small and low set ears, flattened occiput, depressed nasal bridge, clinodactyly of the fifth finger, increased space between the first and second toes, and Brushfield's spots. The presence of six or more of these features on the newborn exam is highly suggestive of Down's syndrome and genetic studies should be performed.

Complications and Management of Down Syndrome

There are numerous **complications associated with Down syndrome**.

- Cardiac problems include ventricular septal defects and endocardial cushion defects.
- Gastrointestinal abnormalities include duodenal atresia and Hirschsprung's disease.
- Individuals with Down syndrome have an increased risk of developing leukemia and Alzheimer's dementia.
- Down syndrome patients have moderate to severe intellectual disability.

Management of a Down syndrome patient requires a team approach. They should be evaluated and followed by a cardiologist, gastroenterologist, and developmental pediatrician. Physical and occupational therapy should also be part of the management plan. The average life expectancy is about 50 years of age.

Possible Complications Associated with Birth Trauma

The most common **traumatic complications of delivery** include caput succedaneum, cephalhematoma, and subgaleal hemorrhage. Retinal and subconjunctival hemorrhages are also seen. Brachial plexus injury, including Erb-Duchenne paralysis (5th and 6th cervical nerve injury) and Klumpke paralysis (7th and 8th cervical nerve injury) are usually the result of excessive traction on the neck during a difficult delivery. Facial nerve injuries are sometimes seen. This is due to compression of the facial nerve against the mother's pelvis or injury from use of forceps. Fractures associated with delivery trauma include skull, clavicle, and extremity fracture. Clavicle fractures are the most common. Birth asphyxia can result from trauma of a complicated birth. This is often due to shoulder dystocia, cephalopelvic disproportion, or breech presentation.

Caput Succedaneum, Cephalhematoma, and Subgaleal Hemorrhage

Caput succedaneum, cephalhematoma, and subgaleal hemorrhage are possible abnormal findings on the newborn examination when examining the head of a newborn.

- **Caput succedaneum** is the presence of edema that crossed the suture lines. It is caused by trauma during the birth process. It is a benign condition that requires no treatment and resolves on its own during the first week of life.
- **Cephalhematoma** is characterized by a scalp swelling that does not cross the suture lines. It is caused by rupture of subperiosteal blood vessels due to trauma during delivery or as a complication of instrument assisted delivery. Jaundice and anemia are possible complications. Cephalhematomas usually resolve on their own; occasionally, phototherapy is needed to treat jaundice.

- **Subgaleal hemorrhage** is usually a complication of vacuum extraction. It presents as a boggy occipital mass that appears 12 to 72 hours after delivery. Subgaleal hemorrhage has the potential to lead to significant blood loss and should be monitored closely.

Neonatal Sepsis

Neonatal sepsis is an overwhelming infection that occurs in the first month of life. Neonatal sepsis can be early onset (birth to 8 days) or late onset (8 to 28 days). Risk factors for early onset sepsis include prematurity, prolonged rupture of membranes, maternal fever during labor, and a history of group B strep colonization. Presenting symptoms include irritability, poor feeding, tachypnea, and temperature instability. The workup should be performed immediately and include CBC, blood culture, chest x-ray, U/A and culture, and CSF cell count and culture. Broad-spectrum antibiotic coverage (ampicillin and gentamicin) should be started, pending culture results. The most common pathogen is group B strep (GBS) followed by gram-negative rods. Late onset sepsis presents with similar symptoms. Pathogens include GBS, gram negatives, *S aureus*, *Enterococcus,* and *Pseudomonas*. The workup is the same as for early onset sepsis.

Neonatal Jaundice

Neonatal jaundice is very common, affecting up to 50% of newborns. The most common cause is physiologic jaundice. Other more serious causes include hemolysis, sepsis, and metabolic disorders. Physiologic jaundice is the result of indirect, unconjugated hyperbilirubinemia. Workup should include direct and indirect bilirubin, CBC, reticulocyte count, exam of peripheral blood smear and type, and Coombs test. It is generally a benign self-limited condition; however, there is a risk of kernicterus with very high bilirubin levels. Phototherapy is the treatment of choice for physiologic jaundice. The level at which to begin phototherapy depends on gestational age, weight of the newborn and age of neonate. The rate of rise of bilirubin levels should not exceed 5 mg/dL per day. In general, phototherapy should be considered in a term neonate who is 24 to 48 hours old and has a bilirubin <15 mg/dL. At a level of 20 mg/dL, exchange transfusion should be considered.

Chromosomal Abnormalities

The following syndromes are all **chromosomal abnormalities**:

- **Edward's syndrome**, or trisomy 18, affects approximately 1 in 6,000 live births. Most affected individuals die within the first year of life. The appearance is variable, but characteristic abnormalities include severe IUGR, severe intellectual disability, and either clubfoot or "rocker-bottom feet."
- **Patau's syndrome**, or trisomy 13, affects approximately 1 in 6,000 births. Congenital abnormalities are severe and most die shortly after birth.
- **Klinefelter's syndrome** (XXY) occurs in approximately 1 in 1,000 births. Characteristics include mildly impaired IQ, gynecomastia, small testes, and decreased facial hair. Treatment includes testosterone replacement.
- **Turner's syndrome** (XO syndrome) occurs in 1 in 10,000 births. Characteristic findings include short stature, shield chest, webbed neck, coarctation of the aorta and amenorrhea. Therapy includes estrogen replacement.

TTN, Meconium Aspiration, and Hyaline Membrane Disease

Transient tachypnea of the newborn (TTN) usually presents shortly after birth. The presenting *symptoms* are increased respiratory rate, often >60 breaths per minute. Risk factors include cesarean section, precipitous delivery, and maternal diabetes. Chest x-ray may show hyperinflation and prominent pulmonary vascular markings. TTN is usually self-limited and treatment is supportive care.

Meconium aspiration occurs when a neonate aspirates meconium-stained fluid during delivery. The most significant risk factor is postdate delivery. If the infant appears healthy and vigorous at delivery, observation is sufficient. If the infant shows signs of distress, suctioning with an endotracheal tube is indicated. Meconium aspiration pneumonia is a very serious condition that requires NICU admission.

Hyaline membrane disease, or infant respiratory distress syndrome, is seen in premature infants as the result of a lack of surfactant. *Treatment* involves respiratory support and surfactant administration via an endotracheal tube.

X-Linked Recessive Disorders

Both are **x-linked recessive disorders**:

- **Duchenne's** affects approximately 1 in 3,500 male births. *Symptoms* usually begin by the age of 5 years and start in the distal muscles and move proximally. Patients present with difficulty getting up and an unsteady waddling gait. Cardiomyopathy and mental impairment are late manifestations. Lab tests show an elevated creatinine kinase (CK). Diagnosis is made by muscle biopsy. *Treatment* involves physical therapy and braces. Most patients die by the age of 20 years.
- **Hemophilia A** (factor VIII deficiency) and **hemophilia B** (factor IX deficiency) are inherited disorders of coagulation. They occur in approximately 1 in 5,000 to 10,000 live births. Patients present with repeated episodes of spontaneous bleeding. *Treatments* include DDAVP for hemophilia A, replacement of clotting factors, and injury avoidance.

Cystic Fibrosis

Cystic fibrosis is an autosomal recessive disorder in which a defect in the CFTR protein (a chloride channel protein) leads to the production of abnormally thick, viscous mucous. It is one of the most common inherited diseases in the United States, affecting mostly individuals of Northern European decent. The *diagnosis* should be suspected in the newborn with meconium ileus. Other symptoms include frequent respiratory infections, failure to thrive, salty taste to the skin, and rectal prolapse. *Staphylococcus aureus* is the most common cause of pulmonary infection early in the disease; *Pseudomonas aeruginosa* is the dominant pathogen in more advanced cystic fibrosis. The diagnosis can be made by a sweat test or genetic testing. Prenatal testing and newborn screening tests are available. At this time, there is no cure for cystic fibrosis. *Treatment* is aimed at slowing the progression and alleviating symptoms. Treatments include mucolytic drugs, bronchodilators, antibiotics, and chest physiotherapy. Lung transplantation is sometimes an option for end-stage disease. Pancreatic enzyme replacement should be administered. End-stage lung disease is the most common cause of death. Life expectancy is 30 to 40 years.

Hirschsprung's Disease

Hirschsprung's disease is a congenital disorder characterized by the absence of ganglion cells in the distal colon. Hirschsprung's disease occurs in about 1 in 5,000 births. It is more common in boys and in patients with Down syndrome. Patients usually present early in life with failure to pass meconium, vomiting, and abdominal distention. Mild cases can present later in childhood with constipation and poor weight gain. The *diagnosis* is suggested by abdominal x-ray showing a dilated proximal colon and absence of gas in the rectum. The diagnosis is confirmed by barium enema. The affected bowel segment will be narrowed and the proximal bowel will appear distended. Manometry and biopsy are also sometimes performed. *Treatment* is surgical removal of the aganglionic segment and subsequent pull-through of normal bowel.

Congenital Hip Dysplasia

Congenital hip dysplasia refers to abnormal hip joint formation leading to a hip that is either unstable or dislocated. Hip dysplasia occurs in about 3 to 4 per 1,000 live births. There is an increased incidence with a positive family history or breech presentation. It is more common in girls and occurs most commonly in the left hip. It can be unilateral or bilateral. Every newborn must be screened for hip dysplasia using Barlow's and Ortolani's maneuvers. Asymmetric thigh or buttock creases may be present. If dysplasia is suspected, an ultrasound should be obtained. The *treatment* of choice is a Pavlik harness.

Metatarsus Varus and Talipes Equinovarus

Metatarsus varus is sometimes seen on the newborn physical exam. It is also known as metatarsus adductus. On exam, the forefoot is twisted inward. It is often due to positioning of the foot in utero and does not require any treatment. On exam, it is critical to determine if the position is flexible and if the foot can be easily manipulated to the midline. If the position is fixed, treatment is required. Treatment options include corrective shoes, serial castings, and corrective bracing. Patients can sometimes also have hip dysplasia. With appropriate treatment, the prognosis is excellent. Talipes equinovarus, or clubfoot, is a congenital structural foot deformity. It may be genetic. Patients present at birth with plantar flexion at the ankle, inversion of the heel, and medial deviation of the forefoot. The position is fixed. *Treatment* is serial casting or surgery.

Nutritional Deficiencies

Scurvy refers to vitamin C deficiency. Presenting symptoms include bleeding from the gums and mucous membranes, poor healing, and failure to thrive. *Treatment* is vitamin C replacement.

Rickets is a vitamin D deficiency. Rickets can also occur as the result of inadequate calcium intake. A lack of sufficient vitamin D leads to inadequate calcium absorption, which will cause bone and muscle abnormalities. *Treatment* is vitamin D supplementation.

Kwashiorkor is defined as an isolated protein deficiency. Patients present with a distended abdomen, edema, and failure to thrive. *Treatment* includes caloric supplementation with slow introduction of protein into the diet.

Marasmus is caused by a severe deficiency of all nutrients. Patients present with severe failure to thrive.

Failure to Thrive

Failure to thrive (FTT) is defined as inadequate physical growth over a period of time. All children should have their height, weight, and head circumference (infants) plotted on a standard growth chart at each visit. If a child's measurements fall such that it crosses two percentile lines, then the child is said to be failing to thrive. Typically, a child's weight will show a decline first, followed by height. Head circumference is rarely involved. Etiologies can be divided into two categories: organic and nonorganic. When a child's height falls off their growth curve, the etiology is more likely to be organic. Nonorganic causes include psychosocial issues and inadequate feeding. There are numerous organic causes; almost any chronic disease can cause failure to thrive. The evaluation must include a thorough history and physical exam. Laboratory tests and further workup should be guided by the findings on the history and physical. Keeping a food diary and observing the parent-child interaction can sometimes be helpful. Occasionally, hospitalization is required.

IPV and Hib Vaccines

IPV

The inactivated polio vaccine is used almost exclusively in the United States. Oral polio vaccine (OPV) is used in countries where wild polio exists. The series is usually started at the two-month visit. The vaccine is contraindicated in individuals with a history of a severe allergic reaction to the antibiotics neomycin, streptomycin, or polymyxin B.

Hib

The Haemophilus influenzae type b (Hib) vaccine is given to all children under the age of 5 years, generally beginning at the two-month visit. Older children who have sickle cell disease, are asplenic, or are immunosuppressed from AIDS or cancer should also be vaccinated. The vaccine should not be given earlier that than 6 weeks of age or to individuals with a history of a significant allergic reaction to the vaccine.

HBV and DTaP Vaccines

HBV

The hepatitis B vaccine is a recombinant DNA vaccine. Universal vaccination of infants is recommended. The first dose is given in the hospital before the newborn is discharged, the second dose is given between 1 to 4 months, and the third dose is given between 6 to 18 months. All children eighteen and under should receive the three-dose series if not previously immunized. The vaccine should be given to high-risk adults. The vaccine is contraindicated in people with a history of an allergic reaction to a previous dose of the vaccine.

DTaP

The vaccine against diphtheria, tetanus, and pertussis (acellular). The vaccine is made using small purified viral proteins. The vaccine series is begun in infants at 2 months of age. It is now recommended that children over the age of 11 years and adults 19 to 64 years receive a single booster dose of the new vaccine Tdap. The vaccine should not be given to an individual with a history of a serious allergic reaction or certain CNS abnormalities.

Influenza and Meningococcal Vaccines

The **influenza vaccine** is recommended annually for children 6 to 23 months of age, adults over the age of 50 years and most individuals with a chronic disease. It is recommended for all healthcare personnel and individuals living with a person at high-risk. It is also recommended before travel to certain areas of the world and before attending college, especially if residing in a dormitory. The vaccine is contraindicated in infants less than 6 months, people who are moderately to severely ill with a fever, and individuals with egg allergies. The nasal mist (live virus) form of the vaccine is contraindicated in children less than 2 years old, adults <50 years, people with a history of asthma or other chronic disease, and pregnant women.

The **meningococcal vaccine** is currently recommended for children at age 11 to 12 years and before starting high school. It is also recommended before college entry and for military recruits. It is contraindicated in individuals with a latex allergy or hypersensitivity to diphtheria toxoid.

MMR and Varicella Vaccines

MMR

The measles, mumps and rubella vaccine is a thimerosal-free live attenuated viral vaccine given in a two-dose series generally at 15 months and at 4 to 6 years of age. The vaccine should not be administered to immunocompromised individuals or people with a history of a gelatin allergy. There is no scientific proof linking the MMR vaccine to the development of autism.

VARICELLA

The Varicella (chickenpox) vaccine is routinely administered at 12 to 18 months of age with a booster at age 4 to 6 years. The vaccine is contraindicated in individuals with allergies to gelatin, neomycin, or a previous dose of the vaccine. It should not be administered to pregnant women or people with T-cell immunodeficiency. The vaccine may not be administered for 5 months following a blood transfusion.

LEAD SCREENING IN CHILDREN AND MANAGEMENT OF INCREASED LEAD LEVELS

Lead poisoning in children remains a common problem. The most common source is exposure to lead paint, which is usually found in homes built before 1950. Contaminated water from lead containing pipes is also a source. Universal screening of children at ages 9 to 12 months is recommended in most communities. Communities with low rates of elevated lead levels in children and a low percentage of homes built before 1950 may be able to do targeted screening. Children at high risk should be initially screened at 6 months. Subsequent screening depends on the initial lead level. A level of >10 mcg/dL is considered abnormal. A careful history should be performed to determine the source of the lead exposure. Counseling the topics of dietary measures, increasing iron, vitamin C and calcium, and avoidance of lead paint should be performed. Acute lead poisoning or levels >45 mcg/dL may require chelation therapy.

ENURESIS

Enuresis (involuntary urination at night) is a very common problem in children.

- **Primary enuresis** is defined as the condition of never having been dry at night.
- **Secondary enuresis** is when a child resumes bed-wetting after a period of being dry of at least 6 months.

Enuresis is more common in boys. The family must be reassured that the problem is very common and most patients will outgrow bed-wetting before the age of 12 years. A screening urinalysis should be performed. *Treatment* is usually just reassurance. In older children who are bothered by the bed-wetting, treatment options include different types of alarm systems to wake a child upon wetting the bed. Medications that are used include DDAVP, imipramine, and oxybutynin.

AUTISM

Autism is a developmental disorder characterized by impaired social interactions and communication abnormalities. Autism is part of a spectrum of disorders known as autism spectrum disorders (ASD) ranging in severity from mild language and behavioral deficits to a complete inability to communicate. Patients are typically diagnosed between 1 to 3 years of age when they present with delayed language skills, lack of interpersonal interactions, and abnormal behaviors. Abnormal behaviors can include repetitive movements like rocking or specific routines or rituals. The cause is still unknown. No study has proven a link between MMR vaccination and autism. It is more common in boys and there appears to be a genetic component. *Treatment* includes behavioral and communication therapies.

ADHD

Attention-deficit hyperactivity/disorder (ADHD) is a commonly diagnosed disorder characterized by inattentiveness, hyperactivity, and impulsivity. In order to be diagnosed with ADHD, a child must exhibit six or more symptoms from at least two of the categories. The symptoms must be present at both home and school. The Conners' ADHD Index and symptom scales are useful in making the diagnosis. Attention-deficit hyperactivity/disorder is typically diagnosed early in childhood, but the disorder also exists in adults. The cause is unknown and there does appear to be a hereditary component. It is more common in boys. It can be associated with other psychiatric disorders such as depression, conduct disorders, and anxiety disorders. Treatment includes medications (stimulants), behavior modification, and psychotherapy.

Slipped Capital Femoral Epiphysis, Leg-Calve-Perthes Disease, and Osgood-Schlatter Syndrome

Slipped capital femoral epiphysis occurs when a growth plate abnormality leads to displacement of the femoral head from the hip joint. It typically affects children ages 11 to 16 years. Boys are affected more often than girls, particularly if they are overweight. Patients present with pain and limp. The diagnosis is made by x-ray. Treatment is surgical pinning.

Legg-Calve-Perthes disease is also known as avascular necrosis of the femoral head. It is typically seen in children ages 4 to 8 years; it is more common in boys. Patients present with pain, limp, and decreased range of motion. Diagnosis is made by x-ray. Treatment is rest and anti-inflammatory medications.

Osgood-Schlatter syndrome is an overuse syndrome where patients present with pain and tenderness over the tibial tuberosity. It typically presents in adolescent athletes. Treatment is rest and pain management. The condition is benign and generally resolves in time.

Heart Murmurs

Heart murmurs are common findings on the pediatric physical exam and approximately 40% are benign. A murmur is more likely benign if it is soft, systolic, and short in duration. The patient should not have any other symptoms of cardiac disease and there should be a normal S1 and S2 on cardiac auscultation. The quality of functional murmurs often changes when a patient changes position from lying to sitting or standing. The presence of failure to thrive, exercise intolerance, or cyanosis are all indications that cardiac disease is present. Still's murmur is a common functional murmur of childhood. It is a soft systolic murmur heard best along the left sternal border. It generally disappears as a child grows. Any suspicion that heart murmur is pathologic requires referral to a cardiologist.

Febrile Seizures

Febrile seizures are a common occurrence in childhood. They usually occur in children between the ages of 6 months and 5 years who have rectal temperatures >102° F.

- A **simple febrile seizure** is generalized, lasts <15 minutes and does not occur more than once during a 24-hour period.
- **Complex febrile seizures** may be focal, last >15 minutes or occur more than once in a 24-hour period.

Simple febrile seizures generally do not need a workup. Parents should be counseled about fever control and the possibility of the child having another febrile seizure. Frequent recurrences of febrile seizure may require use of antiseizure medication. Complex febrile seizures require a complete neurologic workup, including a lumbar puncture.

Kawasaki's Disease

Kawasaki's disease, also known as mucocutaneous lymph node syndrome, is an inflammatory childhood disease of unknown etiology. It typically affects children younger than 5 years of age and is more common in boys. In order for the diagnosis to be made, fever must be present for at least 5 days and the patient must exhibit at least four of the following symptoms: bilateral conjunctivitis, inflammation of the oral mucosa including cracked lips and strawberry tongue, cervical lymphadenopathy, rash and redness, swelling, and ultimately peeling of the hands and feet. The *diagnosis* is made clinically and the *treatment* is with aspirin and IVIG. The most serious complication is coronary artery aneurysm. The patient must be examined and followed by a cardiologist.

Acne Vulgaris

Acne vulgaris is caused by blockage of the pilosebaceous unit. It is extremely common, affecting approximately 85% of teenagers and young adults. Acne is generally divided by degree of severity. Acne is considered mild if there are fewer than 30 total lesions with few inflammatory lesions. Mild acne is generally treated with a topical benzoyl peroxide preparation, a topical antibiotic, or sometimes a mild topical Retin-A® preparation at night. Moderate acne can have up to 100 to 125 total lesions with a higher proportion being inflammatory. Moderate acne is frequently treated with an oral antibiotic as well as topical preparation. Severe acne is characterized by >125 lesions, many inflammatory lesions and the presence of cysts. Severe acne is often treated with oral isotretinoin (Accutane®). If Accutane is used, LFTs must be followed and girls must be counseled regarding the teratogenicity of the medication.

Tanner Stages and Normal Sexual Development

Tanner staging is a system used to describe the stages of sexual development. The stages are as follows:

- **Tanner I** – Prepubescent, no signs of sexual development.
- **Tanner II** – Sparse pubic hair, enlargement of scrotum and testes, breast buds.
- **Tanner III** – Darker, coarser, more curled pubic hair, enlargement of penis in length, enlargement and elevation of breast and areola.
- **Tanner IV** – Pubic hair resembles adult with more limited distribution, increase in length and breadth of penis and darkening of scrotal skin, areola and papilla form secondary mound.
- **Tanner V** – Mature.

Onset of puberty is between ages 9 to 13 years for boys and 8 to 13 years for girls. Signs of puberty at younger ages are considered precocious and should be investigated. Lack of signs of puberty by age 13 years warrants a workup.

Immune System

Allergy Assessment and Presentation

Hypersensitivity Reaction Types

There are four types of **hypersensitivity reactions**:

- **Type I: Immediate.** Occurs minutes to one hour after exposure, and defines "classic" allergies. Ag-specific IgE is cross-linked on mast cells, leading to degranulation, release of immune mediators (especially histamine), and production of others. Complement products can also cause the release of mast cell contents (non-IgE mediated anaphylaxis). Treat type I with IV antihistamines, avoidance of allergen, and epinephrine (SQ if mild, IV if severe reaction), and corticosteroids to diminish relapse or delayed response. Desensitization helps in IgE-mediated reactions only.
- **Type II: Cytotoxic hypersensitivity.** This reaction is mediated by IgG or IgM and results in cell destruction via complement activation and membrane attack complex (MAC), opsonization (C3b), or antibody (Ab)-mediated cytotoxicity.
- **Type III: Immune complex hypersensitivity.** This involves cross-linking of antigens and antibodies. Combination of antibodies with antigens leads to IC formation, which precipitates and activates complement, resulting in inflammation and vasculitis. This may present 1-2 weeks after exposure leading to "serum sickness."
- **Type IV: Cell-mediated hypersensitivity.** T cells become sensitized to an antigen, leading to an inflammatory reaction that peaks in 2-3 day (delayed hypersensitivity). Examples include contact dermatitis and tuberculin sensitivity.

Diagnostic Testing for Allergies

The different types of **allergy testing** include the following:

- **Basic skin testing** is done to observe allergen-specific IgE response. Testing should employ both positive and negative controls and look for wheal and flare after placement of allergen. This is useful and relatively sensitive and specific compared to other testing.
- **DTH** skin testing employs antigen injection and is used to evaluate cell-mediated immunity to antigens, including PPD, toxoid, candida, and others. This test site is observed for induration after 48 hours (similar to PPD induration).
- **Patch skin testing** is just as it sounds. Allergens are applied by patch and examined 2-3 days after application for evidence of a local reaction. This test is excellent to evaluate potential sources of contact dermatitis.
- **RAST** is radioallergosorbent testing, which measures the allergen specific IgE in serum. This is not as sensitive and specific as skin testing, but may be useful if skin disease or anaphylactic sensitivity to the allergen precludes skin tests.

Complement Cascade and Differences Between Classical and Alternative Pathways

The **complement cascade** is a component of the innate immune system divided into the classical pathway and the alternative pathway. Remember: The end result of these pathways is either activation of the membrane attack complex (MAC) or opsonization and removal of the C3-coated entity.

The first key step is activation of C3: The **classical pathway** consists of C1, C2, and C4. C1 subtypes must bind the Fc regions of IgG (two) or IgM (one) for efficient activation of C3. The **alternative pathway** consists of factor B and factor D. Fragments of factor B can stimulate a positive feedback system, which creates high levels of C3b, activating C5.

Conversion of C3 to C3b and activation of C5 leads to formation of the membrane attack complex (C5-C9) and osmotic lysis of the target cell. C3 fragments opsonize targets for removal via phagocytosis. C5a is a potent chemoattractant.

Complement Deficiency

There are **deficiencies of all parts of the complement pathway**, including the (1) classical pathway, (2) C3 and alternative pathway, and (3) membrane attack complex (MAC).

- **Classical deficiency** may include C1 (q, r, s), C2, and C4. This leads to immune complex syndromes and pyogenic infection, such as recurrent sinopulmonary infections with encapsulated bacteria. There is an association with SLE and other rheumatoid diseases. C2 is the most common deficiency in Caucasians in the US.
- **C3 and Alternative complement deficiency** may lead to immune complex syndromes and recurrent infections, such as severe pyogenic infections. It may also be associated with HUS.
- **Membrane attack complex** (MAC) deficiency is aka terminal complement deficiency. This is associated with recurrent Neisseria infections (which can cause meningitis and sepsis) and immune complex disease. The CH50 assay must be checked to determine the activity of the classical pathway. CH50 may also be used to follow disease activity in SLE.

Congenital Immunodeficiencies

Congenital immunodeficiencies include:

- **Common variable immunodeficiency** is primarily an IgG deficiency due to absent plasma cells and B cell differentiation. These patients have increased susceptibility to encapsulated organisms and are more likely to develop bronchiectasis from the recurrent damage. They are also at higher risk for B cell neoplasms, GI malignancy, and autoimmune disease. Test is with functional antibody response and treatment with IVIG.
- **Congenital Agammaglobulinemia** (Bruton's, x-linked) usually leads to a susceptibility to recurrent pyogenic infections and low IgG and no IgA, IgM, IgE, IgD, or B cells.
- **Selective IgA deficiency** is the most common Ig deficiency and leads to recurrent sinopulmonary infections. It has association with recurrent giardiasis, GI malignancy, and autoimmune disorders, including celiac sprue. One should withhold IVIG due to possible anaphylactic reaction to IgA.
- **Wiskott-Aldrich syndrome** is the combination of thrombocytopenia, eczema, and immunodeficiency. It has associated low IgM and elevated IgA and IgE. BMT treats this successfully.

Primary Non-HIV Cellular Immunodeficiency Disorders

Primary immunodeficiency disorders (non-HIV) are caused by genetic mutations and are characterized by abnormal, absent, or inadequate cells:

- **B cell** (humoral immunity): The most common of the immunodeficiency disorder (more than 50%). Interferes with ability to produce antibodies. Includes common variable immunodeficiency, transient hypogammaglobulinemia of infancy, and x-linked agammaglobulinemia. Increases risk of bacterial infections.

- **T cell** (cellular immunity): Includes chronic mucocutaneous candidiasis, DiGeorge syndrome, and x-linked lymphoproliferative syndrome. Increases risk of viral and fungal infections.
- **B and T cell**: Includes ataxia-telangiectasia, hyperimmunoglobulinemia syndrome, and Wiskott-Aldrich syndrome, and severe combined immunodeficiency.
- P**hagocyte**: Impaired movement and ability to destroy cells. Includes chronic granulomatous disease, Chédiak-Higashi syndrome, cyclic neutropenia, ad leukocyte adhesion defects. Impairs ability to destroy pathogens.
- **Complement proteins**: C1, C3, C4, C5. C6, C7, C8 and/or C9 deficiency. Increases risk of recurrent infections and autoimmune disorders.

Causes may include blood disorders (aplastic anemia, leukemia, multiple myeloma, and sickle cell disease), cancers, chromosomal abnormalities (Trisomy 21), diabetes, chronic kidney disease, nephrotic syndrome, SLE, hepatitis, liver failure, asplenia, and infections (varicella, CMV, EBV. Measles). Some medications may also cause immunodeficiency: antiepileptics, immunosuppressives, corticosteroids, chemotherapeutic agents and monoclonal antibodies.

Hereditary Angioedema

Hereditary angioedema is an AD deficiency of C1-esterase inhibitor. It leads to recurrent episodes of angioedema. Patients often have recurring episodes of painless, non-pitting edema, frequently involving periorbital, circumoral, and facial regions. Most important concerns are manifestations, including respiratory distress from laryngeal edema or bronchospasm, systemic vasodilation leading to hypotension and shock, and severe cramping secondary to gastrointestinal tract involvement.

One should consider alternative diagnoses: foods, drugs, insect exposure, drug reactions, physical trauma, or UV exposure, vasculitis, infections including viral hepatitis, fungal disease, and parasitic disease, and underlying neoplasm.

Treatment involves several focuses. Antihistamines may be used initially, including H1 and H2 antagonists. Corticosteroids may not reverse the acute edema but may decrease swelling and prevent worsening or relapse. FFP is used in the short term to replenish the enzyme, and androgens (Danazol®) may help to increase levels and minimize symptoms in the long term. One must remember to maintain airway protection! *Screening* is done by checking C4 levels; and diagnosing, with C1 esterase inhibitor levels of functional assay.

Urticaria

Urticaria, or **hives**, are pruritic, well-circumscribed, red, raised areas of the skin. The wheals are transient and are due to a variety of causes including allergic reactions to foods or allergens, medications, exercise, cold or heat, stress, medical conditions (e.g., autoimmune disease, hypothyroidism, hyperthyroidism) or infections. Urticaria can be **acute** (<6 weeks), **recurrent**, or **chronic** (>6 weeks). Urticaria may result from IgE-mediated (type I hypersensitivity reaction) or non-immune-mediated mast cell and basophil activation. Chronic urticaria can be due to any of the above causes; however, is often idiopathic or associated with chronic medical conditions (e.g., SLE, lymphoma), cholinergic causes (e.g., stress, heat), or autoimmune disorders. A thorough history is necessary; however, it may be difficult to determine the exact trigger. Determine if any bronchospasm or angioedema are present as these require urgent treatment (albuterol or epinephrine respectively). *Diagnosis* is clinical, however further tests are necessary for chronic urticaria (e.g., allergy skin testing, routine labs). Avoid triggers and *treat* with 2nd generation antihistamines (e.g., loratadine, cetirizine, fexofenadine) as these cause less sedation than 1st

generation antihistamines (e.g., diphenhydramine, hydroxyzine). This is especially important in the elderly, as the 1st generation antihistamines can cause confusion and urinary retention. *Complications* include bronchospasm, angioedema, and anaphylaxis.

Drug Allergies

Drug allergies may present with various symptoms, including urticaria, rash, cough, dyspnea, angioedema, wheezing, joint pains, fever, and many others. Only a small number are true allergies with pre-formed IgE and development of rapid urticaria, angioedema, or anaphylaxis. When symptoms of urticaria, fever, and arthralgias are delayed, the development of immune-complex related disorder is suggested. Hemolytic anemia may suggest a type II reaction to the drug.

Some of the most common offending agents include B-lactam antibiotics, sulfonamides, general anesthetics, phenytoin, and NSAIDS.

It is important to elicit a good history to ascertain the temporal relationship to the drug as well as to exclude other possible causes of symptoms. Allergy tests including RAST, provocation testing, Coombs' test, and basic skin testing may be employed to aid in diagnosis.

Treatment includes removal of the offending agent, symptomatic treatment, and if necessary, desensitization.

Anaphylaxis

Anaphylaxis is a term used to describe a rapidly developing, often severe, systemic allergic reaction. An anaphylactic reaction occurs when an individual is sensitized to an allergen and then re-exposed later. Common allergens include insect bites, foods, drugs, and latex. Symptoms usually begin within thirty minutes of exposure and can include urticaria (hives), itching, generalized edema, wheezing, and difficulty breathing. Diagnosis must be made quickly and is usually based on the history and physical exam. *Treatment* must be initiated immediately. First priority is given to stabilizing the patient and the airway, breathing, and circulation (ABC's). The allergen should be removed, if possible. Immediate administration of intramuscular (IM) epinephrine is often required. Drug therapy may also include antihistamines, corticosteroids, and inhaled beta-agonists. Severe cases require endotracheal intubation, mechanical ventilation, and intravenous (IV) administration of epinephrine.

Anaphylactic/Allergic Hypersensitivity Responses

Allergic hypersensitivity responses		
Aspirin idiosyncrasy	Results from abnormal arachidonic acid metabolism. Cyclooxygenase-1 is inhibited and cysteinyl leukotrienes overproduced, causing bronchospasm, rhinorrhea, nasal congestion, and increased airway responsiveness. Patients exhibit asthma and nasal polyps. May occur in 10 to 20% of asthmatics.	Diagnosis is per aspirin challenge, and treatment includes aspirin desensitization. For anaphylaxis, treatment includes: Epinephrine (immediately: Adults—0.2-1mg IV/SC; Pediatrics—0.01-0.1 mg/kg IV/SC), antihistamine, albuterol, cimetidine, bronchodilator, and steroids along with supportive treatment, such as oxygen and IV fluids.
Stinging insect (Venom)	Honeybees, vespids (yellow jackets, wasps, hornets), and fire ants cause most severe anaphylactic reactions, which result from IgE activation that, in turn, activates and degranulates mast cells. This causes vasodilation, increased vascular permeability, contraction of smooth muscles (bronchospasm), and inflammation.	Allergy testing and venom immunotherapy/desensitization is indicated. For anaphylaxis, treatment is as above.
Serum sickness	Reaction to horse serum in antivenin (such as for pit viper). Results in precipitation of antigen-immunoglobulin G (IgG) complexes in kidneys, joints, and skin one to three weeks after receiving serum in about half of patients. Patients may develop arthralgia, urticaria, and glomerulonephritis in addition to hypersensitivity reaction	Diagnosis is per symptoms. Treatment includes epinephrine, corticosteroids, and supportive care.

Common Food Allergies and Treatments

Food allergies	Indications
Milk	(Most common in children under 3. Cross allergy may occur with goat's milk.) GI upset, oral swelling, hives, wheezing, anaphylaxis.
Eggs	(Common in children) Itching, rash, rhinitis, GI upset, hives, anaphylaxis.
Peanuts	Reactions may vary but often severe with anaphylaxis.
Tree nuts	(Common in adults and children. May involve all kinds of nuts, including coconuts and lychee.) Reactions may vary but often severe with anaphylaxis.
Wheat	(Common to age 12. Found in many products, such as hot dogs, candy, beer, and ice cream.) Rash, hives, itching, GI upset, wheezing rhinitis, anaphylaxis.
Shellfish	(Crustacea allergies more common than mollusk.) Reaction may vary but often severe with hives, GI upset, rash, swelling of face, lips, tongue, digits, anaphylaxis
Fish	(Most common allergens include salmon, halibut, and tuna). Reactions may vary with hives GI upset, rhinitis, headaches, asthma, anaphylaxis
Sesame seeds	Reactions may vary with hives, bradycardia, GI upset, oral itching, flushing, anaphylaxis. (Listed as *Sesamum indicum* in non-food items, such as cosmetics and supplements. Increases risk of allergies to other nuts and rye grain. May be undeclared in spice blends and flavorings.)

In all cases of food allergies, avoidance is the primary preventive treatment. For mild reactions, an antihistamine, such as diphenhydramine, may be effective, but for more severe reactions, epinephrine is indicated.

Contrast-Related Allergies

Contrast-related allergies are generally caused by iodinated contrasts. Between 5% and 8% have only mild reactions, such as a feeling of warmth and/or nausea and vomiting. About 1% have moderate reactions with hives, itching, and edema, but only about 0.1% have severe anaphylactic reactions. Contrast-related allergies are not true allergic responses with an antigen/antibody reaction. The contrast media itself releases histamine and other substances from mast cells. Risk factors include:

- Previous reaction.
- Thyroid disorder.
- Heart or kidney disorder.
- Medications: beta-blockers, metformin.

Diagnosis usually occurs after a reaction but can be difficult before as test doses may or may not provoke a reaction. Preventive measures include administration of prednisone or diphenhydramine 60 minutes prior to administration of contrast. Treatment includes immediately discontinuing administration of contrast and monitoring of cardiac status, BP, and O_2 saturation. Mild reactions usually do not require treatment, moderate reactions are treated with diphenhydramine, but severe reactions require epinephrine. Diphenhydramine and cimetidine may also be administered. IV fluids are administered for hypotension.

DESENSITIZATION THERAPY

Desensitization therapy can be used to prevent severe allergic responses/anaphylaxis:

- **Drugs**: Patients are administered tiny amounts (beginning with about 1/10,000 of the dosage) of the drug in slowly increasing increments about every 15 minutes over a number of hours until the patient's optimal dosage is reached. This provides the patient with a non-allergic state that remains as long as the patient takes the medication regularly. The patient reverts back to being allergic if the medication is stopped. Drug sensitization should be used only if patients absolutely need the drug and no other option is available.
- **Allergen specific immunotherapy:** Patients who are allergic to pollens, dust mites, or wasp/bee venom are administered extracts in very slowly increasing dosages to maximal tolerance either by injection or sublingually. Treatment is usually given over a year or longer and then periodically.
- **Food immunotherapy**: Patients severely allergic to food, such as peanuts and tree nuts, take very small amounts of the food allergen orally or sublingually in slowly increasing amounts until they can tolerate the food without a severe reaction. Patients generally do not develop tolerance and must continue the therapy long-term.

SPLENECTOMIZED PATIENT

Asplenic patients are at greater risk for overwhelming infection. A patient can be asplenic resulting from surgical removal of the spleen, or as the result of splenic dysfunction. The most common causes of functional asplenia are celiac disease, liver disease, and alcoholism. The presence of Howell-Jolly bodies on peripheral blood smear is strongly suggestive of functional asplenia. Post-splenectomy sepsis is an overwhelming, rapidly progressive condition that can quickly lead to shock and death. Patients that are either surgically or functionally asplenic should be vaccinated against pneumococcus, *H influenzae*, and meningococcus. Children and adolescents should receive penicillin prophylaxis for three years. Patients should be advised to report any fever to their physician.

Infectious Disease

INFECTION CONTROL PLAN

The **purpose of an infection control/surveillance plan** should be clearly outlined and may be multifaceted, including the following elements:

- Decreasing rates of infection: The primary purpose of a surveillance plan is to identify a means to decrease nosocomial infections, including a notification system and laboratory surveillance.
- Evaluating infection control measures: Surveillance can evaluate effectiveness of infection control measures. (Surgical checklists, handwashing, housekeeping, ventilation).
- Establishing endemic threshold rates: Establishing threshold rates can help to enact control measures to reduce rates.
- Identifying outbreaks: About 5-10% of infections occur in outbreaks, and comparing data with established endemic threshold rates can help to identify these outbreaks if analysis is done in a regular and timely manner.
- Achieving staff compliance: Objective evidence may convince staff to cooperate with infection control measures.
- Meeting accreditation standards: Some accreditation agencies require reports of infection rates.

- Providing defense for malpractice suits: Providing evidence that a facility is proactive in combating infections can decrease liability.
- Comparing infection rates with other facilities: Comparing data helps focus attention and resources.

Proper Protocol for Needlestick Injury and Postexposure Prophylaxis

If the healthcare provider experiences a **needlestick injury**, the individual's initial response should be to wash the wound with soap and water. As soon as possible, the incident must be reported to a supervisor and steps taken according to established protocol. This may include testing and/or prophylaxis, depending on the patient's health history. In some cases, the patient may also be tested for communicable diseases, such as HIV, in order to determine the risk to the healthcare provider. PEP (post-exposure prophylaxis) is available for exposure to HIV (human immunodeficiency virus) and hepatitis B virus (hepatis B immune globulin). However, no PEP is available for HCV (hepatitis C virus) although the CDC does provide a plan for management. PEP should be initiated within 72 hours of exposure. All testing and treatments associated with the needlestick injury must be provided free of cost at a hospital or medical facility.

Importance of Immunization in Disease Prevention

Immunization has an important role in preventing the spread of infection. Immunizations prevent the patient from contracting a disease or lessen the severity of the disease as well as preventing the complications (encephalitis, hearing loss, paralysis) associated with the infectious diseases. Immunizations prevent the spread of infection to infants who are too young to be immunized and to those who are immunocompromised (cancer patients, transplantation recipients). If herd immunity is achieved, then even if there are scatted individual cases of the disease, outbreaks are not likely to occur. Herd immunity is the percentage of the population that must be immunized in order to prevent outbreaks. This percentage may range from 80 to 85% for some disorders, but those that are highly contagious, such as measles, may require a herd immunity of 93 to 95%. People should not avoid immunization and depend on herd immunity for protection because rates of immunization vary from one community to another.

Nosocomial Infections

Nosocomial infections are those that are healthcare-associated or hospital-acquired. Common nosocomial infections include:

- *Enterococci* infections include urinary infections, bacteremia, endocarditis as well as infections in wounds and the abdominal and pelvic areas.
- *Enterobacteriaceae* cause about half of the urinary tract infections and a quarter of the postoperative infections.
- *Escherichia coli* primarily causes urinary tract infections (especially related to catheters), diarrhea, and neonatal meningitis but it can also lead to pneumonia, and bacteremia (usually secondary to urinary infection).
- Group B β-hemolytic *Streptococci* (GBS) has increasingly been a cause of infections in neonatal units, causing pneumonia, meningitis, and sepsis. GBS infections may occur as wound infections after Cesarean sections, especially in those immunocompromised.
- *Staphylococcus. aureus* is a major cause of nosocomial post-operative infections, both localized and systemic, and from indwelling tubes and devices.
- Methicillin-resistant *Staphylococcus aureus (MRSA)* is a common cause of surgical infections.
- *Clostridioides difficile* causes more nosocomial diarrhea cases than any other microorganism.

- *Candida*, a yeast fungal pathogen, can overgrow and lead to mucocutaneous or cutaneous lesions and sepsis.
- *Aspergillus* spp., filamentous fungi, produce spores that become airborne and can invade the respiratory tract, causing pneumonia.

MRSA

Although previously an exclusively hospital-acquired infection, **MRSA** has become increasingly community-acquired. Methicillin-resistant *S aureus* is a strain of *Staphylococcus aureus* that is resistant to antibiotics. Overuse and inappropriate use of antibiotics may be responsible for the emergence of MRSA. Community-acquired infections are most likely spread from asymptomatic carriers. Patients generally present with pustular skin lesions, which can spread rapidly, leading to a life-threatening infection. The diagnosis is made by culture. The *treatment* depends on the sensitivity results of the patient's particular strain of MRSA. Vancomycin is frequently used.

HIV

Human immunodeficiency virus (HIV) is a **retrovirus** (2 types: HIV-1 [most common in the U.S.] and HIV-2) that attacks the T lymphocytes (CD4+ cells) which weakens the immune system. It is spread through blood, semen, genital/rectal fluids, and breast milk. The initial infection may go unnoticed, or 2-4 weeks after exposure, may cause an **acute retroviral syndrome** (fever, fatigue, headache, lymphadenopathy, pharyngitis, rash, and myalgia/arthralgia), and during this time **viral load** is high. Next there is an inactive or latent stage (length varies) and the viral load is lower. Screening (e.g., rapid HIV test) is recommended for those 13-64 years old and pregnant women. *Diagnose* HIV through an antigen/antibody immunoassay or a NAT (nucleic acid test) if it is indeterminate, and confirm with a second test that differentiates between HIV-1 and HIV-2.

AIDS

Acquired immunodeficiency syndrome (AIDS) is a progression of infection with HIV (average time is 11 years) which leads to opportunistic infections and neoplasms. Since patients may not immediately seek medical help, there is a wide range of presenting symptoms, AIDS is diagnosed when these criteria are met:

- HIV infection determined by lab
- CD4 count <200 cells/mm^3
- AIDS defining condition, such as opportunistic infections (cytomegalovirus, tuberculosis), wasting syndrome, neoplasms (Kaposi sarcoma), or AIDS dementia complex.

It is important to review the following: CD4 counts to determine immune status, HIV RNA assay to determine the viral load; WBC and differential for signs of infection; cultures to help identify any infective agents; CBC to evaluate for signs of bleeding or thrombocytopenia; vaccines are up to date; and repeat STD screens and TB tests periodically to determine if there is further exposure to diseases. *Treatment* aims to cure or manage opportunistic conditions, and control underlying HIV infection through highly active anti-retroviral therapy (HAART), ≥3 drugs used concurrently. *Complications* include: opportunistic infections, dementia, neoplasms, wasting, and death. Refer appropriately.

Common Infections and Malignancies Associated with HIV and AIDS

The **AIDS patient** is highly susceptible to many bacterial, viral, fungal, and parasitic **infections** as well as certain types of **cancers**, such as Kaposi's sarcoma, central nervous system lymphoma, and non-Hodgkin's lymphoma. **Bacterial infections** include streptococcus pneumonia, atypical mycobacterial disease (cause pulmonary infection) which include *Mycobacterium avium* intracellulare (MAI) and *Mycobacterium avium* complex (MAC), tuberculosis (TB), salmonellosis, syphilis, and bacillary angiomatosis. **Viral infections** include cytomegalovirus (CMV), viral hepatitis, herpes simplex virus (HSV), human papillomavirus (HPV), and progressive multifocal leukoencephalopathy (PML). **Fungal infections** include *Candida albicans, Histoplasma capsulatum,* cryptococcal meningitis, and *Pneumocystis jiroveci* pneumonia (PJP) (previously *Pneumocystis carinii,* PCP) which is the most common opportunistic infection in those with HIV. **Parasitic infections** include toxoplasmosis, and cryptosporidium. The rate of contracting these types of infections in AIDS patients far exceeds the rates found within the general population. The AIDS defining illnesses typically appear when the CD4 count is <200 /mm^3.

HIV/AIDS Post-Exposure Prophylaxis (PEP)

The goal of **post-exposure prophylaxis** is to reduce the chance of HIV infection in an individual following a potential exposure. Post-exposure prophylaxis is generally initiated after an occupational exposure or following unprotected sexual intercourse with a potentially HIV positive individual. The specific regimen depends on the type of exposure, but usually involves taking two or more antiretroviral medications for a period of four weeks. Prophylaxis must be initiated as soon as possible after the exposure. The potential benefits of post-exposure prophylaxis must be weighed against the possibility of significant side effects of the medications. Issues of compliance with the regimen and increasing HIV drug resistance as are also of concern.

Current Treatment Regimens for HIV/AIDS

There is currently no cure for AIDS. **Treatment goals** include suppressing the viral load, and delaying immunosuppression and symptoms for as long as possible. The current treatment approach is known as highly active antiretroviral therapy (HAART). This regimen aims to reduce a patient's level of HIV as much as possible, ideally to an undetectable level. Treatment generally begins as soon as a patient is symptomatic or has a CD4 count less than 200 to 350 cells/mm^3. Treatment includes a combination of antiretroviral drugs. There are six different classes of antiretroviral drugs: nucleoside analogue reverse transcriptase inhibitors (NRTIs), protease inhibitors (PIs), non-nucleoside reverse transcriptase inhibitors (NNRTIs), nucleotide reverses transcriptase inhibitors (NtRTIs), fusion inhibitors, and integrase inhibitors. A typical treatment regimen will consist of three different drugs. Treatment also involves prophylaxis against opportunistic infection in patients with low CD4 cell counts.

Tetanus

Tetanus (lockjaw) is a disease caused by the neurotoxin released by the bacteria *Clostridium tetani* whose spores can be found in soil, dust, and animal feces. Spores thrive in anaerobic conditions and usually enter the body through a wound (especially puncture wounds; most often stepping on a nail). *Symptoms* usually start within 5-10 days of exposure and include headache, jaw stiffness or spasms, trismus (lockjaw), a fixed smile, dysphagia, and eventually generalized, painful muscle spasms, and even death. *Treatment* includes antitoxin, tetanus immune globulin (TIG), metronidazole (first-line) or penicillin, benzodiazepines for muscle rigidity, and airway support. Tetanus cases have decreased due to the immunization (DTaP for pediatrics and Td or Tdap for adults). Postexposure prophylaxis includes TIG and a tetanus booster (if last tetanus vaccine ≥5 years).

Bacterial Diarrhea

The following **bacteria cause diarrhea** (sometimes due to travel) and are confirmed with stool cultures:

- ***Campylobacter jejuni*** can cause crampy abdominal pain, watery and bloody diarrhea, and also systemic disease (e.g., fever). It is usually contracted by eating undercooked poultry; incubation is 2-5 days. It usually resolves spontaneously, but may be treated with erythromycin or azithromycin.
- **Cholera** produces a profuse, watery diarrhea due to the saltwater-living bacteria, *Vibrio cholerae*. It is transmitted through the fecal-oral route (usually through ingesting contaminated water or food); and incubation is short, usually 1-3 days. Rehydration is the primary goal.
- ***Escherichia coli*** (E. coli) is a gram-negative rod normally found in the GI tract, yet certain strains cause diarrhea and even bloody diarrhea (O157:H7) due to toxins they produce. It is transmitted through water or food (ground beef). *Symptoms* start in 1-10 days with the O157:H7 strain and include severe cramping, bloody/watery diarrhea, and usually no fever; it can be complicated with hemolytic uremic syndrome (1-2 wks. after onset). *Treatment* involves supportive care (hydration).
- **Salmonellosis** is a disease caused by *Salmonella*. It can be spread via contaminated foods (poultry, eggs, beef) or animals (reptiles), and incubation is 6-72 hours. *Symptoms* include fever, abdominal pain, and watery diarrhea. *Treatment* is supportive. Sepsis can be a complication.
- **Shigellosis** (bacillary dysentery) is a disease caused by gram-negative bacteria, genus *Shigella*. It is spread through the fecal-oral route and incubation ranges from ½ -4 days. *Symptoms* include high fever, N/V, severe abdominal cramps, and a watery and bloody diarrhea. *Treatment* is supportive.

CMV Infection

Cytomegalovirus (CMV) is a **herpesvirus** (human herpesvirus 5). After the initial infection, CMV, like other herpes viruses, remains in the body in a latent phase. If contracted, CMV usually causes only mild disease and can even go unnoticed. CMV is one of the congenital **TORCH infections** which can cause birth defects. More severe disease usually only affects the immunocompromised. It is spread through direct contact via **body fluids**, including by way of sexual contact, blood, and human milk. Those at increased risk of getting CMV include health and childcare workers, pregnant women, transplant recipients, and those with HIV (immunocompromised). CMV can affect any organ system. Patients may be asymptomatic, present with mild flu-like symptoms, mononucleosis-type symptoms, with community-acquired pneumonia, or with fever of unknown origin; or if immunocompromised, may have severe disease including retinitis, encephalitis, esophagitis, and colitis. *Diagnosis* is through serology tests, PCR, or viral cultures. Patients typically do not require *treatment* unless there is severe disease. Ganciclovir is the first-line treatment. *Complications* include birth defects, CMV relapse, hepatitis, Guillain-Barré syndrome, myocarditis, and anemia/cytopenias.

Epstein-Barr Infection

Epstein-Barr virus (EBV) is a herpesvirus (human herpesvirus 4) and is responsible for causing **infectious mononucleosis**. After the initial infection, it remains latent in B cells and epithelial cells. It has been linked to certain epithelial and lymphatic neoplasms (e.g., nasopharyngeal carcinoma, Burkitt lymphoma, Hodgkin lymphoma). It is transmitted through **body fluids** like saliva, hence is often referred to as the 'kissing disease." This is most common in teenagers or college-age young adults and incubation is typically 30-50 days. *Symptoms* of EBV infection range from being asymptomatic to swollen painful lymph nodes, pharyngitis (can mimic strep pharyngitis), extreme fatigue, fever, and possibly hepatosplenomegaly. The WBC count is elevated (~10,000-20,000 cells/mL) with 10-30% atypical lymphocytes in the differential. Confirm *diagnosis* with a Mono Spot test or EBV antibody serology tests. *Treatment* is supportive, and antibiotics are not helpful in treating this viral infection. Therefore, avoid unnecessary antibiotics in those with EBV, especially since administration of ampicillin or amoxicillin is often associated with a pruritic, maculopapular rash. Analgesics, warm salt water gargles, increased fluid intake, and rest will help to relieve some of the symptoms. Symptoms may last for several weeks and fatigue may last even longer. Patients should avoid contact sports for up to 2 months. *Complications* include hepatitis, cytopenias (e.g., thrombocytopenia), Guillain Barré syndrome, and splenic rupture.

HSV-1 and HSV-2

There are 2 types of the **herpes simplex virus (HSV),** human herpesvirus 1 and 2.

HSV-1 usually causes a **gingivostomatitis** (often referred to as "cold sores" or "fever blisters") and is transmitted through **close contact**. **HSV-2** usually causes painful **genital lesions** through sexual contact. Either may be found in other areas of the body. Incubation time is ~2-12 days. The primary infection is usually more severe (causes systemic symptoms) than the reactivated infection, but it may be asymptomatic. After the primary infection, the virus remains dormant in the nerve ganglia, and can be reactivated especially during times of stress, illness, immunosuppression, or sun exposure. While patients are most contagious during times of active lesions, the disease may be spread while asymptomatic. The frequency of the outbreaks usually decreases over time. HSV lesions are grouped vesicles with an erythematous base. They are usually painful, and a prodrome of tingling, pain, or burning sensations may be felt hours to a couple days before the eruption. Lesions last for approximately 2-3 weeks in primary infection (up to 4 weeks with genital HSV), and 1-2 weeks in recurrent infections. *Diagnose* clinically and confirm with a + culture, PCR test, or HSV antibody tests (HSV-1 or HSV-2: IgM= active or recent infection; IgG= previous infection). Symptomatic *treatment*, proper wound care, and antivirals (acyclovir, valacyclovir, or famciclovir) may be given. *Complications* include perinatal infection, keratitis, herpetic whitlow, herpes gladiatorum, secondary infections, and encephalitis.

Measles, Mumps, and Rubella

Measles (rubeola) virus is highly contagious, is spread through **respiratory secretions** (incubation is 7-14 days), and peaks in late winter to spring. It causes a prodrome of high fever (4-7 days), cough, congestion, conjunctivitis; then Koplik spots (pathognomonic), and finally a maculopapular rash (spreads cephalocaudally). Report suspected cases immediately to the health dept. *Diagnose* with a + IgM antibody test (collected after 3 days of rash), viral culture, or PCR. *Treatment* is supportive.

Mumps (parotitis) is a viral infection that is spread via **saliva** (incubation is 12-24 days), and often occurs during winter and spring. It causes painful swelling of the salivary glands (parotid). Report to health dept. Supportive *treatment*. *Complications*: orchitis (infertility), pancreatitis, meningitis.

Rubella (German measles) is a virus that spreads via **respiratory droplets** (incubation is 2-3 weeks), and peaks in the spring. There is a mild prodrome (fever, aches, sore throat, conjunctivitis, swollen nodes [esp. suboccipital, postauricular, & posterior cervical]), then a maculopapular rash (face 1st then down). Report to health dept. Confirm with rubella antibodies IgM or IgG. Symptomatic care.

Roseola and Erythema Infectiosum

Roseola is a herpesvirus (human herpesvirus 6 or 7) that is spread by **saliva** (incubation 5-15 days) and may occur any time of the year. It causes a high fever (3-5 days) then a fine pink/red maculopapular rash appears as the fever leaves (starts on trunk; lasts 2-3 days). *Treat* symptoms.

Erythema infectiosum (Fifth disease) is caused by parvovirus B19, is spread via **respiratory secretions** (incubation is 4-21 days), and usually peaks late winter to early spring. It causes a mild prodrome, then a "slapped cheek" appearance, then finally a lacey rash appears (patient is not contagious at this point). *Treatment* is supportive as this is self-limited. Pregnant women should avoid contact with those with this virus (may cause stillbirth/hydrops fetalis).

Influenza

Influenza is a highly contagious viral infection that affects the entire **respiratory system** from the nose to the lungs. There are 3 types of influenza virus: **A** (causes epidemics), **B** (only in humans), and **C**. Types A and B are seen most often and the ones the annual flu vaccine is most effective against; and type C is not as common and much less severe. Prevention is key and annual, age-appropriate influenza vaccines should be given to those ≥6 months and older; 2 vaccines are required in first-time vaccine patients if 6 mo. through 8-year-olds (separated by 28 days). Incubation is 1-4 days and it is spread via respiratory droplets. Though symptoms can be very similar, the flu and the common cold differ in that the flu has a very sudden onset. *Symptoms* of influenza include a high fever (may last up to 5 days), headache, myalgias, dry cough, rhinorrhea, and fatigue. There may also be vomiting and diarrhea, although children are more prone to this. Clinical judgement, community patterns, and rapid influenza tests (high specificity, but lower sensitivity) aid in diagnosis, but RT-PCR or viral culture definitively confirm the *diagnosis*; pulse oximetry and CXR as needed for pulmonary issues. Antibiotic treatment is not effective unless there is a secondary bacterial infection (e.g., pneumonia). Look for signs of secondary infections (e.g., dyspnea, cyanosis, fever that goes away and returns, confusion/lethargy). Supportive *treatment* with rest, fluids, and analgesics. Antivirals should be considered in those who are at high risk (<5 years old, elderly, pregnant, chronic conditions). These are most effective if initiated within 24-48 hours of symptom onset. The neuraminidase inhibitors (oseltamivir, zanamivir) treat type A, type B, and avian H5N1. There is extensive resistance to the adamantanes (amantadine, rimantadine) so they are rarely used. *Complications* include pneumonia, ARDS, and death.

Varicella

Varicella (chickenpox) and **Herpes-zoster** (shingles) are both caused by a **herpes virus** (human herpesvirus 3), referred to as **varicella-zoster virus**. Incubation is 10-21 days from initial exposure, and patients are contagious 2 days before the cutaneous eruption and until all lesions have crusted.

Varicella is the acute, initial infection with varicella-zoster virus and usually presents with a prodrome of fever, headache, and malaise which is followed by (in 2-3 days) pruritic lesions that become vesicles with an erythematous base. *Diagnosis* is clinical and confirmed with a Tzanck smear or viral culture. *Treatment* is symptomatic; secondary infections are common. The first dose of the varicella vaccine is recommended at 12-15 months and the second at 4-6 years.

Herpes-Zoster Infection

Herpes-zoster infection, or **shingles**, can be a very painful condition. It is caused by the same virus that causes chickenpox in children. The virus lies dormant in the **dorsal root ganglia** until increased stress or an immunocompromised state causes the virus to be reactivated, resulting in shingles. Patients may complain of burning pain and paresthesias 2-3 days before the lesions appear. Lesions most often erupt in the thoracic area, in a dermatomal pattern, though they can occur anywhere, including the face and eyes (trigeminal nerve; refer to optometrist). Vesicular lesions will open and eventually crust over. Patients may be left with chronic pain (*post-herpetic neuralgia*). *Diagnose* per clinical evaluation, and a viral culture of vesicular fluid or polymerase chain reaction assay (PCR) can help confirm. *Treating* with antivirals within 48 hours of rash onset (e.g., acyclovir, valacyclovir, famciclovir) may reduce the length, severity, and complications. Topical analgesics or anesthetics (e.g., Capsaicin or lidocaine patch) may help reduce the pain; anticonvulsants (gabapentin) and tricyclic antidepressants may help with the lasting pain of post-herpetic neuralgia. Immune globulin (VZIG) is given for post-exposure prophylaxis to those who are at high risk. Two doses of the shingles vaccine (Shingrix®) 2-6 months apart is recommended for all those >50 years old, regardless of previous shingles or vaccination with Zostavax®. *Complications* include disseminated infection (especially in immunocompromised), and visceral organ involvement (presents rapidly and includes encephalitis, hepatitis, and pneumonia).

CRYPTOCOCCOSIS

Cryptococcosis is an infection resulting from inhaling the **fungus** *Cryptococcus neoformans,* which is found worldwide in soil (can be associated with bird droppings), or *Cryptococcus gattii,* which is associated with certain trees in the Northwest. Cryptococcosis is most often due to *C. neoformans*, is found more often among those with compromised immune systems, and is an **AIDS-defining opportunistic infection**. Healthy patients may be asymptomatic and the only finding may be pulmonary lesions on CXR that resolve spontaneously. The fungus can disseminate and cause meningitis, encephalitis, cutaneous lesions, and affect long bones and other tissues. *Symptoms* are based on the area of involvement. Patients may experience cough, pleuritic chest pain, weight loss, and fever if there is pulmonary involvement; headache, double vision, light sensitivity, N/V, and confusion if CNS involvement; cutaneous lesions (papules, pustules, nodules, ulcers) if the skin is involved. *Diagnosis* includes microscopic analysis, culture (gold standard), or an antigen test (highly sensitive; good for detecting early infection) for *Cryptococcus* using CSF, tissue, sputum, blood, or urine. Check CSF by India ink (limited sensitivity) or culture so meningitis can be ruled out. Confirm that no mass lesion is present by CT or MRI before LP is performed. Mild cases may only require monitoring to ensure that the infection does not spread. In more advanced cases, the infection is *treated* with different antifungal medications (e.g., fluconazole for pulmonary infections, amphotericin B ± flucytosine for meningitis). The patient should also be monitored for CNS infection and medication side effects. AIDS patients may need lifelong antifungals. *Complications* include cryptococcal meningitis, neural deficits, optic nerve damage, and hydrocephalus.

HISTOPLASMOSIS

Histoplasmosis is an infection caused by inhalation of **spores** from the fungus *Histoplasma capsulatum* that is found in soil and is associated with bird and bat droppings (e.g., chicken coops, caves). Healthy patients are usually asymptomatic and those with symptoms are typically immunocompromised or those who've had a heavy exposure to spores. The primary pulmonary infection occurs 3-17 days after exposure and can present with flu-like symptoms. It is typically self-limited but may become chronic. Histoplasmosis can also spread through the blood and can cause progressive disseminated disease in the immunocompromised (high mortality rate); this is an **AIDS-defining illness**. *Diagnose* through antigen tests (urine, serum), histopathology, or cultures; order a CXR. Mild and even moderate acute pulmonary histoplasmosis may resolve on its own. If needed, *treat* mild to moderate infections with itraconazole and severe illness with amphotericin B.

Pneumocystis

Pneumocystis jiroveci is a **fungus** (previously known as *Pneumocystis* carinii) that causes **pneumonia** (PJP, previously PCP) in the immunocompromised. Most people have been exposed to this by the age of 3 or 4. Symptoms of PJP include a dry nonproductive cough, fever, dyspnea, and weight loss. CXR may show diffuse bilateral infiltrates or it may be normal; and pulse oximetry may be low, especially on exertion. *Diagnosis* is confirmed with sputum histopathology using sputum induction or bronchoalveolar lavage. *Treat* immediately with TMP-SMX (trimethoprim/sulfamethoxazole) for 21 days if HIV + and for 14 days in other cases. Steroids may be added for HIV patients with severe PJP. HIV/AIDS patients with CD4 counts <200/μl should receive PJP prophylaxis with TMP-SMX. Dapsone and pentamidine are alternatives. *Complications* include ARDS and death.

Malaria

Malaria is a **blood-borne disease** caused by a **parasite** from the genus *Plasmodium and* found in tropical areas. There are 4 known to cause disease in humans (*P. malariae*, *P. vivax*, *P. ovale*, and *P. falciparum*). These protozoa are transmitted by the **female *Anopheles* mosquito**. They travel to the **liver** where they multiply, are released, and then infect the RBCs, where they continue to multiply. Incubation time varies from 9 days to 1 month or even years based on the species of the infecting parasite. *Signs and symptoms* include headache, high fever with shaking chills and sweating (rigors; occurs when merozoites, an immature form of the parasite, are released from RBCs), jaundice, anemia, and hepatosplenomegaly. Take a thorough history including recent travel. *Diagnose* with 3 thin and thick blood smears (gold standard) stained with Giemsa (preferred) and obtained 12-24 hours apart. Labs typically show elevated LDH, thrombocytopenia, and atypical lymphocytes. Rapid antigen tests are also available as well as PCR. *Treat* with chloroquine. If travelling, chemoprophylaxis depends on the area of travel due to species and resistance patterns, and may include chloroquine, primaquine, mefloquine, Malarone®, or doxycycline. Report infections to your local or state health department. *Complications* include severe anemia and hemolysis, organ failure (liver, spleen, kidneys), cerebral malaria, ARDS, and death.

Travel Prophylaxis

Specific prophylaxis for travel depends on the individual patient's health status and the travel destination. If a patient is traveling to a country with a risk of malaria, appropriate prophylaxis must be prescribed. Depending on the level of risk of the particular country, prophylaxis may include taking precautions to avoid mosquito bites, as well as different combinations of antimalarial drugs. The drugs used for **malarial prophylaxis** include mefloquine, doxycycline, Malarone, chloroquine, and proguanil. The specific regimen depends on the type of malaria and the resistance patterns of the location to be traveled. Mosquito bite avoidance is about 85% effective and chemoprophylaxis is about 75% to 95% effective in preventing malaria. A patient frequently does not exhibit symptoms of malaria until returning home.

Helminth Infestations

Helminth infestations (worms) include **roundworms** [nematodes: *Ascaris*, hookworms (cause anemia), **filariae** (cause elephantiasis)] and **flatworms** [tapeworms (cause weight loss); **flukes** (intestinal or liver)]. **Pinworms** are a type of roundworm that cause enterobiasis and is the most common helminth infestation. Pinworms are more prevalent in warmer areas of the country and infestations occur more frequently in children. The worms lay eggs within the digestive tract and then travel to the anal area where they are usually found. Pinworms are highly contagious. As a patient itches the anal area where the eggs are located, the eggs cling to the fingers and can easily be transmitted to other people either directly or through food or surfaces. The eggs can survive for

2-3 weeks on inanimate objects. Patients may be asymptomatic or have intense anal itching that is usually worse at night and can cause insomnia. Abdominal pain, nausea, and vomiting can also occur. *Diagnose* with the "tape test" which involves pressing cellophane tape over the perianal area to pick up eggs or worms and examine under the microscope. Most other helminth infestations can be diagnosed with a stool sample for ova and parasites; filariasis requires a blood smear or antigen test. Anthelmintic medications are given in a single dose and repeated in 2 weeks to kill the pinworms and their larvae (mebendazole, albendazole, or pyrantel pamoate). The entire family and close contacts should be *treated* simultaneously since pinworms are so contagious.

Toxoplasmosis

Toxoplasmosis is an infection caused by the **parasite** *Toxoplasma gondii* and is found in the soil. This is widespread and transmitted through cat feces; however, it also may be contracted by eating undercooked meat (especially pork, lamb, or venison) or poorly washed vegetables. Toxoplasmosis can cause serious disease and can affect various organs; and immunocompromised and pregnant women and their unborn babies are especially likely to have side effects of the disease (the "T" in congenital TORCH infections). Healthy patients are usually asymptomatic; however, once infected the parasite can remain latent until the patient becomes immunocompromised and the parasite is reactivated causing *symptoms*. The disease can cause a flu-like illness with fever, myalgias, and lymphadenopathy. More serious effects include retinochoroiditis, brain lesions, and encephalitis. Congenital toxoplasmosis may cause retinochoroiditis, microcephaly, hydrocephalus, intellectual disabilities, and possibly miscarriage or stillbirth. *Diagnose* with serology for *Toxoplasma* antibodies IgM and IgG. Also, PCR may be used to test amniotic fluid, CSF, or tissue. *Treat* with pyrimethamine (preferred) plus folinic acid or sulfadiazine plus folinic acid. Pregnant women should avoid high-risk practices like changing the cat litter and should avoid sand boxes.

Lyme Disease

Lyme disease occurs from a bite from a **deer tick** (blacklegged tick) infected with the **spirochete bacterium** *Borrelia burgdorferi*. It is the most common tick-born disease in the U.S. and is more prevalent in heavily wooded areas. Adult ticks are more active during colder times whereas the nymphs (<2mm in size) are more active in the warm, spring or summer months. Once the tick bites, it stays attached, however it takes about 36-48 hours for nymphs and about 48-72 hours for adult ticks before the spirochete is transmitted to the person. Incubation is 3-30 days. There are 3 stages to this disease: early localized, early disseminated, and chronic disseminated. **Stage 1** 75% have the characteristic expanding red rash (erythema migrans; can be large, ~30cm) which can progress to have central clearing (bull's eye), headache, fever, chills, myalgias, and fatigue. **Stage 2** occurs weeks to months after initial infection and involves systemic symptoms (flu-like), neck stiffness, headaches, migrating pain in muscles and joints, rashes, paresthesias, Bell's palsy, confusion, fatigue, myocarditis, and heart palpitations. **Stage 3** occurs months to years after initial infection and involves neurologic (e.g., encephalitis) and rheumatologic issues, especially arthritis of large joints (e.g., knee).

Review Video: Lyme Disease
Visit mometrix.com/academy and enter code: 505529

Diagnosis and Treatment of Lyme Disease

Diagnose Lyme disease using 2-tiered testing: antibodies (IgM, IgG), then Western blot. Antibiotic *treatment* for localized Lyme disease involves 2-3 weeks of doxycycline, amoxicillin, or cefuroxime axetil is started immediately after diagnosis. IV antibiotics may be needed for severe disease (e.g., IV ceftriaxone). Prevention is key by wearing clothes covering the skin, using tick repellents, showering soon after being outdoors in tick-prone areas, and thoroughly checking for ticks (especially in hard to see areas by using a mirror). The Lyme vaccine is no longer available and previous vaccine recipients are still at risk of contracting the disease as protection decreases over time. *Complications* are prevalent with untreated Lyme disease and include chronic arthritis, fatigue, chronic musculoskeletal issues, acrodermatitis chronica atrophicans, and memory and concentration issues. Report cases to the local health dept.

Rocky Mountain Spotted Fever

Rocky Mountain Spotted Fever (**RMSF**) is a disease caused by a bite from a **tick** carrying the bacteria *Rickettsia rickettsii*. This can be found in all parts of the U.S. and especially in eastern and central states. This is the most common tick-born illness leading to death. Prevention is key. Incubation is 3-12 days. Patients usually present with the sudden onset of fever, myalgias, headache, N/V, abdominal pain, and a rash that usually appears within 2-4 days of the start of the fever, however the rash may appear later. A maculopapular pink rash usually begins on the wrists, forearms, palms, soles, and ankles and spreads centrally and to the extremities. Typically, the rash becomes darker red and petechial as the disease progresses; however, the rash is highly variable or even absent leading to misdiagnosis. The disease can lead to severe illness including encephalitis, myocarditis, uveitis, and gangrene. *Diagnosis* can be difficult and is based on clinical findings and labs (e.g., thrombocytopenia, anemia, reduced Na^+). RMSF can be confirmed with immunofluorescent antibody tests, however it may take weeks to confirm. It is vital to start empiric antibiotic *treatment* when RMSF is suspected since and lab tests may be falsely negative in the first 7-10 days and since mortality is decreased if treatment is begun within the first 5 days of symptom onset. Treat with doxycycline. Hospitalization is often required. *Complications* include pulmonary edema, renal failure, shock, seizures, encephalopathy, hearing loss, DIC, and death. Report cases to the local health department.

Zika Virus in Pregnant Women

Zika virus is a **flavivirus** that is transmitted by the *Aedes* mosquito and through sexual contact. This virus can be passed on to an unborn baby causing severe congenital defects while causing mild or no disease in the mother. It is advised that all pregnant women avoid traveling to areas with the Zika virus (e.g., Central and South America, Mexico, Caribbean, Africa). Incubation period is 3-14 days and symptoms may last 4-7 days. The virus has been found to remain longer in semen than in other body fluids. If symptoms are present, they may include fever, headache, myalgias, arthralgias, a maculopapular rash, and conjunctivitis. Congenital defects include severe microcephaly, severe brain abnormalities, macular scarring, hearing loss, motor disabilities (e.g., hypertonia), and contractures. Women should be screened for Zika exposure at each prenatal visit. *Diagnostic* testing is recommended for all asymptomatic pregnant women who have continued exposure to Zika and for all symptomatic pregnant women who have possibly been exposed to the Zika virus. Testing includes RNA NAT testing on serum and urine, and serum IgM Zika antibody testing. Prenatal ultrasound helps determine if the effects of Zika are present. Report cases to the state health department; and the CDC can be consulted. There is no *treatment* or cure for the Zika virus.

Syphilis

Syphilis is caused by the **spirochete** *Treponema pallidum* and is passed on through direct contact with a syphilitic sore by vaginal, oral, or anal sex or through the placenta to an unborn baby. The disease has 4 phases, with an average incubation period of about 3 weeks (10-90 days):

Primary: Chancre (painless) in areas of sexual contact, persisting 3 to 6 weeks. **Secondary**: General flu-like symptoms (sore throat, fever, headaches) and red papular rash on trunk, flexor surfaces, palms, and soles, and lymphadenopathy occur about 3 to 6 weeks (up to 3 months) after end of primary phase and eventually resolves. **Latent**: In the early latent phase (within 1 year of infection) the patient has a positive RPR, VRDL, or antibody test (FTA-Abs), no symptoms, and is contagious; but in late latent phase (>1 year from infection) is not contagious, except to an unborn baby. **Tertiary**: Affects about 30% and includes CNS and cardiovascular symptoms 3 to 20 years after initial infection. Gummas (granulomatous lesions) may be widespread.

Neurosyphilis may occur at any stage of this disease. Early neurosyphilis occurs weeks to a few years after the exposure and presents as meningitis. Late neurosyphilis occurs 10-30 years after exposure and involves dementia, nerve damage causing weakness and paralysis. *Diagnosis* is made by dark-field microscopy (primary or secondary) or serologic testing. An LP is needed in all patients with neurologic symptoms. *Treatment* for primary, secondary, and early latent is benzathine penicillin G 2.4 million units IM in 1 dose. For late latent or tertiary, treatment consists of benzathine penicillin G 2.4 million units IM weekly for 3 weeks (7.2 million units total). *Complications* include dementia, meningitis, neuropathy, hearing loss, ocular syphilis, thoracic aneurysm, aortic aneurysm, stroke, and cardiac valve disease. Report cases to the local health dept.

GONORRHEA, *CHLAMYDIA*, AND TRICHOMONIASIS

Gonorrhea, Chlamydia, and trichomoniasis are all sexually transmitted infections. They are often asymptomatic, or patients may present with a history of a purulent vaginal discharge. Gonorrhea and Chlamydia cause a mucopurulent discharge and friable cervix. Both can lead to pelvic inflammatory disease. The diagnosis can be made using amplified DNA probe testing or culture. Treatment of gonorrhea is with ceftriaxone or cefixime. Chlamydia should be treated with a single dose of azithromycin 1 g PO for one dose followed by a 7-day course of doxycycline. Trichomoniasis typically causes a watery green-yellow vaginal discharge. The diagnosis is made by wet mount examination. The treatment is metronidazole.

VAGINITIS

Vaginitis is an **inflammation of the vagina** that is not necessarily due to an infection. Though infection from bacteria (bacterial vaginosis), viruses, or yeast (vaginal candidiasis) can cause this inflammation, it can also be due to decreased estrogen levels following menopause (atrophic vaginitis), causing the vaginal walls to be drier and easily irritated. The *symptoms* will depend upon the cause of the inflammation, but all types will usually cause vaginal itching or burning and pain with sexual intercourse. **Bacterial vaginosis** causes a foul-smelling, fishy discharge that may be grayish in color; shows clue cells under the microscope. **Vaginal candidiasis** causes a white curd-like discharge; hyphae are seen under the microscope/KOH prep.

SYMPTOMS AND TREATMENT

Trichomoniasis is an STD caused by the parasite *Trichomonas vaginalis*, that can cause a greenish-yellow, frothy vaginal (or penile) discharge. It is often asymptomatic in both men and women. A wet-mount microscopic specimen will show protozoan flagellate motile organisms. **Atrophic vaginitis** causes itching and irritation of the vagina and painful intercourse. There may be pain present during urination, as well. *Treatment* varies, depending on the cause of the inflammation. Appropriate antibiotics or antifungals are necessary for infections: Bacterial vaginosis = Metronidazole 500 mg bid x 7 days OR topical gel; Vaginal candidiasis = Clotrimazole 1% cream x 7-14 days; OR Clotrimazole vaginal tablet x 7 days OR fluconazole 150mg po x 1; Trichomoniasis (also treat all sex partners) = 2 gram of metronidazole OR tinidazole PO x 1 dose; Atrophic vaginalis = estrogen cream or tablets helps with the postmenopausal vaginal dryness. *Complications* of trichomoniasis include urethritis, cystitis, cervical neoplasia, PID, infertility, preterm birth, and it increases susceptibility to HIV. Screen for other STDs as needed and treat partners accordingly. Counsel patients to avoid douching.

PID

Pelvic inflammatory disease (**PID**) is a condition of inflammation and infection in the **upper female reproductive tract** that can lead to infertility. It begins from an infection that moves up from its original source, usually the **cervix or vagina**. The typical causative agents include *Chlamydia trachomatis, N. gonorrhoeae*, and *Gardnerella vaginalis* (and other organisms that are found in bacterial vaginosis). PID is often polymicrobial. Risk factors for PID include young women <25 who engage in unprotected sex, and have multiple sexual partners. *Signs and symptoms* include lower abdominal pain and cramping that is worse after sex/motion, fever, bleeding after sex, vaginal discharge, and possibly N/V. Pelvic exam shows cervical motion tenderness and tenderness throughout the reproductive tract, inflammation, and abnormal discharge. This may be *diagnosed* clinically or may be definitively diagnosed laparoscopically. Test for STDs and order a pregnancy test; rule out an ectopic pregnancy. *Treat* with empiric antibiotics to cover gonorrhea and chlamydia (ceftriaxone 250 mg IM x 1, PLUS doxycycline 100 mg po bid x 14 days, and possibly with metronidazole 500 mg po bid x 14 days); hospitalization may be required to receive IV antibiotics and to monitor the patient. It is important to treat PID to lower the possibility of *complications* like infertility, future ectopic pregnancies, chronic pain, and tubal or ovarian abscesses.

TORCH

TORCH stands for:

- **T**oxoplasmosis (avoid contact with cat feces)
- **O**ther (syphilis, varicella-zoster, parvovirus B19 [erythema infectiosum], human immunodeficiency virus [HIV], Zika virus)
- **R**ubella
- **C**ytomegalovirus
- **H**erpes simplex virus – type 2 (HSV-2)

These **congenital infections** are known to cause **sequelae** in unborn babies while usually only causing mild disease in the mother. The sequelae depend on the disease and includes microcephaly, seizures, hearing loss, cataracts/blindness, neurologic deficits, intellectual disabilities, encephalitis, hydrocephalus, pneumonitis, prematurity, small for gestational age/growth delay, jaundice, anemia, cardiac defects, miscarriage, and stillbirth. It is important to screen for and counsel pregnant women on prevention of these diseases.

Blood and Lymphoreticular System

Anemia and Transfusion Reactions

Iron Deficiency Anemia

Iron deficiency anemia is the most common form of anemia and causes a **microcytic, hypochromic anemia** due to a **lack of iron**. This can be caused by inadequate intake, impaired absorption, or bleeding. Iron is absorbed in the **duodenum and upper jejunum**, transported by **transferrin**, and is stored as either **ferritin** (available for immediate use by the body) or **hemosiderin**. Iron requirements increase during times of growth (infancy through adolescence), during menstruation, and in pregnancy. Many patients are asymptomatic but may present with fatigue, weakness, cold intolerance, glossitis, cheilosis, koilonychia (concave nails), SOB, or signs of pica. *Diagnose* with CBC, TIBC, serum iron and ferritin (reflects iron stores), retic count, and peripheral smear. These show reduced H & H, reduced MCV, elevated RDW, elevated TIBC, reduced iron, reduced ferritin, normal retic; and as the anemia progresses, the smear shows hypochromic, microcytic RBC's with anisocytosis (unequal size), and poikilocytosis (shape variations). *Treat* with oral iron supplements; ferrous iron salts (e.g., ferrous sulfate, ferrous gluconate, ferrous fumarate); and are best absorbed when taken on an empty stomach and with vitamin C, which increases absorption. The underlying cause should be determined and corrected as well as any source of bleeding. Iron supplements are usually given during pregnancy. *Complications* include pregnancy issues, and hypoxemia resulting in irregular heart rate and CHF.

Anemia of Chronic Disease

Anemia of chronic disease or anemia of chronic inflammation produces a microcytic or normocytic anemia due to an acute or chronic **activation of the immune system**. Causes include infections, cancer, autoimmune diseases (e.g., RA, SLE, DM, IBD), chronic kidney disease, or even severe trauma. The disease triggers the immune system and in turn, several processes occur: The liver releases hepcidin which decreases iron absorption in the duodenum and decreases the release of iron from macrophages. Old RBCs are degraded and macrophages sequester and store more iron due to increased ferritin levels. Erythropoietin production in the kidneys is also decreased due to the inflammatory response. These processes all result in decreased iron availability and decreased RBC production, resulting in anemia. Patients may present with nonspecific *signs and symptoms* including fatigue, weakness, dizziness, cold intolerance, and pallor as well as signs and symptoms of the disease triggering the anemia. *Diagnose* with CBC with peripheral smear, serum iron, TIBC and ferritin, and retic count. These show reduced H & H (moderately low), reduced TIBC, reduced iron, elevated ferritin, reduced retic, and a normochromic or microcytic anemia on the smear. *Treating* the underlying disorder is the primary goal. In severe cases, erythropoiesis-stimulating agents (ESAs: epoetin alfa, darbepoetin alfa) may be used by hematologists or nephrologists (due to black box warnings), especially in those with CKD or patients undergoing chemotherapy for cancer; or blood transfusions may be necessary. Iron supplements are typically not used, but may be if there is a concomitant iron deficiency anemia in patients with CKD if not on dialysis. Experimental therapies are under investigation. *Complications* include hypoxia, and increased mortality from cardiovascular disease and CKD.

Thalassemia

Thalassemia is a group of **autosomal recessive disorders** that affects **hemoglobin (Hgb) formation** causing a mild to severe **microcytic, hemolytic anemia**. This mostly affects those of African, Mediterranean, or South Asian descent. There are two main types: *α-thalassemia* and *β-*

thalassemia. Both forms can produce a silent carrier state, a mild form called *thalassemia trait (thalassemia minor)* which is often diagnosed when a mild microcytic anemia does not respond to iron supplements, an intermediate form (Hgb H disease in α), and a severe form of the disease (*thalassemia major*: hydrops fetalis in α, Cooley anemia in β). Symptoms usually start appearing after 6 months of life when fetal hemoglobin starts being replaced by adult Hgb. *Symptoms*, if present, can include pallor, fatigue, jaundice, scleral icterus, and splenomegaly. *Diagnose* with CBC, peripheral smear, and hemoglobin electrophoresis (usually normal in α-thalassemias, except Hgb H is elevated in Hgb H disease; elevated Hgb A2 and/or Hgb F in β-thal. trait; and elevated Hgb F in β-thal. major). Peripheral smear varies according to severity and ranges from a mild microcytic anemia, to Heinz bodies (Hgb H disease), or to target cells, nucleated RBCs, and basophilic stippling (β-thalassemia trait, β-thalassemia intermedia, β-thal. major). *Treatment* varies according to the severity of the disease. Patients who are carriers do not require treatment, those with the trait or intermediate disease may need blood transfusions, and those with Cooley anemia depend on blood transfusions and iron chelation throughout their lifetime. Iron supplements are avoided. Splenectomy may be required and a bone marrow transplant may be considered. Refer patients to genetic counseling. *Complications* include iron overload (r/o hemochromatosis), increased risk of infection, splenomegaly, bone deformities, heart failure, and death if severe thalassemia.

Hemolytic Anemia

Hemolytic anemia results from destruction of **red blood cells (RBC)** and this is either inherited or acquired. It can be due to **intrinsic causes** (defect within the RBC itself) or **extrinsic causes** (from outside the RBC). Examples of intrinsic causes include sickle cell anemia, thalassemia, G6PD deficiency, TTP, and hereditary spherocytosis. Extrinsic causes include drugs, toxins, autoimmune disorders (warm antibody hemolytic anemia or cold agglutinin disease), infections, hypersplenism, and prosthetic heart valves. Hemolysis can be acute, chronic, or sporadic; and can occur intravascularly or extravascularly. *Signs and symptoms* depend on the underlying disorder causing the hemolysis, but may include pallor, fatigue, tachycardia, dyspnea, jaundice, ecchymosis, and dark urine from hemoglobinuria. *Diagnose* with CBC with differential, peripheral smear, reticulocyte count, indirect bilirubin, haptoglobin, serum LDH, and a direct Coombs test (aka direct antiglobulin test, DAT). The retic count is elevated in hemolysis and lower if the bone marrow is suppressed (e.g., aplastic anemia); the peripheral smear helps differentiate the cause (e.g., spherocytes, sickle cells, schistocytes); reduced haptoglobin, elevated indirect bilirubin, elevated LDH are present in hemolysis; a positive DAT shows that antibodies or complement are present on RBC membranes which indicates an immune-mediated cause (e.g., autoimmune, drugs, *transfusion reaction*). *Treatment* is directed at the underlying cause and may include steroids, blood transfusions, and a splenectomy or bone marrow transplant. Folic acid supplements are needed since folate is depleted during times of hemolysis; however, iron is usually not depleted during hemolysis but is recycled and therefore can be harmful if given. Avoid causative agents. *Complications* include bilirubin gallstones, heart failure, and death.

Autoimmune Hemolytic Anemia

With **autoimmune hemolytic anemia**, autoimmune antibodies react with RBCs, causing destruction, either at temperatures ≥37°C (warm antibody HA) or <37°C (cold agglutinin disease):

- **Warm antibody HA** is most common with destruction of RBCs occurring primarily in the spleen and may be primary or secondary to autoimmune disease (such as SLE) or drugs (levodopa, cephalosporins, sulfonamides). Warm antibody HA causes severe hemolysis and may be fatal. Autoantibodies are typically IgG. Symptoms are those of anemia: pallor, weakness, syncope, chest pain, and heart failure (if severe).

- **Cold agglutinin disease** may be idiopathic or associated with infection or lymphoproliferative disorders in which the body produces antibodies against I antigen, which is located on the RBC cell membrane. Hemolysis occurs primarily in the liver and spleen and may be acute or chronic. Anemia is typically mild but other diseases affected by cold, such as Raynaud syndrome, may be present. Autoantibodies are typically IgM. Symptoms may include acrocyanoses and occlusive disease associated with cold exposure.

Diagnosis is per direct and indirect antiglobulin (Coombs) test. Treatment may include identifying and eliminating triggers, blood transfusions, IV immune globulin, corticosteroids (DOC for warm antibody HA), and monoclonal antibodies.

Microangiopathic Hemolytic Anemia

Microangiopathic hemolytic anemia (MAHA) refers to various conditions with fragmented RBCs (schistocytes) and small vessel disease (damage to endothelial layer causing platelets to aggregate and fibrin deposits), such as thrombotic thrombocytopenic purpura and hemolytic uremic syndrome (HUS). Blood traveling through the damaged vessels fragments, and these fragments are destroyed in the spleen. MAHA may be primary or secondary to disorders of pregnancy (HELLP, DIC, abruptio placentae, fatty liver), cardiovascular disease (malignant hypertension, hemolysis associated with heart valves), cancer, rheumatologic disorders (SLE, scleroderma renal crisis, antiphospholipid syndrome, or medications (chemotherapeutic agents, immunosuppressants). Symptoms include fatigue, jaundice, and anemia. Diagnosis is per laboratory findings: decreased hemoglobin, schistocytes present, increased LDH, indirect bilirubin, urine urobilinogen, and reticulocyte count and decreased haptoglobin. Treatment includes identifying and treating underlying problem as treatment will vary depending on the cause and associated disorders, plasma exchange (emergent treatment) and supportive care. With HUS, patients may require renal dialysis. Platelet transfusions are usually avoided as they may promote further clotting.

Transfusion Reaction

Transfusion reaction is an adverse reaction after a **blood transfusion** which can be immune-mediated or non-immune-mediated and hemolytic or non-hemolytic. The reaction can be acute or delayed (>24 hours to 2-3 weeks). Often the reactions are not serious and include febrile nonhemolytic reactions and allergic reactions. Hemolysis is serious and often fatal if due to ABO/Rh incompatibility. Patients with previous transfusions and multiparous women are at a higher risk of immune-mediated transfusion reactions due to the formation of alloantibodies. Transfusion-related acute lung injury (TRALI) is another possible serious complication of a transfusion. *Signs and symptoms* of a transfusion reaction may include fever, chills, flushing, hypotension, dyspnea, wheezing, N/V, anxiety, flank pain, and dark urine. Signs and symptoms of allergic reactions can include urticaria, pruritus, and wheezing. Blood typing and crossmatching before any transfusion helps decrease these reactions, but should retype if a transfusion reaction occurs. Also use a DAT (direct antiglobulin test, aka direct Coombs test), which tests for antibodies directly attached to RBCs, to determine if the hemolysis is due to an immune-mediated process. The patient's plasma and centrifuged urine will appear pink or red if intravascular hemolysis/hemoglobinuria is present. Immediately D/C the transfusion, give appropriate *treatment* (e.g., antihistamines, acetaminophen), and properly report if a transfusion reaction occurs. *Complications* include DIC, TRALI, pulmonary edema, renal failure, volume overload, and anaphylaxis.

G6PD Deficiency

Glucose-6-phosphate dehydrogenase deficiency (G6PD) is an X-linked **genetic disorder** in which the red blood cells undergo hemolysis causing **hemolytic anemia**. This is due to an **enzyme deficiency** that affects RBC metabolism, and variants of the deficiency result in different levels of hemolysis. Many people will not ever experience symptoms or complications from the disorder. G6PD is the most common enzyme deficiency worldwide and is more common in males, and in those of African, Mediterranean, or Asian descent. This condition is not constant, but occurs during times of oxidative stress or certain triggers. Hemolysis may result from infection/fever, medication (e.g., acetaminophen, salicylates, sulfa drugs, Pyridium, chloroquine), or other triggers like fava beans or mothballs. Hemolysis begins 24-48 hours after the oxidative stress and spontaneously resolves in 8-14 days. The patient may present with pale skin, jaundice, splenomegaly, dark urine, complaints of extreme fatigue, difficulty breathing, and an increased HR. *Diagnose* the condition with a G6PD blood test (do not test during an episode of hemolysis due to high likelihood of false negatives). During hemolysis there is an elevated reticulocyte count, elevated LDH, and elevated indirect bilirubin. CBC shows anemia; and peripheral blood smear shows Heinz bodies and bite cells. *Treatment* is supportive during hemolysis since the episodes are self-limiting. Avoid triggers. *Complications* include chronic anemia and possible need of a transfusion (rare).

Sickle Cell Disease and Anemia

Sickle cell disease (**SCD**) is an **autosomal recessive disorder of chromosome 11**, causing hemoglobin (Hgb) to be defective so that red blood cells (RBCs) are sickle-shaped and inflexible, resulting in their accumulating in small vessels and causing painful blockage (**sickle cell crisis**). While normal RBCs survive 120 days, sickled cells may survive only 10 to 20 days, stressing the bone marrow that cannot produce fast enough and resulting in **chronic hemolytic anemia**. There are variations of sickle cell disease, with homozygous Hgb S being the most common in the U.S. (60-70%), affecting mostly African Americans. Sickle cell trait (Hgb A/S) occurs in 8-10%, is much less severe, and does not cause anemia. Different types of crises occur in SCD (aplastic, hemolytic, vaso-occlusive, and sequestrating) and can be brought on by stress, dehydration, and hypoxic states. Pain, pallor, jaundice, swelling in the extremities, weakness, and fatigue are common symptoms. Newborn screening is required in the U.S. and prenatal diagnosis is possible. *Diagnosis* is per electrophoresis (Hgb S is present), PCR, or direct DNA testing. Hematology studies show: Hgb 5-9 g/dL, reduced Hct, elevated WBC, elevated reticulocyte count, elevated platelets; and sickle, target cells, and possibly Howell-Jolly bodies on peripheral smear. *Treatment* is supportive during a crisis (hydration, O_2, analgesics); blood transfusions, iron chelation, and erythrocytapheresis may be necessary. Daily folate supplements (to prevent a megaloblastic anemia), penicillin prophylaxis (2 months to 5+ years old), and hydroxyurea therapy are also used. Stem cells transplantation is the only curative treatment and is about 85% effective. *Complications* of SCD include hemolytic anemia, aplastic crisis, avascular necrosis, organ damage, stroke, MI, acute chest syndrome, sequestration syndrome (spleen), chronic pain, increased risk of infection from encapsulated organisms, priapism, blindness, and pulmonary HTN.

Aplastic Anemia

Aplastic anemia is a **pancytopenia** where hematopoietic stem cells fail to make adequate **RBCs, WBCs, and platelets**. This is a rare, but treatable condition. This can be genetic or acquired and can occur at any age; however, it is more common in the younger years and in the elderly. Genetic conditions that result in aplastic anemia include Fanconi anemia, familial aplastic anemia, and dyskeratosis congenita. Most cases of aplastic anemia are acquired and can be caused by radiation, chemotherapy, toxins, medications, viral infections, or can be idiopathic (most common). The mechanism that causes aplastic anemia is thought to be either the direct damaging effects of an exposure or an immune-mediated response to various triggers (autoimmune). The onset of *signs and symptoms* is insidious and may include pallor and fatigue, increased infections, and easy bleeding and bruising. *Diagnose* with a bone marrow biopsy. *Treatment* depends on the severity of the disease and may be supportive or may include immunosuppressive agents (e.g., antithymocyte globulin, cyclosporine), blood transfusions, or hematopoietic stem cell transplants (HLA-matched sibling donors are preferred). Patients should be referred to a hematology expert. *Complications* include increased risk of infection and death.

Hypoproliferative Anemias

Hypoproliferative anemia	Characteristics	Diagnosis and treatment
Sideroblastic anemia	Acquired (drugs, toxins, vitamin B6 deficiency) or congenital disease in which bone marrow produces abnormal ringed sideroblasts instead of healthy erythrocytes.	Diagnostic tests include CBC, reticulocyte count, blood smear (peripheral), serum iron, serum ferritin, transferring saturation, and bone marrow examination. Treatment includes identifying and eliminating cause, vitamin or mineral supplementation and (for congenital cases) pyridoxine.
Lead intoxication/ poisoning	Exposure to lead causes slow build up in body. Children may experience developmental delay, learning disabilities, pica, GI problems, hearing loss, weight loss, and seizures. Adults may have hypertension, impaired cognition, headache, mood disorders, abdominal pain, arthralgia, myalgia, reduced sperm count, miscarriage and stillbirth, and mood disorders	Diagnosis is per blood test for lead levels. Treatment includes identifying source of exposure and eliminating. Severe cases (≥45 mcg/dL may require chelation therapy or EDTA chelation therapy.

Blood Transfusions

Indications for **blood transfusions** with RBCs include hemorrhage (>30% loss of volume), severe symptomatic anemia (≤7 g/dL), and sickle cells crisis. FFP may be used to reverse anticoagulation (INH >1.6 with bleeding), and platelets to those at risk of severe bleeding because of thrombocytopenia. Cryoprecipitate may be used for severe hemorrhage or coagulopathy with hypofibrinogenemia. Complications include:

- **Urticaria**: Allergic response with itching and red, elevated wheals, and flushing. Transfusion should be discontinued and antihistamine administered. If the symptoms recede, the transfusion may be restarted if the patient is carefully monitored.
- **Anaphylaxis**: Severe life-threatening allergic reaction with fever, shock, bronchospasm, ARDS, laryngeal edema. The transfusion must be discontinued immediately and epinephrine administered. Other treatments may include antihistamine, albuterol, cimetidine, bronchodilator, and steroids along with supportive treatment, such as oxygen and IV fluids.
- **Transfusion-related acute lung injury**: Antibodies in the plasma of the donor may stimulate leukocytes in the patient's blood, causing them for form aggregates in the pulmonary vasculature, resulting in fever, chills, pulmonary edema, and ARDS (without LV failure). Pulmonary infiltrates are present bilaterally. Transfusion must be immediately discontinued and supportive treatment provided, such as oxygen, diuretic therapy, and intubation and mechanical ventilation.

Clotting Disorders

Factor VII Deficiency and Factor VIII Deficiency

Factor VII deficiency can be genetic or acquired, is due to a lack of factor VII (proconvertin), is activated when combined with tissue factor, is necessary to complete the clotting cascade in both the intrinsic and extrinsic pathways, and is vitamin K-dependent. A prolonged PT and normal aPTT will be present. *Treat* with infusions of fresh frozen plasma (FFP) and recombinant factor VIIa.

Factor VIII deficiency *(hemophilia A; classic hemophilia)* is an X-linked recessive disorder causing a deficiency in factor VIII which results in easy bruising and bleeding. It is typically genetic, but rarely may be acquired (autoantibodies). PT and platelets are normal, aPTT is prolonged, and there is reduced factor VIII; rule out Von Willebrand disease. *Treat* prophylactically before procedures and use replacement therapy with recombinant or concentrated factor VIII.

Factor IX Deficiency, Factor XI Deficiency, and Von Willebrand Disease

Factor IX deficiency (*hemophilia B or Christmas disease*) is an X-linked disorder, so it affects males more, and is less common than hemophilia B. Factor IX is vitamin K-dependent. A prolonged PTT, normal PT and platelets, and reduced factor IX assay will be present. *Treat* with infusions of factor IX (purified or recombinant).

Factor XI deficiency *(Hemophilia C or Rosenthal syndrome)* is an autosomal disorder (males and females equally affected) and is more common in the Ashkenazi Jewish population. A prolonged PTT and normal PT are present. Infusions of fresh frozen plasma (FFP) are the primary *treatment.*

Von Willebrand disease is the most common bleeding disorder, it is usually autosomal dominant, and causes a deficiency of von Willebrand factor (VWF) resulting in platelet malfunction and low factor VIII. Labs show normal platelets and slightly prolonged aPTT. *Diagnose* with plasma VWF antigen, VWF ristocetin cofactor, and plasma factor VIII. *Treatment* may include desmopressin, recombinant VWF, and VWF/Factor VIII concentrates.

Coagulation Factor Disorders

Primary hypercoagulable states	Characteristics	Diagnosis and treatment
Antithrombin (AT) III deficiency	Acquired (DIC, HUS, sepsis, microangiopathic hemolytic anemias, oral contraceptives) or inherited (autosomal dominant or recessive). AT is a protease (not vitamin K dependent) that inhibits coagulation and is potentiated by heparin. Deficiency increases risk of thrombosis (usually venous).	Diagnosis is per PT, aPTT, antithrombin assays, protein C and S tests, Factor V Leiden test, homocysteine level, and anticardiolipin antibodies. Imaging may include echocardiography, Doppler US, and V/P scan. Treatment may include antithrombin III concentrate, FFP, enoxaparin to prevent thrombi, and anticoagulation (warfarin) if clots have formed
Activated protein C resistance	One of primary inherited (autosomal dominant) risk factors for VTE. May also be acquired if Factor VIII concentrations are high. Results in inadequate response to anticoagulant activity of protein C and thrombus formation (pulmonary emboli, stroke)	Diagnosis is per activated protein C resistance ratio (normal is >2.1. Treatment is per anticoagulation (heparin, LMWH, warfarin) and lifestyle changes (exercise, weight loss, smoking cessation).

Hypercoagulable States and Virchow's Triad

Hypercoagulable states are a group of inherited or acquired disorders or conditions causing **increased coagulation** that lead to an increased risk of **thromboembolic events** (venous or arterial). The risk of thrombosis has been described by **Virchow's triad**: hypercoagulability, endothelial injury, and stasis. The states of hypercoagulation include cancer, pregnancy, elevated estrogen (e.g., oral contraceptives, hormone replacement therapy), elevated or dysfunctional platelets, clotting disorders (e.g., *Factor V Leiden*, prothrombin G20210A mutation, protein C or S deficiency, antithrombin deficiency), antiphospholipid antibodies, surgery or trauma, and blood stasis (e.g., immobilization, CHF, AFib). These increase the risk of venous thrombosis and pulmonary embolism (PE) which can be fatal. Routine coagulation studies include: CBC with platelet count, PTT (intrinsic and common coagulation pathways), PT (extrinsic and common pathways), TT (thrombin time; only common pathway), and fibrinogen. A 1:1 mixing study helps determine whether the prolonged PT ot PTT is due to a clotting factor disorder (clotting time corrects when mixed with normal pooled plasma) or due to the presence of inhibitors like heparin or autoantibodies (clotting time does not correct). Specific coagulation disorder studies include: Factor V Leiden and Prothrombin 20210 mutation tests, Protein C or S activity tests, and antithrombin activity or antithrombin antigen tests. The presence of specific autoantibodies can be tested with a Lupus anticoagulant, antiphospholipid antibody, or, cardiolipin antibody test. A negative D-dimer along with clinical judgement helps rule out thrombosis.

ITP

Immune (or idiopathic) thrombocytopenic purpura (ITP), also called **immune thrombocytopenia**, is a disorder causing bleeding and bruising due to a reduced number of **platelets** (thrombocytopenia). This is an autoimmune disorder (antiplatelet antibodies) which can be acute or chronic (>6 months), is seen in both children and adults, and can be initiated by triggers including viruses, medication, or pregnancy. Children usually have acute ITP that is mild and self-limited, whereas adults usually have chronic cases of ITP. Consult a hematologist. *Signs and symptoms* include petechiae, purpura, bruising, and bleeding, but with a normal spleen size and no systemic symptoms. This is a *diagnosis* of exclusion; rule out leukemia, myelodysplastic syndrome, SLE, and other secondary causes of thrombocytopenia (e.g., HIV, Hep C). Thrombocytopenia is defined as platelets <150,000/mm^3, but bleeding is not usually seen until platelets are <50,000 mm^3. Diagnose with CBC, platelets, and a peripheral smear; a bone marrow biopsy may be necessary to rule out other illnesses if the patient is unresponsive to treatment. Children with acute ITP usually do not require treatment. *Treat* with corticosteroids and possibly IV RhIG (e.g., RhoGAM®) if Rh-positive, or IVIG (immune globulin IV) if Rh-negative. Other treatments include monoclonal antibodies (e.g., Rituximab®), other immunosuppressants, and thrombopoietin receptor agonists. Platelet transfusion may be necessary if severe bleeding, and a splenectomy may be necessary if the response to the initial treatment is inadequate. Avoid drugs that affect platelet function (e.g., ASA, NSAIDS). *Complications* include intercranial hemorrhages, GI bleeds, and recurrent disease.

TTP

Thrombotic thrombocytopenic purpura (TTP) is a rare **blood disorder** with the formation of multiple thromboses (blood clots) in the small vessels which results in a **low platelet count**. It is a medical emergency. It can be inherited or acquired (more common). The exact cause is unknown, but it can be triggered by drugs, pregnancy, hemorrhagic *E. coli*, and deficiency of the ADAMTS13 enzyme appears to be involved in some. *Signs and symptoms* can include microangiopathic hemolytic anemia, thrombocytopenia causing petechiae and purpura, fever, abnormal kidney function (however, not as severe as HUS, hemolytic uremic syndrome), and neurologic symptoms (e.g., altered mental status, paresthesias). *Diagnosis* consists of the following:

- CBC will show low platelets (20,000 -50,000/µL) and low RBCs.
- Blood smear will show broken and torn RBCs (schistocytes).
- Coagulation studies, negative DAT (Coombs), BUN, creatinine, elevated serum bilirubin, and elevated lactate dehydrogenase.

The first line of *treatment* is plasma exchange, in which the patient's own plasma is removed and replaced with healthy plasma from a matching donor through transfusion. If the disease remains unresponsive to this treatment, immunosuppressive medications may be prescribed and a splenectomy may be necessary. *Complications* include stroke, kidney impairment, and recurrence.

Primary Polycythemia

Primary polycythemia (polycythemia vera) is a rare, chronic **myeloproliferative disorder** where there is an increase in all three **myeloid cell lines** (RBCs, granulocyte WBCs, and platelets). This is due to a mutation (usually the JAK2 gene) in a **hematopoietic stem cell** and is usually diagnosed later in life (~50-70 years old). The blood volume expands and becomes hyperviscous due to the increased quantity of RBCs. Polycythemia vera places patients at an increased risk of thromboses and bleeding. *Signs and symptoms* include headache, vision issues, pruritus (often noted after a warm bath), reddish skin, fatigue, GI and gum bleeding, splenomegaly, HTN, and SOB. *Diagnosis* is initially suspected with CBC findings (elevated Hct, Hgb, and RBCs). Secondary causes of elevated peripheral RBCs must be ruled out (e.g., disorders causing chronic hypoxemia, dehydration, tumors secreting erythropoietin). The primary *treatment* is phlebotomy. Consult with and/or refer to a hematologist.

THROMBOCYTHEMIA (THROMBOCYTOSIS)

Primary thrombocytosis is a chronic **myeloproliferative disorder** marked by an increase in **platelets**. This is more common in the elderly and is rare in pediatrics. The cause is unclear, but seems to be due to mutations. Patients are at an increased risk of **thromboses and bleeding**. Patients are often asymptomatic, but *signs and symptoms* include headache, paresthesias, signs of thromboses, and bleeding or bruising. *Diagnose* initially with CBC (platelets >600,000/mm^3) and peripheral smear; rule out other causes (secondary thrombocytosis= iron deficiency, infection, inflammation, neoplasms) since this is a diagnosis of exclusion. *Treatment* may include ASA. Refer to a hematologist.

Blood and Lymphatic Cancers

LEUKEMIA

Leukemia is a condition in which the proliferating malignant **hematopoietic cells** compete with and cause the suppression of normal **blood cell formation**. This results in several consequences, regardless of the type:

- Decrease in production of erythrocytes (RBCs), resulting in anemia.
- Decrease in neutrophils, resulting in increased risk of infection.
- Decrease in platelets, with subsequent decrease in clotting factors and increased bleeding.
- Increased risk of physiological fractures because of invasion of bone marrow that weakens the periosteum.
- Infiltration of liver, spleen, and lymph glands, resulting in enlargement and fibrosis
- Infiltration of the CNS, resulting in increased intracranial pressure, ventricular dilation, and meningeal irritation with headaches, vomiting, papilledema, nuchal rigidity, and coma progressing to death.
- Hypermetabolism that deprives cells of nutrients, resulting in anorexia, weight loss, muscle atrophy, and fatigue.

Leukemia occurs when one type of WBC proliferates with immature or inadequately functioning cells, with the defect occurring in the **hematopoietic stem cell**, either lymphoid (lympho-) or myeloid (myelo-). With **acute leukemia**, WBC count remains low because the cells are halted at the immature blast stage and the disease progresses rapidly. **Chronic leukemia** progresses more slowly and most cells are mature, yet don't function properly. Risk factors include exposure to ionizing radiation or chemicals (e.g., benzene), previous chemotherapy, viruses, and chromosomal mutations.

ALL AND CLL

Acute lymphocytic (lymphoblastic) leukemia (ALL) is the most common type of **pediatric cancer** in the U.S. (may be seen in adults) and involves the proliferation of lymphoid precursors (lymphoblasts → T-cells, B-cells). Risk is increased with Down syndrome. Symptoms depend on if there is primarily bone marrow involvement or if organs have been infiltrated (e.g., spleen, liver, lymph nodes, thymus, CNS, gonads) with blasts. *Signs and symptoms* include sudden onset of fever, fatigue, pallor, easy bleeding and bruising, petechiae, lymphadenopathy, and bone pain. *Diagnosis* is made with CBC (elevated WBCs) with peripheral smear and bone marrow biopsy (pancytopenia with >20% blasts). Refer to hematologist-oncologist. The cure rate is high in children.

Chronic lymphocytic leukemia (CLL) is the most common leukemia in **adults** (usually >60-70 years old) and involves the accumulation of mature but incompetent neoplastic lymphocytes (usually B-cells). Incidence of CLL is increased in males. Risk factors include exposure to certain chemicals (e.g., Agent Orange) and a positive family history. CLL has an insidious onset and patients may be asymptomatic when diagnosed (incidental finding). *Signs and symptoms* may include enlarged lymph nodes, hepatosplenomegaly, signs of anemia, and increased infections. *Diagnose* with CBC with peripheral smear (lymphocytosis, smudge cells), and bone marrow biopsy. Refer to hematologist-oncologist.

AML AND CML

Acute myelogenous leukemia (AML) is a disease which originates in the **bone marrow** and involves the acute proliferation of **malignant myeloid precursor cells** (immature granulocytes and monocytes). AML is the most common **adult acute leukemia**. It may occur at any age but usually affects those >50 years old, and affects men more than women. Risk is increased if the patient has myelodysplastic syndrome or previous chemo/radiation. *Signs and symptoms* may include fatigue, fever, SOB, and gum issues (infiltrates, swelling, bleeding). *Diagnose* with CBC/peripheral smear, and bone marrow biopsy (>20% myeloblasts; Auer rods). Refer to hematologist-oncologist.

Chronic myelogenous leukemia (CML) is a chronic disease originating in the **bone marrow** and is almost always due to a **genetic mutation** (Philadelphia chromosome). CML involves the malignant production of granulocytes (neutrophils, eosinophils, basophils) and their precursors. It may occur at any age, but is usually seen in adults. CML has an insidious onset and may present with general, nonspecific *symptoms* (e.g., fatigue, weight loss), splenomegaly (common), fever, night sweats, and signs of anemia. *Diagnose* with CBC, peripheral smear, and bone marrow biopsy (elevated WBCs; Philadelphia chromosome in bone marrow). Refer to hematologist-oncologist.

HODGKIN LYMPHOMA

Lymphomas are cancers of the **lymphatic system**. The 2 primary types are Hodgkin and Non-Hodgkin lymphoma. **Hodgkin lymphoma** (previously, Hodgkin Disease) is a painless lymphoma usually in the cervical (most common), supraclavicular, mediastinal, or inguinal nodes. It is more common in males and in those 15-34 years old or >55 years old. Patients may present with fever, night sweats, weight loss (>10% body weight), dry cough, pruritus, splenomegaly, and palpable nodes. Some patients experience pain at the involved site when consuming alcohol. *Diagnosis* involves a biopsy and identifying Reed–Sternberg cells (a type of B cell). If caught in the early stages, most cases of Hodgkin lymphoma are curable. It spreads first to other nearby lymph nodes and may sometimes, eventually spread to the lungs, liver, or bone marrow. *Treatment* includes chemotherapy and/or radiation. Patients may desire to preserve fertility (egg or sperm banking).

NON-HODGKIN LYMPHOMA

Non-Hodgkin lymphoma is a group of **lymphocyte cancers**, is much more common than Hodgkin lymphoma (7th overall most common cancer), and can start in either T or B-cell (more common) lymphocytes. It may occur anywhere in the lymphatic system and often spreads beyond (e.g., bone marrow, GI), even by the time of diagnosis. It is more common in males and is usually diagnosed in those ≥65 years old. Risk factors include environmental exposures, some viruses (e.g., EBV), immunodeficiency conditions (e.g., HIV), and chronic inflammation. *Signs and symptoms* include painless peripheral lymphadenopathy that may cause compression symptoms; systemic symptoms are less common than Hodgkin lymphoma. Biopsy enlarged nodes for *diagnosis*. *Treatment* involves chemotherapy, radiation, and monoclonal antibodies. Refer all lymphoma patients.

Multiple Myeloma and Myelodysplasia

Multiple myeloma is a cancer of the **plasma cells** and includes a range of diseases. The cancer cells invade the nearby **bone tissue** and destroy it. This affects men slightly more than women, is increased in African Americans, and incidence increases with age. *Symptoms* vary widely and patients may be asymptomatic or may experience bone pain (especially in the back or ribs), osteoporosis, pathological fractures, symptoms of anemia, and increased infections. *Diagnose* with CBC (elevated Ca^{++}), serum and urine protein electrophoresis, and x-rays; confirmed with bone marrow biopsy. *Treatment* includes high dose chemotherapy and autologous stem cell transplantation. The disease is progressive and prognosis is poor. **Myelodysplasia** (or myelodysplastic syndrome) is an abnormality in the development of **hematopoietic progenitor cells** (myeloid cell lines = RBCs, granulocytes, and megakaryocytes) and include a wide range of **neoplastic disorders** depending on which cell line is affected. More dysplastic blasts are formed and this causes a hypercellular (rarely it is hypocellular) bone marrow, but with peripheral cytopenia. This can be a precursor to acute myelogenous leukemia (AML). Risk factors include increasing age (>60 y/o), previous chemotherapy, radiation, and chemical exposure (e.g., benzene). *Signs and symptoms* depend on which cell line is affected. Decreased RBCs causes signs of anemia (pallor, fatigue, SOB), decreased neutrophils causes an increase in infections, and decreased platelets causes easy bleeding and bruising (e.g., bleeding gums). *Diagnosis* starts with CBC, peripheral blood smear, and bone marrow biopsy. Rule out other disorders causing a macrocytic anemia (e.g., vitamin B_{12} deficiency, folate deficiency). Refer to a hematologist-oncologist.

Behavioral Health

Anxiety Disorders

Panic Disorder

Panic disorder is a chronic condition in which people experience **unexpected panic attacks** that may become severe enough to affect their lives and level of functioning. Patients must experience >1 month of continued worry and behavioral changes (avoidance) regarding thoughts of a future panic attack in order to be *diagnosed* (DSM-5-TR). These panic attacks may vary in intensity and frequency and are not caused by medications or other medical disorders. It is 2 to 3 times more likely to affect females, more likely to start in late teens to early adulthood, it is likely to occur in families, and it is also common to be associated with other psychiatric disorders like major depression, OCD, and phobias. It may occur with other medical conditions like asthma, IBS, and migraines. The panic attacks experienced with panic disorder give patients a sense of extreme anxiety with rapid HR or palpitations, chest pain, paresthesias, chills or hot flashes, sweating, dyspnea, a choking feeling, shaking, dizziness, abdominal distress/nausea, derealization or depersonalization, and fear of dying or going crazy/losing control (must meet 4 of the 13 criteria). Patients may also have a fear of leaving their homes or encountering crowds of people (*agoraphobia*). Refer to a mental health professional. Evidence-based *treatment* for panic disorder includes flooding or implosion therapy, implemented through in vivo exposure and response prevention. Flooding is typically accompanied by cognitive therapy, relaxation, breathing training, or pharmacotherapy. **Antidepressant medications** are often prescribed to relieve the symptoms of panic disorder. If stand-alone drug treatment is used, the risk of relapse is very high.

Generalized Anxiety Disorder

Generalized anxiety disorder (GAD) is a condition in which a person **worries** all the time about situations or conditions. This worry or stress is out of proportion with the general reaction of most people and patients are unable to control the anxiety/worry. Also, it cannot be caused by medications or due to other medical conditions. This must be present for most days over a 6-month period over different situations or conditions. This is more common in females and often begins in childhood or adolescence. It is thought that an imbalance in the neurotransmitters **serotonin** and **norepinephrine** may play a role in the development of GAD. GAD causes a generalized state of unrest or feeling keyed up with muscle tension, irritability, fatigue, difficulty concentrating/mind goes blank, and insomnia (must meet ≥3 criteria for diagnosis, DSM-5-TR). On exam, patients may appear very restless with SOB, elevated HR, diaphoretic, and they may complain of somatic symptoms such as nausea, diarrhea, difficulty swallowing, clammy hands, or headache. The *treatment* for generalized anxiety disorder usually entails a **multicomponent cognitive-behavioral therapy (CBT)**, occasionally accompanied by pharmacotherapy. **SSRI** antidepressants and the anxiolytic buspirone have both demonstrated success in diminishing the symptoms of generalized anxiety disorder. CBT can be used to address **cognitive distortions** that accompany generalized anxiety disorder, including all-or-nothing thinking (e.g., "I'll always be destined for failure"), catastrophic thinking (e.g., "This breakup means I'll be alone forever"), and mind reading (e.g., "She didn't return my text because I am 'nobody' to her").

Phobias

Phobias can be specific or social phobias. In both, the phobia cannot be caused by another medical condition or better defined by another mental disorder. In both the fear and anxiety brings much distress and patients greatly desire to avoid these objects or situation and will only endure them under immense distress. These fears must be present >6 months and are more common in women. A **specific phobia** is a persistent, intense, disproportionate fear or anxiety regarding a certain **object or situation** that causes immediate distress when exposed to and interferes with how patients function as they try to avoid the object or situation. Some examples include fears of snakes, spiders, heights, water, weather, needles, medical procedures, and blood. The primary *treatment* involves exposure therapy. Occasionally, short-term use of benzodiazepines is used in certain unavoidable situations. In **social phobias**, or **social anxiety disorder**, the object of the intense fear or anxiety is **public situations** where the patient may be scrutinized (e.g., speaking in public, performing, social interactions, eating, or using public restrooms). Patients worry that they will be looked down on or that they will offend others with their actions. *Treatment* involves cognitive-behavioral therapy and pharmacotherapy. SSRI's are first line; and β-blockers may be added to help decrease the physical symptoms caused by performance anxiety.

Adjustment Disorder and Normal Bereavement/Grief Reactions

An **adjustment disorder** is a stress-related condition that occurs in response to some **change or stress** in a person's life. The behavioral and emotional symptoms begin within 3 months of the stressor and stop within 6 months after the stressor ends. The reaction to the stressor(s) is disproportionate to what is regularly expected and interferes with regular functioning. Therefore, this does not include normal bereavement/grief reactions that involve normal stages (e.g., denial, blame/anger, bargaining, sadness, acceptance). Examples of adjustment disorder stressors include relationship issues/divorce, work or money problems, becoming a parent, moving, illness, and natural disasters. *Signs and symptoms* may include anxiety, depressed mood, sleep disturbances, sadness, irritability, withdrawing, feeling hopeless, or even thoughts of suicide. Patients may exhibit behavior changes and have conduct issues like abusing drugs or alcohol, getting into trouble, and destroying property. Children with adjustment disorder may have failing grades or may skip school. *Treatment* consists of psychotherapy to help work through the stress caused by the change in their lives and to develop healthy coping skills. Sometimes short-term antidepressants or benzodiazepines are added and may be helpful in relieving the symptoms of depression, anxiety, or insomnia.

PTSD

Posttraumatic stress disorder (**PTSD**) occurs following direct involvement in, witnessing, or by indirectly learning a close friend or relative was exposed to an **extremely traumatic event** or the threat of such an event. This can also include first-responders or other professionals who repeatedly see or hear about traumatic events. But this does not include things only witnessed in photos, tv, or other electronics. PTSD can occur after sexual or physical abuse or attacks, from accidents, war, or from experiencing a natural disaster. *Symptoms* of PTSD usually begin within 3 months of the triggering event but may occur up to years later. Patients may have sudden, recurrent, unwanted, and disturbing memories or flashbacks of the trauma, nightmares, insomnia, irritability, difficulty concentrating, anger, guilt, and possibly self-destructive behavior. Small internal or external reminders of the trauma can send patients into an episode of severe distress, anger, fear, and intense physical reactions. There is avoidance of internal or external reminders, an increased startle response, and there can be feelings of hopelessness and helplessness. Children <6 may experience different symptoms including reenacting the trauma through play, regression, and delayed development. For establishing a *diagnosis*, symptoms must last >1 month, including 1 or more "intrusion" symptoms, avoidance of triggers, 2 or more negative changes in "mood and cognitions," and 2 or more changes in "arousal and reactivity," and can't be due to a substance or other medical condition. *Treatment* involves psychotherapy and SSRIs (sertraline or paroxetine). Medical treatment can vary, depending on the predominant symptom a patient is experiencing (e.g., prazosin for insomnia).

Mood Disorders

Bipolar Disorder

Bipolar disorders are chronic and characterized by **mood swings** that range from **major depression to mania**. The severity of the disorder varies among patients, but it usually greatly affects a person's life. The exact cause of bipolar disorders is unknown, but a positive family history, imbalances in the brain's neurotransmitters, and some environmental factors may play a role in its development. It can be classified as **bipolar I** (must have 1 manic episode with a hypomanic or major depressive episode), **bipolar II** (at least 1 hypomanic and 1 major depressive episode), and **cyclothymic disorder** (2 years of hypomanic and depressive "periods," not episodes). **Rapid cycling** refers to 4 or more mood episodes in a year; and bipolar I or II can have mixed features. The "**low**" points of bipolar disorder cause the classic symptoms of major depression (must be present in the same 2 week period and have ≥5, with at least 1 of the 1st 2 symptoms, to be classified as a major depressive episode): anhedonia, depressed mood most of the day, fatigue, sleep disturbances, psychomotor restriction or agitation, decreased concentration/ability to think or indecisiveness, weight loss or gain, feelings of worthlessness or guilt, and suicidal ideation or an attempt. The "**high**" points occur during the manic phase (symptoms must be present for 1 week) and include (must have ≥3 to be classified as a manic episode): restlessness, racing thoughts, distractibility, lack of sleep, agitation or increase in goal-centered activities, pressured speech, inflated self-esteem (grandiosity), and increased involvement in high-risk activities. It is termed **hypomania** if ≥3 of the above manic symptoms last for 4 consecutive days. Medical *treatment* depends on the main symptoms and includes mood stabilizers (lithium is first line), antipsychotics (haloperidol, risperidone), anti-anxiety (lorazepam, clonazepam), anticonvulsants (carbamazepine, valproate), and antidepressants (may heighten mania or suicide risk). Also include psychotherapy and ongoing monitoring.

Major Depressive Disorder

Major depressive disorder (**MDD**) is a condition in which a depressed mood and/or anhedonia are present for most of the day for 2 weeks (usually lasts longer) and greatly affect a patient's ability to function. This affects women more than men and usually presents in adolescence or young adult years. At least 5 of the following *symptoms* must be present in the same 2 week period, with at least 1 of the 1st two symptoms, to be classified as MDD: anhedonia, depressed mood most of the day, fatigue, sleep disturbances, psychomotor restriction or agitation, decreased concentration/ability to think or indecisiveness, weight loss or gain, feelings of worthlessness or guilt, and suicidal ideation or an attempt. Certain specifiers can be added to the *diagnosis* including with anxious distress, mixed features, melancholic features, psychotic features, catatonic features, peripartum onset, and seasonal pattern. Major depressive disorder has the specifiers of:

- With anxious distress
- With melancholic features
- With peripartum onset
- With seasonal pattern
- With psychotic features (mood congruent or mood incongruent)
- With catatonia
- With atypical features
- With mixed features

Clinicians should screen for depression and there are multiple screening questionnaires including the Beck Depression Inventory (BDI), Patient Health Questionnaire-9 (PHQ-9), and the Zung Self-Rating Depression Scale. On physical exam patients often have a normal appearance, but may have poor grooming and hygiene as the symptoms worsen. Patients often have a flat affect and speech may be slow or monotone. Rule out other causes of the symptoms including drug-induced depression or other conditions. MDD is usually *treated* with both psychotherapy and medication. SSRI's are typically first line and other antidepressants include SNRI's, tricyclics, and MAOI's. If drugs are ineffective, ECT (electroconvulsive therapy) or phototherapy (for seasonal pattern) may be used.

Review Video: Major Depression
Visit mometrix.com/academy and enter code: 632694

Persistent Depressive Disorder

Persistent depressive disorder (dysthymia) is a **DSM-5-TR diagnosis** that combines the previous DSM diagnoses of **chronic major depressive disorder and dysthymia**. This usually has an insidious onset in childhood, adolescence, or young adulthood (referred to as early onset if diagnosed before 21 years old). The causes include a positive family history, imbalances in the neurotransmitters in the brain, and possibly environmental factors, such as tragedy in one's life. Patients are at an increased risk of personality disorders, anxiety disorders, and substance abuse. Depression is a common illness, and most patients experience more than one major depressive episode in a lifetime. But patients with persistent depressive disorder have **continuous depressive symptoms** for ≥2 years (≥1 year in children/adolescents) for most of the day and for more days than not. Plus ≥2 of the following symptoms: decreased appetite or overeating, insomnia or hypersomnia, decreased energy/fatigue, low self-esteem, decreased concentration or a hard time making decisions, feeling hopeless. This is chronic, can be debilitating, and can be difficult to treat. *Treatment* includes a combination of psychotherapy and antidepressant medications (SSRI's). In-patient treatment may be necessary in those contemplating suicide. *It should be noted that suicide rates tend to be higher in patients as they are "coming out of" a major depressive episode, when their mood and outlook on life seem to be improving.*

Postpartum Major Depression

Postpartum depression is defined as a significant episode of depression occurring in the postpartum period. It is extremely common in up to 10% of postpartum women. The onset can be anywhere from one day to several months post-delivery. Postpartum major depression must be distinguished from "baby blues," which is a mild transient form of postpartum depression that generally begins about 4 days following delivery and resolves by day 10. The diagnosis is generally made clinically after a thorough psychiatric evaluation. Treatment options include counseling and antidepressant medications. Selective serotonin reuptake inhibitors (SSRIs) and tricyclic antidepressants (TCAs) can be used; however, they are excreted into the breast milk, and therefore caution should be used with breast-feeding mothers. Complications include postpartum psychosis. This affects approximately 0.2% of postpartum women. Postpartum psychosis increases the risk of the mother harming herself or her baby and is a psychiatric emergency.

ADD/ADHD

Diagnostic Criteria

Attention deficit hyperactivity disorder (ADHD) can be diagnosed if a child displays at least six symptoms of inattention or hyperactivity-impulsivity in more than one setting (e.g., home, school). Their onset must be before the age of 12, and the symptoms must have persisted for at least 6 months.

Inattentiveness Symptoms (must have six for diagnosis in children)	Impulsivity/Hyperactivity Symptoms (must have six for diagnosis in children)
• Forgetful in everyday activities • Easily distracted (often) • Makes careless mistakes and does not give attention to detail • Difficulty focusing attention • Does not appear to listen, even when directly spoken to • Starts tasks but does not follow through • Frequently loses essential items • Finds organizing difficult • Avoids activities that require prolonged mental exertion	• Frequently gets out of chair • Runs or climbs at inappropriate times • Frequently talks more than peers • Often moves hands and feet or shifts position in seat • Frequently interrupts others • Frequently has difficulty waiting on turn • Frequently unable to enjoy leisure activities silently • Frequently "on the go" and seen by others as restless • Often finishes other's sentences before they can

Subtypes

There are three subtypes of ADHD:

- **Predominantly inattentive type** is diagnosed when a child has six or more symptoms of inattention and fewer than six symptoms of hyperactivity-impulsivity.
- **Predominantly hyperactive-impulsive type** is diagnosed when there are six or more symptoms of hyperactivity-impulsivity and fewer than six symptoms of inattention.
- **Combined type** is diagnosed when there are six or more symptoms of both hyperactivity-impulsivity and inattention.

Prevalence

Worldwide, ADHD occurs in just more than 7% of children and 2.5% of adults. Males are more likely to receive the diagnosis than females, with a **2:1 male-to-female ratio** among children. Females are more likely to present as predominantly inattentive, and many females are underidentified and underdiagnosed. The rates of ADHD among adults appear to be about equal for males and females.

Prognosis and Etiology

The behavior of children with ADHD is likely to remain consistent until **early adolescence**, when some may experience diminished overactivity but continue to exhibit attention and concentration problems. Adolescents with ADHD are much more likely to participate in antisocial behaviors and engage in substance use. More than half of all children who are diagnosed with ADHD will carry the diagnosis through to adulthood. Adults with ADHD are more susceptible to divorce, work-related trouble, accidents, depression, substance abuse, and antisocial behavior. Children with ADHD who are co-diagnosed with conduct disorder are especially likely to have these problems later in life.

There is significant evidence suggesting that ADHD is a **genetic disorder**. ADHD occurs at a slightly higher rate among biological relatives than among the general population, and there are higher rates among identical twins, rather than fraternal twins. However, like many neurodevelopmental disorders, ADHD can be attributed to a combination of genetics, environment, and epigenetics.

ADHD is associated with structural abnormalities in the brain, such as subnormal activity in the frontal cortex and basal ganglia and a relatively small caudate nucleus, globus pallidus, and prefrontal cortex. Prenatal care also contributes to ADHD. Children exposed to alcohol and nicotine in utero have higher instances of ADHD, as well as those with viral infections and nutritional deficiencies.

TREATMENT

Treatment for ADHD is a combination of behavioral therapy and medication. Children with ADHD tend to exhibit trouble in school because executive functioning interferes with planning and organization and their impulsivity and inattention interfere with focusing and retaining information. This is compounded by low frustration tolerance, lability, and difficulty with peers. Research has consistently shown that **pharmacotherapy** works best when it is combined with **psychosocial intervention**. Many teachers use basic elements of **classroom management (e.g., behavioral modification)** to assist children with ADHD. This involves providing clear guidelines and contingencies for behavior so that students do not have to speculate on what will happen in class or what they should be doing. Treatment is most effective with **parental involvement.**

Stimulants and nonstimulant medications are the pharmacologic therapies approved for ADHD. Somewhat counterintuitively, central nervous system stimulants such as **methylphenidate (Ritalin)** and **amphetamine (Dexedrine)** control the symptoms of ADHD. Side effects include headaches, gastrointestinal upset, anorexia, sleep difficulty, anxiety, depression, blood sugar increases, blood pressure increases, tics, and seizures.

Nonstimulant medication options include antidepressants (e.g., atomoxetine, bupropion) and alpha agonists (e.g., clonidine, guanfacine). The trigeminal nerve stimulation system is a US Food and Drug Administration (FDA)-approved nonpharmacological treatment effective in children with mild to moderate symptoms and those whose primary symptoms involve executive functioning impairments.

AUTISM SPECTRUM DISORDER

Autism spectrum disorder is a **neurodevelopment disorder** in which there are **deficits in social interaction and communication** as well as **restricted or repetitive behaviors** that significantly affect how patients interact and function. This appears in early childhood and affects boys more than girls. The cause is unknown but may be affected by genetics, prenatal/obstetric complications (e.g., congenital rubella), and toxic exposure.

There are two categories of symptoms necessary for a diagnosis of autism spectrum disorder (ASD). The first category is **deficits in social interaction and social communication**, which include:

- Absence of developmentally appropriate peer relationships
- Lack of social or emotional reciprocity
- Marked impairment in nonverbal behavior
- Delay or lack of development in spoken language
- Marked impairment in the ability to initiate or sustain conversation
- Stereotyped or repetitive use of language or idiosyncratic language
- Lack of developmentally appropriate play

The other category of symptoms necessary for diagnosis of ASD is **restricted, repetitive patterns of behavior, interests, and activities**. These include:

- Preoccupation with one or more stereotyped and restricted patterns of interest
- Inflexible adherence to nonfunctional routines or rituals
- Stereotyped and repetitive motor mannerisms
- Persistent preoccupation with the parts of objects

OCD and Related Disorders

Obsessive-compulsive disorder (**OCD**) is a condition, according to the DMS-5-TR, in which a person has **intrusive and unwanted obsessions** (recurrent and persistent urges, thoughts, or images) and/or **compulsions** that compel them to perform repeated activities or mental acts (e.g., counting, praying) that must be rigidly followed and completing it allows them to lower their anxiety and stress levels. These obsessions and compulsions cause distress (patients try to suppress or neutralize the obsession with a thought or action), are time-consuming (>1 hour/day), and interfere with their daily lives. Examples of obsessions include fear of contamination, desire for safety, forbidden or aggressive thoughts including harm to self or others, and needing symmetry or order. The condition frequently begins during adolescence, affects males and females equally, and may be due to several factors including environmental (e.g., abuse, traumatic events), genetic, and low serotonin levels may also play a role. There is some research that indicates there may be a link between Group A streptococcal infections and OCD. Excessive stress can worsen OCD. *Treatment* is psychotherapy (e.g., cognitive behavior therapy), and SSRI antidepressants (e.g., Prozac, Paxil®, Zoloft®) or clomipramine (a tricyclic with serotonergic effects). These medications help to elevate serotonin levels in the brain. OCD patients are at an increased risk of suicide. Other OCD-related disorders include: body dysmorphic disorder, hoarding d/o, trichotillomania, and excoriation d/o.

Dissociative and Personality Disorders

Dissociative Disorders

Dissociative disorders are a group of disorders, according to the DSM-5-TR, in which there is a disruption/discontinuity in the way people normally **integrate** consciousness, identity, memory or perception, their body representation, motor control, emotions, and their behavior. These usually appear due to **intense trauma** in a person's life. These disorders include: **dissociative identity disorder** (formerly multiple personality disorder; usually due to extreme trauma in childhood), **dissociative amnesia** (autobiographic memories are forgotten usually surrounding a traumatic event), and **depersonalization/ derealization disorder** (disordered perception usually due to severe stress). All of these dissociative disorders may not be due to a substance, other medical condition (e.g., seizures), or other mental disorder that better describes the symptoms. These patients are at a high risk of self-harm and suicide. These are clinical *diagnoses* and *treatment* involves psychotherapy (sometimes medications for symptoms) and it is important that patients feel safe.

Paranoid Personality Disorder

Paranoid personality disorder is characterized by **odd or eccentric behavior** that interferes with daily living due to a **pervasive distrust/suspicion of others**, and so interpret others' motives as bad. There may be a genetic component to this disorder and environmental factors, such as a history of child abuse or neglect, may also play a role in developing this disorder. *Symptoms* of paranoid personality disorder include 4 or more of the following: without proper evidence they suspect that others are out to harm, exploit, or deceive them; preoccupied with doubts that people are untrustworthy or disloyal; reluctant to confide in others due to fear that the information will be used against them; reads hidden meanings in innocuous comments or events; unforgiving/bears grudges; quick to angrily react to perceives attacks on their character and then counterattacks; have recurring suspicions about the faithfulness of their spouse/partner. This personality pattern begins by early adulthood, is chronic, goes against the social norm, and is present in all settings (socially and work). These patients may find criticism in even the most innocent remark, have difficulty maintaining healthy relationships, and do not work well with others. *Treatment* of paranoid personality disorder is with a combination of psychotherapy (cognitive-behavior therapy, group therapy) and sometimes medications (antidepressants, antianxiety, and antipsychotics may be helpful in controlling some of the symptoms. Therapy can be difficult because of patients' inability to form trusting relationships with therapists.

Schizoid Personality Disorder

Schizoid personality disorder is a condition in which people are **detached, withdraw from society, have difficulty expressing emotions, and avoid interaction with others**. This affects males slightly more than females and usually appears before adolescence and definitely by young adulthood. They often find relationships too distressing and feel more comfortable when they are isolated. The cause is thought to be genetic. *Symptoms* of schizoid personality disorder include ≥4 of the following: doesn't enjoy or desire close relationships (e.g., being part of a family); prefers solitary activities; little to no interest in sexual activities with others; little to no pleasure in activities; lack close friends (except maybe a 1st degree relative); indifference to praise or criticism; emotionally cold, have a flat affect, show very little emotion, or are detached. These patients may be poor students and seem to have no direction in life. Psychotherapy is the mainstay of treatment with schizoid personality disorder. This is focused on developing social skills and helping patients find pleasure from interacting with others. Medications may be used to help treat some of the concomitant symptoms of depression or anxiety. This is difficult to *treat* since patients lack interest in others, and therefore, have little desire to change.

Schizotypal Personality Disorder

Schizotypal personality disorder is a chronic condition in which people **isolate themselves from social situations** because of extreme anxiety when interacting with others due to **distortions in their perceptions and thinking**. The main risk factor is a family history of schizophrenia and patients are at increased risk of major depressive disorder and substance abuse. *Symptoms* of schizotypal personality disorder include ≥5 of the following: ideas of reference (interpret ordinary events as having special meaning); odd beliefs, superstitions, magical thinking, or powers (e.g., mental telepathy...); experience unusual perceptions; odd thinking and speech; suspicious or paranoid ideation; inappropriate and restricted facial expressions; odd/eccentric appearing behavior; lack close friends (except for 1st degree relatives)/ have problems relating with others; anxious in social settings/ social anxiety/ have paranoid fears about the intentions of others. Stress can cause brief psychotic episodes but only last minutes to hours and therefore, does not meet diagnostic criteria for a psychotic disorder. *Treatment* is with a combination of psychotherapy (cognitive behavior therapy and skills training) and medications (atypical antipsychotics may help to relieve some of the symptoms of this condition as well as antidepressants). Therapy can be difficult because of patients' inability to develop trusting relationships with therapists.

Antisocial Personality Disorder

Antisocial personality disorder is a pervasive pattern of **disregard for the rights of others and society's rules**, so they often repeatedly break the law, lie, cheat, steal, or harm others. The condition is often noticed during the teenage years and symptoms tend to decrease as a person approaches middle age. It is much more common in males, has a genetic component, and may develop in those who suffer child abuse or neglect especially if they already have conduct disorder. They are at an increased risk of other personality disorders (e.g., narcissistic, borderline), suicide, substance abuse, pathologic gambling, and becoming homicidal. *Symptoms* include ≥3 of the following (these symptoms must be present by 15 years old, however this cannot be *diagnosed* until 18 y/o): fails to conform to societal norms by repeatedly breaking the law; repeated deceitfulness/lying/conning others; impulsiveness/doesn't plan ahead; irritable and aggressive/ often gets into fights/assaults; reckless disregard for the safety of self or others; and lacks remorse. They don't like to be bored, are often poor parents, and are frequently imprisoned for their actions.

Oftentimes, these people appear to be charming at first. Antisocial personality disorder is very hard to *treat* and controversy surrounds if it is even a treatable condition. A combination of psychotherapy (cognitive behavior therapy) with antidepressants (SSRIs) or mood stabilizers (lithium, valproate) may help to control some of the symptoms (e.g., aggressiveness).

Borderline Personality Disorder

Borderline personality disorder is a condition in which a person is **unstable in their relationships, self-image, and mood**, and are **impulsive**. They are constantly in a **conflicting state** in which they cannot regulate their emotions. This condition is much more prevalent in women (75%), begins by young adult years, and is thought to occur due to a combination of genetics and environment (e.g., child abuse or neglect is common). They are at an increased risk of suicide and comorbid conditions like bipolar d/o, bulimia, substance abuse, and other personality disorders. *Symptoms* of borderline personality disorder must include ≥5 of the following (DSM-5-TR): frantic efforts to avoid abandonment, either real or imagined; unstable and intense relationships that oscillate between idealizing the person and then devaluing them; unstable self-image; impulsive in at least 2 areas that can be harmful (e.g., substance abuse, overspending, reckless driving); recurrent suicidal or self-mutilating behaviors; reactive mood and affect; chronically feel empty; difficulty controlling anger or angry outbursts; temporary paranoid ideation or dissociative symptoms that are related to stress. The rollercoaster of mood swings makes relationships very difficult; they may be happy with their life situation one day and hate it the next, and they frequently change jobs. *Treatment* of borderline personality disorder is with a combination of various forms of psychotherapy and medications. Mood stabilizers (lamotrigine, topiramate), atypical antipsychotics, and SSRI's may help control some of the symptoms. Do not use benzodiazepines in these patients since they are prone to substance abuse and overdose. Hospitalization is necessary if patients are at imminent risk of harming themselves.

Histrionic Personality Disorder

Histrionic personality disorder is a condition in which a person is **extremely emotional and attention seeking**. The condition seems to be similar or slightly more common in women than men, and the cause is not completely understood though it may be due to a combination of genetic and environmental factors. This appears by early adulthood and they are at an increased risk of comorbid somatoform disorders and major depressive disorder. *Symptoms* of histrionic personality disorder are present in a variety of settings and include ≥5 of the following (DSM-5-TR): they are uncomfortable when they are not the center of attention; often act provocatively towards others; rapidly changing and shallow emotions; use their appearance to draw attention to themselves; speech lacks details; expresses emotions in a dramatic, theatric, and over-the-top way; suggestible and easily influenced by others or by their circumstances; they consider relationships more intimate than they truly are. *Treatment* of histrionic personality disorder is usually with psychotherapy, but this can be difficult since patients may exaggerate symptoms and form inappropriate attachments to the therapist. Antidepressants and antianxiety medications may help with possible comorbid conditions.

Narcissistic Personality Disorder

Narcissistic personality disorder is a condition in which people feel that they are **superior to others, need to be admired, and have no regard for others**. It occurs more frequently in males than females, symptoms often become evident in early adulthood, and they are at an increased risk of comorbid depressive disorders, substance abuse, and other personality disorders. Narcissistic personality disorder may be caused by multiple factors (neurobiologic and environment), but is not yet understood.

Symptoms of narcissistic personality disorder occur in a variety of situations and must include ≥5 of the following (DSM-5-TR): grandiose sense of self-importance; preoccupied with fantasies of unlimited success, power, influence, intellectual superiority, beauty, or ideal/perfect love; believe they are special and can only truly be understood by those who are equally special (e.g., high-status); needs to be excessively admired; entitled; exploits others; lacks empathy for others; envies or thinks others envy him/her; has arrogant or haughty attitudes or actions. Criticism from others can be devastating, but these patients will often put down those who do not praise them or counterattack. They belittle others and have difficulty maintaining healthy relationships since take advantage of others to get what they want. The primary treatment for narcissistic personality disorder is psychotherapy. If there is underlying depression or anxiety, medications to treat these conditions may be helpful.

Avoidant Personality Disorder

Avoidant personality disorder is a condition in which a person feels **inadequate** and so is very anxious or fearful of **social situations where they may be criticized**. The cause is not fully understood, but social, biological/genetic, temperament (e.g., shy and fearful), and environmental factors may play a role in the development of this disorder. This occurs equally in males and females, begins by early adulthood, and they have an increased risk of depressive, anxiety, bipolar, and dependent personality disorder. *Symptoms* must include ≥4 of the following (DSM-5): avoids work-related activities due to fears they will be criticized or rejected; avoids relationships with others unless they think they will be liked; is restrained in intimate relationships due to fear of being shamed or ridiculed; preoccupied with thoughts of being criticized/rejected in social settings; inhibited in new social situations due to feeling inadequate; has low self-esteem/feels inferior; doesn't want to be embarrassed so is reluctant to take risks/be a part of new activities. *Treat* with a combination of psychotherapy and antidepressants or antianxiety meds.

Dependent Personality Disorder

Dependent personality disorder is a condition where there is an **extreme need to be cared for**, which causes patients to be **submissive and overly clingy**. It may be slightly more common in women, appears by early adulthood, and there is an increased risk for anxiety and adjustment disorder. ≥5 of the following must be present (DSM-5): can't make decisions on their own; need others to be responsible for most parts of their life; find it hard to disagree with others; has a hard time initiating things on their own; go to great lengths to get other's support; feel helpless and fearful of being alone since they don't think they can care for themselves; seeks relationships with people who will care for them; preoccupied with fears of being alone and unable to care for themselves. *Treatment* primarily involves psychotherapy (cognitive behavior therapy) and sometimes antidepressants (SSRI's). Therapists need to be careful not to encourage dependent attachments of the patient.

Obsessive-Compulsive Personality Disorder

Obsessive-compulsive personality disorder is a persistent preoccupation with organization and mental or interpersonal control. At least four of the following symptoms are required for diagnosis of obsessive-compulsive personality disorder:

- Preoccupation with rules and details
- Perfectionism that interferes with progress
- Excessive devotion to work
- Counterproductive rigidity about beliefs and morality
- Inability to throw away old objects
- Reluctance to delegate authority to others
- Rigid or stubborn
- Hoards money without spending

Delusional Disorder

Delusional disorder is a condition in which a person develops a very **strong, fixed belief** (delusion; must be present ≥1 month) in a specific situation that is **not true**, to the point that they alter their behaviors and life around this idea. However, there are no psychotic symptoms as in schizophrenia. This disorder may be caused by a combination of environmental or genetic factors though no specific cause is understood. Delusional disorder can take different forms. Patients may have **delusions of grandeur** (*grandiose type*), believing that they are above everyone else and in a much higher standing than they really are. They may have **persecutory delusions** (*persecutory type*) that others are out to hurt, cheat, spy on, or conspire against them. They may have a belief that **someone is in love with them** (*erotomanic type*) or that their **partner is unfaithful to them** (*jealous type*). They may also have delusions that **something is wrong with their body** like an odor or a sensation that bugs are crawling on them or they have an infection (*somatic type*) when there is nothing medically wrong. *Treatment* can be challenging since many don't go seek medical help since they don't think anything is wrong; but may include a combination of supportive psychotherapy and medications (antidepressants and antipsychotics may help to control the symptoms). Treatment can be difficult since patients firmly believe in their delusions; therefore, the medical provider must work to develop an alliance with the patient.

Schizophrenia and Schizoaffective Disorders

Schizophrenia

Schizophrenia is a chronic disorder where there is the presence of ≥2 of the following and at least 1 of the first 3 (most of the time in a 1-month period): delusions; hallucinations; disorganized speech; grossly disorganized/ bizarre or catatonic behavior; negative symptoms like reduced expression of emotions. These psychotic *symptoms* (delusions and hallucinations) greatly affect how patients function. Signs of the disturbance are present for ≥6 months and can include the certain stages of schizophrenia (prodromal, active phase, residual periods). This condition usually appears in late adolescence and affects males and females equally. *Treatment* includes antipsychotics (1st generation (cause extrapyramidal side effects): haloperidol, chlorpromazine; 2nd generation (cause weight gain and glucose/lipid issues): clozapine. Early treatment is key. Suicide risk is increased in this.

Schizoaffective Disorder

Schizoaffective disorder is a combination of **schizophrenic symptoms** (≥2 schizophrenic symptoms) with **mood symptoms** (either major depressive or manic). These patients may have hallucinations and delusions with depression or mania; specify if patient is bipolar type or depressive type). The cause is unknown but may be due to imbalances of brain neurotransmitters. *Symptoms* may become severe enough that patients can be at risk for harming themselves or others. Treatment consists of a combination of psychotherapy and medications to control the symptoms. Antidepressants (SSRI's) and antipsychotics in depressive types; mood stabilizers (e.g., lithium, carbamazepine, valproic acid) and antipsychotics in manic types. Hospitalization may be necessary for in-patient treatment, especially if patients are at risk of hurting themselves or others.

Eating Disorders

Anorexia Nervosa

Anorexia nervosa is an **eating disorder** in which patients have a considerably **below normal body weight** due to food intake that's under the necessary requirements, an intense fear of weight gain/being fat, and misperceptions of their body weight and/or shape. Patients avoid eating, exercise a lot, purge, and some even binge then purge. This usually affects adolescent females. The cause is complex and not completely understood, but there is a genetic component. Those at higher risk include those with perfectionistic or obsessive tendencies, low self-esteem, a positive family history, conflict resolution difficulties, and a difficulty expressing negative emotions. Patients are at a higher risk of having OCD tendencies, bipolar disorder, depressive disorders, and anxiety disorders. On physical exam the patient may appear emaciated and have orthostatic hypotension, bradycardia, hypothermia, dry skin, thinning or brittle hair and nails. Amenorrhea and osteopenia may be present, and cardiac dysrhythmias often develop which increases mortality and the risk of sudden death. Lab results can show anemia, decreased WBC, decreased platelets, increased LFT's, hypoglycemia, hyponatremia, hypochloremia, hypokalemia, increased blood urea nitrogen (BUN), and either acidosis (from overusing laxatives) or alkalosis (from vomiting). Patients may need to be admitted to closely monitor while refeeding is slowly started; and treatment also includes various forms of psychotherapy to help patients develop a better self-image and learn healthy coping methods. Medication is typically only used for medical complications, but SSRI's may help with some of the anorexia symptoms. Close medical monitoring is necessary to detect any possible life-threatening effects of anorexia.

Bulimia Nervosa

Bulimia nervosa is an **eating disorder** characterized by episodes of **binging and purging**. Patients feel out of control and eat excessive amounts over a certain timeframe (2-hour period) then compensate through activities like inducing vomiting, over-exercising, or using laxatives/diuretics. The DSM-5-TR states that this must occur once a week for most weeks over a 3-month period to be diagnosed. This usually affects adolescent or young adult females. It is not entirely clear what causes bulimia, but a family history of eating disorders, along with a low self-esteem, anxiousness, depressive symptoms, and concerns over weight can contribute. Also, there are links between bulimia and low levels of the endogenous opioid beta-endorphin and the neurotransmitters serotonin and norepinephrine. Patients with bulimia are at an increased risk of having other mental disorders. Suicide risk is increased in both anorexia and bulimia nervosa. Patients with bulimia usually appear normal in size to overweight and may have bilateral parotid gland enlargement. A positive Russell sign (callouses or scarring on the knuckles from inducing vomiting), esophagitis, and dental caries or dental erosion (especially noted on the front teeth) can occur because of damage from stomach acids during vomiting. Dehydration, hypotension, electrolyte abnormalities (hypokalemia, hyponatremia, hypochloremia), metabolic alkalosis (vomiting), metabolic acidosis (laxative and diuretic abuse), and cardiac dysrhythmias may also occur and may be life-threatening. *Treatment* often involves **CBT techniques** such as self-monitoring, stimulus control, cognitive restructuring, problem solving, and self-distraction. Some antidepressants, such as imipramine, have been effective at reducing instances of binging and purging.

Nervous System and Special Senses

Nervous System Disorders

Cranial Nerves I-VI, Their Function, and Physical Exam Test(s) That Check for Each CN

	Name	Function	PE Test
I	Olfactory	Smell	Test olfaction
II	Optic	Visual acuity	Snellen eye chart; Accommodation
III	Oculomotor	Eye movement/ pupil	Pupillary reflex; Eye/eyelid motion
IV	Trochlear	Eye movement	Eye moves down & out
V	Trigeminal	Facial motor/ sensory	Corneal reflex; Facial sensation; Mastication
VI	Abducens	Eye movement	Lateral eye motion
VII	Facial	Facial expression; Taste	Moves forehead, closes eyes, smile/frown, puffs cheeks; Taste
VIII	Vestibulo-cochlear (Acoustic)	Hearing; Balance	Hearing (Weber/Rinne tests); Nystagmus
IX	Glosso-pharyngeal	Pharynx motor/sensory	Gag reflex; Soft palate elevation
X	Vagus	Visceral sensory, motor	Gag, swallow, cough
XI	Accessory	Sternocleidomastoid and trapezius (motor)	Turns head & shrugs shoulders against resistance
XII	Hypoglossal	Tongue movement	Sticks out tongue

Cluster Headaches

Cluster headaches are a type of **trigeminal-autonomic cephalgias** (TACs) that are characterized by periods of severe unilateral orbital/periorbital or temporal pain with ipsilateral autonomic symptoms (e.g., lacrimation or conjunctival injection, rhinorrhea, miosis, ptosis) that occur frequently, perhaps for a few days or months, and then go into remission without headaches for a period of time. They can be classified as **episodic** (last 7 days to 1 year with pain-free periods lasting ≥3 months) or **chronic** (last ≥1 year without remissions or remissions <3 months). There is no definite known cause of cluster headaches though dysfunction of the **hypothalamus** may play a role. They are more common in males over 30 years old who are heavy drinkers and smokers. Cluster headache triggers may also include nitroglycerine, temperature extremes, and histamine. These headaches last for 15-180 minutes and may recur from 8 times a day to every other day. Patients will not have an aura before the headache. Cluster headaches are extremely severe, described as a stabbing or sharp pain, and are more likely to occur at night or in the early morning. Patients are restless and prefer to pace rather than lie still. Patients may describe nasal congestion at the time of the headache, possibly with swelling around the eyes. *Diagnose* clinically. Abortive first-line *treatment* includes 100% oxygen, triptans (Imitrex®, injection or nasal spray), or ergot alkaloids (e.g., dihydroergotamine). Some patients respond well to lidocaine administered nasally. Also, short-term use of corticosteroids and occipital nerve injections may help with episodes. Preventative first-line treatment includes the Ca^{++} channel blocker verapamil and the mood stabilizer lithium. Anticonvulsants (e.g., Depakote®) may also help with prevention.

Tension Headaches

Tension headaches, now referred to as tension-type headaches (**TTH**). are the most common type of headache and are described as a **generalized, mild to moderate headache** that does not become worse with regular physical activity. It can be classified as **episodic** (frequent or infrequent) or **chronic**. It was previously thought to be mostly due to muscle contractions, but now is believed to result from many factors. Stress and poor sleep may affect these headaches. Patients will describe bilateral head pain that usually feels like a band squeezing around the skull and may report difficulty concentrating. The pain typically starts towards the frontal or occipital regions and then spreads to the whole head. There can be muscular tightness and pain in the neck or upper back. There is no prodrome and no N/V or light or sound sensitivity. *Diagnose* clinically. The neuro exam will be normal. NSAIDs (ibuprofen is usually the first choice) and other pain relievers may help as well as relaxation techniques. Decreasing stress, sufficient sleep, and other lifestyle changes like avoiding alcohol and caffeine and quitting smoking may help control chronic TTH. Excessive use of NSAIDs can contribute to medication overuse headaches (rebound headaches) and GI bleeds. Other *complications* include dependence on narcotic meds or those containing caffeine, and patients with tension-type headaches are 4 times more likely to be diagnosed with epilepsy.

Migraine Headaches

Migraine headaches are moderate to severe usually unilateral and throbbing headaches with nausea, photophobia, and phonophobia that recur and becomes worse with regular physical activity. They can be classified as **migraines w/o aura** (previously common migraine), **migraines with aura** (previously classic migraine), or **chronic migraines**. These are fairly common, have a genetic component, and occur much more frequently in women. Several factors may trigger a migraine: changes in hormone levels during the menstrual cycle, stress, sleep disturbances, weather changes, smoking, red wine, MSG, and caffeine. Patients may describe a prodrome hours to a day or 2 before the migraine begins (e.g., fatigue, irritability, nausea, yawning). About 25% of patients describe an aura which usually starts before the migraine begins, but may occur after it starts. The aura lasts from minutes to an hour and is usually visual (flashes of light, dark spots, scotomas, bright zigzag lines), but may include a tingling sensation or other sensory/motor symptoms. The headache is severe, usually unilateral, throbbing, and may be accompanied by photophobia, phonophobia, or N/V. They typically last for 4-72 hours, and patients prefer being in a dark and quiet room. The postdrome (fatigue, mood changes) lasts about 24-48 hours after the migraine has resolved. *Diagnose* clinically; neuro exam is typically normal. Rule out other disorders that may mimic a migraine (e.g., ruptured brain aneurysm or SAH if a "thunderclap" headache, dissecting carotid artery, cancer, meningitis, giant cell arteritis). Triptan medications at the 1st sign of a migraine can help to abort it or lower the pain intensity and help in moderate to severe cases. Pain relievers (i.e. NSAIDs, Tylenol®, or ASA if mild), ergot medications, and anti-emetics can also help. Prophylactic meds, such as β-blockers and antiepileptics can also help to lower the incidence of migraines. *Complications* include seizures and strokes.

Delirium

Delirium is an acute, usually reversible **decline in mental function** due to a medical condition, substance, or withdrawal that causes the disturbance in attention, awareness, and cognition. This state fluctuates during the day and can be due to multiple factors.

Risk factors for delirium include but are not limited to older age, diabetes, underlying brain conditions (e.g., stroke), human immunodeficiency virus (HIV), renal impairment, and substance or medication withdrawal. Delirium may be caused by systemic infection or toxins, metabolic disorders, postoperative states, head trauma, and immobility.

There are **three types** of delirium:

- **Hyperactive**—increased psychomotor activity (e.g., agitation, restlessness)
- **Hypoactive**—decreased psychomotor activity (e.g., stupor, slowness, extreme fatigue)
- **Mixed**—normal or rapidly changing psychomotor activity

MAJOR AND MILD NEUROCOGNITIVE DISORDERS

Cognitive decline is divided into major and mild neurocognitive disorders in the DSM-5-TR. Specifiers for major and mild neurocognitive disorder should include severity (mild, moderate, or severe), cause (Alzheimer's disease, frontotemporal degeneration, Lewy body disease, vascular disease, traumatic brain injury, HIV, substance/medication use, prion disease, Parkinson's disease, Huntington's disease, or another medical condition/etiology), and whether it is with or without behavioral disturbance.

MAJOR NEUROCOGNITIVE DISORDER

Individuals with major neurocognitive disorder find it difficult to independently manage activities of daily living due to a **substantial decline** in cognitive functioning. Clinicians can better understand a client's cognitive functioning from informant reports, such as those received from significant others, family members, or caretakers. The impairment can also be determined by a comprehensive clinical assessment, such as the Mini-Mental State Examination, or standardized testing, including the Montreal Cognitive Assessment. This diagnosis cannot occur in the presence of delirium or must not be better explained by another mental disorder.

Individuals with major neurocognitive disorder exhibit **cognitive deficits**, including memory impairment, aphasia, apraxia, agnosia, or impaired executive functioning. Depending on the etiology of the neurocognitive disorders, these deficits may remain stable or may become progressively worse. There may be a decrease in **language skills,** specifically manifested in an inability to recall the names of people or things. Individuals may also need help performing routine motor programs, and they may be unable to recognize familiar people and places. Abstract thinking, planning, and initiating complex behaviors may also be challenging.

MILD NEUROCOGNITIVE DISORDER

The diagnosis of mild neurocognitive disorder is marked by a **modest decline** in cognitive functioning. Individuals with mild neurocognitive disorder exhibit moderate difficulty with memory, planning, organization, attention, learning, or processing social cues. However, these difficulties are often managed with the use of **compensatory strategies**, such as keeping a written schedule, the use of mnemonics, assistance with organization, and related accommodations. Much like the diagnostic criteria for major neurocognitive disorder, the decline can be measured by an informant's report, a comprehensive clinical assessment, or standardized testing. The deficits cannot occur in the context of delirium, nor can they be better explained by another mental disorder.

Individuals with neurocognitive disorders, such as those caused by Alzheimer's disease, could have **anterograde** and **retrograde amnesia**, meaning that they find it difficult to learn new information and recall previously learned information. Clinicians must be careful when differentiating between other forms of amnesia, such as those caused by trauma, transient global amnesia, and dissociative amnesia. Other forms of amnesia will generally improve over time or when underlying causes are addressed. Delirium, major depressive disorder, and learning disorders also serve as differential diagnoses.

MENINGITIS

Meningitis is an infection of the **meninges** that surround the **brain and spinal cord**. It is most often due to a **virus** which is self-limited but can be fatal if a **bacterium** is the cause. It may also be due to a fungus, parasite, amoeba, or noninfectious cause (e.g., cancer, medication). It is referred to as **aseptic meningitis** when a source cannot be found (usually due to a virus). According to the CDC, the most common bacterial cause is *Streptococcus pneumoniae* which may especially affect the young and elderly. In newborns, Group B *Streptococcus* is a common cause in that 1st week. **Meningococcal meningitis** is caused by the bacteria *Neisseria meningitidis*, most often affects 16-23-year-olds, and is known to cause outbreaks on college campuses. *H. influenzae* type b and *Listeria monocytogenes* may also cause meningitis. Common viral causes include: non-polio enteroviruses (most common), measles, mumps, influenza, arboviruses (e.g., West Nile), and herpesviruses. The young, elderly, and immunocompromised are more at risk of developing meningitis. Patients usually present with a severe headache, stiff neck (nuchal rigidity; may have a positive Kernig or Brudzinski sign), and fever. They may also have lethargy, photophobia, confusion, and possibly seizures. Rashes may be present in viral or meningococcal (petechiae and purpura) meningitis. *Diagnose* with a lumbar puncture and CSF analysis (Bacterial: high opening P, elevated WBC, decreased glucose, elevated protein; Viral: normal opening P, elevated WBC, normal or slightly decreased glucose, normal or slightly elevated protein) with gram stain and culture and C & S. If focal deficits or signs of elevated ICP, perform a head CT before the LP. While awaiting lab results, immediately start empiric IV antibiotics: ceftriaxone OR cefotaxime AND vancomycin, AND if >50, add ampicillin. If viral, supportive treatment is all that is necessary, and it usually resolves within 7-10 days. Prevention is important with available vaccines. *Complications* are more common with bacterial meningitis (e.g., seizures, hearing loss, blindness, cerebral edema, coma, and death).

Bacterial Meningitis

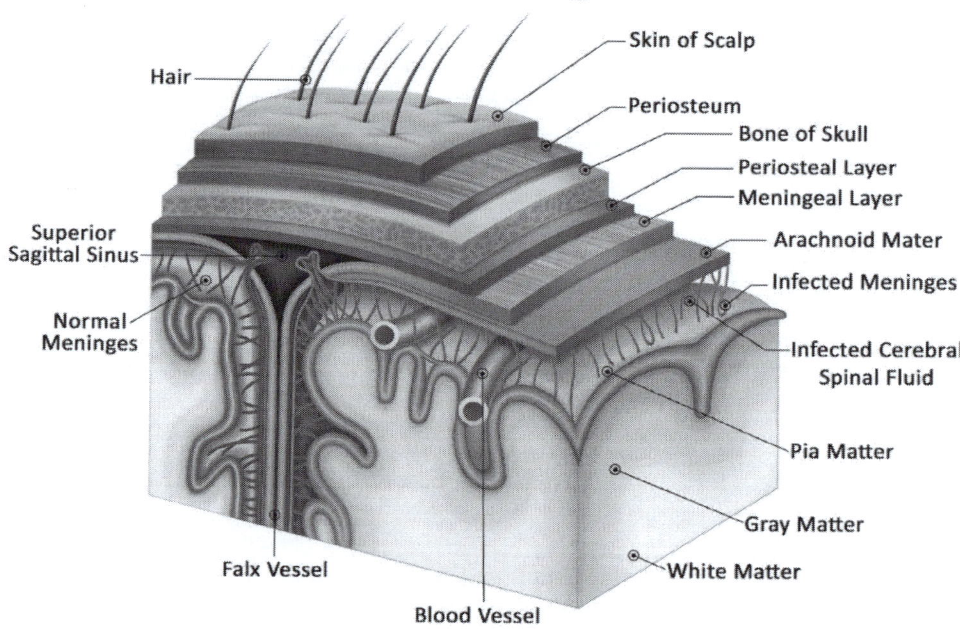

Additional CNS Infections

CNS infections	Characteristics	Diagnosis and treatment
Brain abscess	A space-occupying (pus-filled) lesion in the intracranial area, usually caused by nasal or ear infection, systemic infection, trauma, or surgical intervention. Causative agents commonly include streptococci, staphylococci, and anaerobic bacteria. Symptoms include nausea, vomiting, headache, lethargy, confusion, seizures, increasing intracranial pressure, and focal deficits.	Diagnosis is per CT, MRI (preferred), and arteriography. Treatment includes IV antibiotics for 6 to 8 weeks and then oral antibiotics for up to 3 months, surgical aspiration and drainage, and dexamethasone.
Epidural abscess	Space-occupying (pus-filled) lesion in the epidural space of the brain and spinal cord, usually from *Staphylococcus aureus* and associated with bacterial rhinosinusitis, otitis media, osteomyelitis, or epidural injection. Edema may cause swelling and pressure on the spinal cord. Symptoms include headache, altered consciousness, fever, lack of coordination, general weakness, paralysis of arms or legs, back pain, incontinence, nausea and vomiting, and grogginess.	Diagnosis is per CT or MRI, aspiration and C&S, and CBC and blood cultures. Treatment is similar to brain abscess (above).

Progressive Multifocal Leukoencephalopathy

Progressive multifocal leukoencephalopathy (PML) is a demyelinating disorder of the CNS caused by reactivation of a polyomavirus (John Cunningham virus) that causes childhood infections, resulting in lytic infection of oligodendrocytes. Reactivation typically occurs in immunocompromised adults, such as those with AIDS or idiopathic CD4 lymphopenia syndrome. It may also occur with lymphoproliferative or myeloproliferative disorders and rheumatic disorders (SLE, RA) and in those who have undergone hematopoietic cell transplantation. PML may also be triggered by medications, such as monoclonal antibodies (natalizumab, rituximab). Symptoms may vary depending on the part of the CNS involved but may include alterations of mental status, ataxia, aphasia, paresis or paralysis, visual field disturbance, and seizures (18% of those infected). Diagnosis is per isolation of JCV in cerebrospinal fluid (PCR) and MRI. Treatment includes decreasing immunosuppression (transplant patients), ART treatment (HIV/AIDS patients), cidofovir (non-AIDS patients), and plasma exchange (natalizumab-associated). Other treatments may include risperidone and mirtazapine.

Encephalitis

Encephalitis is inflammation of **brain tissue** and may be a primary infection or secondary (postinfectious). This is usually due to a **viral infection**; however, often the source cannot be identified. Viruses that cause encephalitis include enteroviruses (most common), herpes viruses (herpes simplex 1 & 2, Epstein-Barr, CMV, varicella-zoster, roseola), measles, mumps, rabies, and arboviruses (e.g., Eastern and Western equine encephalitis, West Nile encephalitis, Zika virus). Other causes are bacterial, fungal, parasitic, and autoimmune. The viral prodrome is followed by a few symptoms of encephalitis or the disease may be severe. Patients may present with a fever, severe headache, neck stiffness, N/V, photophobia, focal neurologic deficits, lethargy, personality changes, confusion, altered mental status, and seizures may be present. *Diagnose* with an LP/CSF analysis including viral titers and gram stain, head CT or MRI, EEG, and blood cultures and viral cultures as needed (head CT *before* LP if focal deficits or signs of elevated ICP). Viral CSF results show: normal opening P or slightly elevated, elevated WBC, normal or slightly reduced glucose, normal or slightly elevated protein. Definitive diagnosis is with a brain biopsy. While waiting for lab results immediately begin *treatment* with empiric IV acyclovir. If herpes simplex or varicella-zoster encephalitis is confirmed, continue acyclovir for 14-21 days. May also start patients on empiric antibiotics as needed. Otherwise, treatment is mainly supportive. Anticonvulsants (benzodiazepines) may be necessary if patients are having seizures. *Complications* include epilepsy, memory issues, personality changes, balance/movement issues, coma, and death.

Brain and Spinal Cord Tumors

Brain tumors may be benign or malignant and primary or secondary (metastases). Even **benign tumors** cause problems since they compress adjacent tissues within the skull. **Primary brain tumors** are more common in children while **metastases** are more common in adults. Most metastases come from lung cancer, but also are often from breast cancer, malignant melanoma, colon cancer, and renal cancer. **Pituitary adenomas** are common and are almost always benign. Brain tumors are classified according to where they arise. The most common types of brain and spinal neoplasms are **gliomas** (from glial cells in the brain or spinal cord; includes astrocytomas, oligodendrogliomas, ependymomas, medulloblastomas), **metastases**, **meningiomas** (from the meninges, so may appear anywhere along the brain or spinal cord; benign and usually in adults), **pituitary adenomas**, and **acoustic neuromas** (from Schwann cells). **Glioblastoma multiforme** is the most common and the most aggressive primary brain tumor. Tumors are classified from Grade I (slowest growing and non-invasive) to Grade III or IV (fastest growing).

Signs and Symptoms and Best Imaging Study for Initial Diagnosis

Patients with brain or spinal cord tumors have **signs and symptoms** based on the type and location of the tumor and may include: headache (most common), vision/hearing problems, speech issues, N/V, weakness/motor issues, changes in personality/mood, difficulty concentrating, and seizures. Deficits caused by tumor location: Frontal lobe- personality, memory, learning, speech, motor; Temporal-memory, hearing, understanding language; Parietal- spatial awareness; Occipital-vision; Cerebellum/Brainstem- coordination/voluntary movement, cranial nerve palsies. Look for signs/symptoms of elevated ICP: headache, N/V, diminished mental status, diplopia, papilledema, abnormal pupillary light reflexes, and Cushing's triad (decreased RR, decreased pulse, and elevated BP). Initial *diagnosis* is usually made with a head CT after a thorough neurologic exam. An MRI may be obtained. Refer to neurosurgery.

Cervical Root Disease

Cervical root disease (AKA cervical radiculopathy), most often at C6 and C7, is most commonly associated with herniated disk or spondylitis and pain in the neck, shoulder, and/or arm. Arthritic bones spurs and changes associated with age may result in nerve compression. Patients may have decreased sensation along the nerve path and weakness and tingling in the hand and fingers. Neck pain is typically unilateral. Tests for cervical root disease should be carried out in the presence of neck and/or shoulder pain. Spurling's sign (pain on extension and rotation of the neck) is positive with cervical root disease, but raising the arm over the head tends to relieve compression. Diagnosis is per MRI or CT myelography. Treatment may include corticosteroids or NSAIDs, PT (cervical traction, exercises, manipulation), cervical collar for temporary immobilization, and nerve blocks. In some cases, surgery to decompress the nerve root may be indicated.

Peripheral Neuropathies

Peripheral neuropathies	Characteristics	Diagnosis and treatment
Meralgia paresthetica	Painful paresthesias/numbness of upper lateral thigh (usually unilateral) from entrapment of the lateral femoral cutaneous nerve, resulting from pregnancy, tool belts, body armor, prolonged lying in fetal position, and neoplasms (rare). Other causes include trauma, ischemia, and stretch injury. Sitting relieves symptoms.	Diagnosis per physical examination, may be confirmed with nerve conduction studies. Treatment includes weight loss, comfortable loose clothing, nerve block (for severe pain), and anticonvulsants (carbamazepine, gabapentin). Surgical decompression may be done if nonresponsive to other treatments.
Postherpetic neuralgia	Chronic severe burning pain that persists for 3 months are longer following herpes zoster (shingles) infection, primarily in patients over 50. Skin may be sensitive to touch, and some may experience itching and numbness.	Diagnosis is per symptoms. Treatment includes lidocaine skin patches, capsaicin skin patches, anticonvulsants (typically gabapentin), TCA, intrathecal/epidural steroids, and opioids.
Toxin induced peripheral neuropathy.	Associated with medications, drug abuse, and chemical exposure, resulting in axonal degeneration. Characteristics may vary according to the toxin but include pain, tingling and numbness of feet, hypo/hyperhidrosis, GI disorders, urinary incontinence and retention, blurred vision, sexual dysfunction, tachycardia, labile BP, stocking-glove sensory loss, ataxic gait (stiff-leg).	Diagnosis is per history and physical, sensory testing, EMG, and nerve conduction tests, and various lab tests, such as GTT, Vit-B-12 level, and immunofixation. Treatment includes identifying and eliminating causative agent, cool compresses, massage, TCAs, anticonvulsants, opioids, and topical capsaicin cream.
Peroneal nerve injury (Foot drop)	Movement and sensation of the lower extremity impaired because of traumatic injury, prolonged immobility, fracture, or disease (Parkinson's, ALS, MS). Characteristics include foot and ankle weakness, slapping or abnormal gait, and numbness and tingling.	Diagnosis is per history and physical, confirmed by EMG, nerve conduction tests, MRI, and/or nerve US. Treatment includes PT, orthotics, braces, splints, or surgical decompression of the nerve.

Bell's Palsy

Bell's palsy, now called idiopathic facial nerve palsy, is a condition in which the muscles supplied by the **7th cranial nerve** (CN VII; facial nerve) are unilaterally weakened or paralyzed. The etiology of the 7th CN impairment is unknown, but risk factors include a current or recent viral infection (most often due to herpes simplex or varicella-zoster), pregnancy, and diabetes mellitus. CN VII is a mixed motor/sensory nerve that has motor fibers that innervate the muscles of **facial expression** including the forehead, and **sensory fibers** to the anterior 2/3 of the tongue. Patients may notice a tingling and rather rapid onset of weakness on one side of the face that may occur quite suddenly over a few hours to a couple days. Both upper and lower parts of the face will be unilaterally affected and may cause difficulty closing the eye, blinking, smiling, frowning, wrinkling the forehead, and taste disturbances may be present. Some patients may experience posterior ear pain which may occur a couple days before the palsy sets in. Thoroughly test the cranial nerves and perform a thorough neurologic exam (motor and sensory; impaired motor, but sensory is intact). This is a clinical diagnosis that is made after other causes are ruled out (e.g., infection, autoimmune disorder, CNS disease). If the onset is gradual, rule out a tumor. If only the upper or lower half of the face is affected, rule out a CVA. Bell's palsy is almost always a self-limited condition that lasts from a week to a few months. *Treatment* involves giving corticosteroids early on (start within 72 hours of symptom onset) which helps improve the outcome. If a virus is suspected, antiviral medications may be used (if given with steroids); however, their effectiveness is still being studied. Lubricating eye drops and/or ointment and eye patches, especially at night or if there is a corneal erosion or abrasion, may help the affected dry eye. Refer to neurology or ophthalmology as needed.

Seizures

Seizures are broadly classified as either focal, generalized, or an unknown onset.

Focal seizures (previously referred to as partial seizures) are miss-firings of the electrical signals of the brain that are localized to a particular part of the brain. Focal seizures can be **simple** (conscious) or **complex** (impaired awareness). These may have motor, sensory (e.g., visual, auditory, olfactory, or taste), and autonomic (e.g., diaphoresis, flushed face) components including an aura. Congenital defects, head trauma, disease, infection, or a stroke may increase the risk of developing a seizure disorder. **Epilepsy** is the term used when >1 non-physiologic seizure has occurred (e.g., it cannot be due to a fever). **Simple (aware) focal seizures** do not cause a loss of awareness, but rather a change in how things appear, taste, or smell and can last for seconds to minutes. **Complex (impaired awareness) focal seizures** will cause a change in consciousness or loss of awareness (interruption in behavior or staring) with some motor changes, such as arm movements, lip smacking, repeated swallowing, or yelling out and usually last for 1 to 1 ½ minutes. Postictal confusion may last for a short time or for days. *Diagnose* clinically and with an EEG (electroencephalogram); rule out other causes. *Treatment* is with anticonvulsants (e.g., carbamazepine, divalproex sodium), but it may take several trials of drugs to find the most effective treatment for patients. Monotherapy at the lowest dose is the goal, but 2 or more medications may be required. Rarely, surgery is chosen if the seizures are unresponsive to medications.

Generalized seizures occur when **both hemispheres of the brain** are immediately affected by **abnormal electrical signals** which results in a loss of consciousness. According to the 2017 International League Against Epilepsy generalized seizures can be classified as motor or non-motor. These seizures include **tonic** (rigid), **clonic** (rhythmic jerking), **tonic-clonic** (grand mal), **myoclonic** (muscle group twitching or nonrhythmic jerking), **atonic** ("drop attacks"), and **absence** (petit mal; starring episodes usually lasting about 30 secs.). These generalized seizures all involve a loss of consciousness or loss of awareness and a post-ictal state of varying degrees. Head trauma, congenital malformation, infection, stroke, a tumor, and genetics may increase the chances of developing a seizure disorder. Generalized seizures vary greatly. The mildest of these would be an absence seizure, or petit mal, in which patients stare blankly or have very subtle movements. The other end of the spectrum is a tonic-clonic seizure, or grand mal, in which there is LOC or loss of awareness with generalized jerking and possibly loss of bowel or bladder control. *Diagnose* clinically and with EEG and MRI; rule out causes (e.g., febrile seizures, infection). *Treat* with anticonvulsants (e.g., valproic acid, topiramate; ethosuximide or Depakote® for absence), but it may take several trials of drugs to find the most effective treatment for patients and sometimes multiple medications are necessary. Rarely, surgery is used if the seizure activity unresponsive to anticonvulsants.

Status Epilepticus

Status epilepticus is a condition in which the **seizure does not stop in 5 or more minutes** or if there are repeated seizures (>2) where the patient remains **unconscious for 5 or more minutes**. It may be **generalized convulsive or nonconvulsive**. This is considered a medical emergency because of the physiologic effects of sustained seizures, especially with the convulsive type (e.g., elevated HR, elevated temperature, elevated catecholamines, nerve cell death, pulmonary edema) and risk of asphyxiation or respiratory arrest during the seizure. Status epilepticus is most often due to patients not taking their **seizure medications** correctly or due to **changes in these medications** but can also occur in acute illnesses such as meningitis, encephalitis, very high fevers, or decreased glucose levels, alcohol withdrawal, or head trauma. Patients exhibit signs of a tonic-clonic seizure persisting >5 minutes. There may be a known diagnosis of epilepsy or another illness. *Diagnose* clinically and begin *treatment* before labs are back; obtain stat glucose, CBC, LFTs, BUN/Cr, ABG, anticonvulsant levels, and a toxicity screen. Check ABCs, give oxygen, and the airway of patients should be protected, intubation may be necessary, and obtain an IV access. According to the 2016 guidelines from the American Epilepsy Society the following is recommended: Give a benzodiazepine as first-line treatment (i.e. IV lorazepam, IV diazepam, or IM midazolam); If the seizure persists >20 minutes begin a second medication (i.e. IV fosphenytoin, IV valproic acid, or IV levetiracetam); More studies are necessary to determine the best way to handle seizures persisting longer than 40 minutes. If the cause of the seizure is not immediately known, an EEG and other testing should be done. If an acute illness is suspected, a lumbar puncture with CSF analysis and blood cultures should also be drawn to assess for sepsis. *Complications* include acidosis, rhabdomyolysis, hyperthermia, respiratory failure and death.

Cerebral Palsy

Cerebral palsy is a **movement disorder** that develops due to permanent brain damage that occurs during **prenatal or postnatal neural development**, or during **birth**. It affects a child's motor development and may or may not be accompanied by intellectual disabilities or seizures. It is diagnosed before 2 years old and may be classified as **spastic** (movement difficulties/ stiffness; most common), **dyskinetic** (involuntary movements), or **ataxic** (balance issues). It can result from a variety of incidents including prenatal/postnatal infections, prenatal/ postnatal exposures to toxins, trauma/intracranial hemorrhage, prematurity, or anoxia during or after birth. Parents will notice their children are not reaching developmental milestones, like sitting up, crawling, speaking, or walking, as they should. Cerebral palsy affects **motor function** usually by causing the muscles to be flaccid and weak early on and then rigid and spastic. The limbs will appear under-developed and flaccid or more commonly, stiff, rigid, and with contractures. The child will be uncoordinated, hyperreflexic, and primitive (newborn) reflexes may still be present. *Diagnosis* is made clinically and confirmed with an MRI. Rule out possible metabolic or neurologic causes. There is no cure for cerebral palsy, but physical therapy and kinesiotherapy can help with stretching the muscles and preventing contractions due to rigidity. Botulinum toxin, baclofen, and other muscle relaxants can be given to help decrease spasticity. Braces and surgery may also be used. If there are learning impairments, special education should be utilized to maximize the child's learning potential.

Multiple Sclerosis

Multiple sclerosis (**MS**) is chronic disorder of the **CNS** in which inflammation, demyelination, and damage to **axons** occurs. The cause is unknown but there may be genetic factors, viral, or other triggers to this autoimmune disease. This affects women more than men, is more common in temperate climates, and is usually diagnosed between 20-40 years of age. The 4 different types include: **Relapsing-remitting** (most common, 85%); **Primary or Secondary Progressive**; and **Progressive-relapsing MS**. **Clinically isolated syndrome** is an episode that presents with at least

24 hours of one of the symptoms of MS which may or may not eventually lead to a diagnosis of MS. Common presenting symptoms may include optic neuritis (vision loss, blurred vision, scotomas, eye pain), diplopia, focal sensory loss/paresthesias/weakness (usually in arms, hands, legs, face), muscle spasms, balance issues, urinary incontinence, cognitive problems, and depression. Typically, these episodes last from days, weeks, or months and are followed by periods of remission which may last from months to years. **Attacks** are defined as lasting at least 24 hours and must be 1 month from the last attack. Clinical findings and MRI are used to *diagnose* this condition and to follow the progress of the disease. To diagnose MS the MRI needs to show plaques or damage in at least 2 different areas that occurred at different times (lesions separated in "time and space"); or 1 area of damage plus oligoclonal bands in CSF. *Treatment* involves corticosteroids for attacks or exacerbations as well as disease-modifying agents (e.g., interferon) for long-term treatment.

Review Video: Multiple Sclerosis (MS)
Visit mometrix.com/academy and enter code: 417355

Chorea, Athetosis, and Tremor

Chorea is an involuntary movement disorder characterized by rapid, irregular movements of the hands and feet. Movements are often "dance-like". Explosive and inappropriate speech is sometimes present. Symptoms do not occur during sleep.

Athetosis is an involuntary movement disorder characterized by slow, writhing movements, generally of the hands or feet. The movements can be brought on by emotional stress or during specific activities. There are no symptoms during sleep.

A **tremor** is an involuntary movement disorder characterized by rhythmic or oscillatory movements. A postural tremor occurs when there is a sustained posture of an extremity, for example, an outstretched arm for example. An intention tremor occurs when a purposeful movement is being attempted, such as touching a finger to the tip of one's nose for example. A resting tremor is a tremor that occurs at rest. Parkinson's disease is characterized by resting tremors.

Essential Tremors

Essential tremor is an **involuntary shaking disorder** that usually occurs in older adults and typically affects the hands, forearms, head, chin, or even the voice. This is the most common tremor, prevalence increases with age, and this affects men and women equally. These tremors are not accompanied by any other symptoms, as seen with the tremor of Parkinson's disease, but can be debilitating if severe. Most patients have a family history of essential tremors (autosomal dominant), but it is not known what causes the tremors. Patients usually complain of gradually progressive tremors in the hands or other areas. The tremors occur when maintaining posture against gravity or during voluntary movements. Tremors are most pronounced when performing simple activities such as eating, drinking, and writing. The tremors usually stop when patients are resting and not moving, but restart when performing activities. Tremors worsen during periods of stress and are absent when sleeping. In some cases, alcohol can temporarily decrease the amplitude of the tremor. Muscle tone is normal and reflexes remain intact. *Diagnose* clinically. Rule out other causes of tremors: medications, caffeine, alcohol withdrawal, vitamin B_{12} deficiency, hyperthyroidism, and Parkinson's. *Treat* with the β-blocker propranolol or the anticonvulsant primidone, which can help control the tremors in most patients. When the tremor is severe and not responding to medical management, a thalamotomy may be performed or a deep brain stimulator can be surgically implanted to try to control the tremor.

Parkinson's Disease

Parkinson's disease is a **movement disorder** that involves progressive damage and destruction of neurons in the **substantia nigra** that produce dopamine. The **basal ganglia** and the neurotransmitter **dopamine** are responsible for allowing the body to move smoothly and without rigidity or jerkiness. *Symptoms* result from an imbalance between dopamine-activated and acetylcholine-activated neural pathways in the basal ganglia. The exact cause of Parkinson's is not clearly understood, but it is thought to be due to genetic and environmental factors as there is an increased incidence in people with chronic exposure to herbicides, pesticides, and well water. This affects men more than women and symptoms usually start after the age of 60 but may begin earlier. The onset is insidious and usually starts with a unilateral resting tremor in the hand, wrist, or fingers ("pill rolling") which improves with intentional motion. Other symptoms include gait disturbances with decreased arm swing on the affected side, soft voice, flat affect, and sometimes dementia. Rigidity, "cogwheel" movements, bradykinesia, akinesia, poor posture, and lack of balance and coordination, cause increasing problems with mobility, talking, and swallowing. Some patients experience sleep disturbances, depression, and mood changes. *Diagnose* clinically; be sure to rule out drug-induced symptoms. *Treat* symptoms with levodopa (precursor to dopamine) and carbidopa. Other drugs like ropinirole, safinamide, bromocriptine, and amantadine may be used in specific situations like early or late disease or to help with medication side effects. A deep brain stimulator may be surgically implanted to help with the movement disorders associated with Parkinson's.

TBI and Intracranial Hemorrhages

Traumatic brain injury (TBI) is an injury that is caused by external forces that may cause temporary or permanent **brain impairment**. This may be from a variety of causes which include falls, motor vehicle accidents (MVA) or other crashes, sports injuries, or gunshots/assaults. Helmet wearing, seatbelts, and child safety seats have helped reduce the incidence of TBI, but this continues to be a common cause of morbidity and mortality. This may be an open or closed head injury. Those with moderate and severe injuries may present with seizures, dilated pupils, and may be unresponsive. Increased intracranial pressure can cause what is known as the **Cushing triad**: HTN, bradycardia, and irregular respirations. **Basilar skull fractures** should be suspected if rhinorrhea (possible CSF), the Battle sign (postauricular ecchymosis), raccoon eyes (orbital ecchymosis), or hemotympanum. **Subdural hematomas** result from a venous bleed, may have symptoms that rapidly progress, or may have a more insidious onset, especially if chronic. **Epidural hematoma** patients often have LOC then a period of lucidity, then rapid deterioration. **Subarachnoid hemorrhages** usually present with a severe "thunderclap" headache with N/V, and altered consciousness. Assess Glasgow coma scale within 48 hours of the injury: Eye opening (1-4 points); Verbal response (1-5 points); Motor response (1-6 points). Mild TBI = 13-15; Moderate TBI = 9-12; Severe TBI = 3-8. Evaluation and *treatment* involve ABC management to stabilize the patient, a Glasgow coma scale, and obtaining a head CT. Mannitol may be used to help reduce ICP. Admit and refer to neurology or neurosurgery as needed.

TIA

A **transient ischemic attack (TIA)** occurs when blood flow to an area of the brain, spinal cord, or retina is temporarily interrupted, causing **focal neurologic dysfunction**, but without causing tissue damage. This can occur due to atherosclerosis in an artery, arterial inflammation, emboli/thrombi, a hypercoagulable state, drugs (e.g., cocaine), or anything that causes a **temporary decrease in oxygen to a certain portion of the brain**. Risk factors for a TIA include a positive family history of TIA or CVA, African American or Hispanic descent, male, >55 years old, HTN, DM, hypercholesterolemia, and smoking. About one-third of patients who have a TIA will eventually have a stroke, with most of those occur in the next days or weeks post-TIA. Patients will have *symptoms* similar to a stroke with possible hemiparesis, paresthesias, garbled speech, dizziness, cranial nerve dysfunction, and loss of vision in one eye. The difference between a stroke and a TIA is that, with a TIA, the symptoms will resolve spontaneously, within 24 hours and often much less (minutes). This is a clinical *diagnosis* with a thorough history and PE (thorough neuro and cardiac exams, listen for carotid bruit), as there is no tissue damage to be seen on imaging. However, to rule out a cerebral infarct or hemorrhage, an MRI (diffusion weighted is most sensitive) or a CT must be obtained. Also rule out other causes (e.g., AF, carotid stenosis) with appropriate labs, ECG, and imaging studies (e.g., carotid ultrasound, echo). After a hemorrhage has been ruled out, patients who have had a TIA should be started on daily antiplatelet meds (e.g., low-dose aspirin, clopidogrel, dipyridamole). Anticoagulants are started for cardiogenic TIAs (e.g., AF). Lifestyle changes should be implemented, including eating foods lower in fat and cholesterol, quitting smoking, and losing weight, if necessary. The primary *complication* is a CVA.

CVA

A stroke or **cerebrovascular accident (CVA)** occurs when **damage and death of brain cells** occurs from ischemia or a hemorrhage and is a medical emergency. Neurons die within minutes without having a blood supply, so early intervention is critical. According to the American Heart Association (AHA), most CVAs are caused by **arterial blockage causing ischemia** (87%) while bleeding of a vessel only accounts in about 13% of all CVAs. These 2 main types are termed ischemic and hemorrhagic strokes, respectively. **Ischemic strokes** can be due to a thrombus or embolus; a **hemorrhagic stroke** can be intracerebral or subarachnoid. Within the US, strokes are the fifth leading cause of death. The extent of the damage, presenting symptoms, and mortality are dependent upon the location and size of the vascular compromise. Common *symptoms* include weakness, loss of voluntary movement (ataxia), paralysis, or a loss of sensation on one side of the body. The damage can result in problems with speech (aphasia), swallowing, increased drooling, impaired balance, and vision or breathing issues; hemorrhagic patients typically appear sicker. If damage is extensive, unconsciousness or death may occur. Obtain a fingerstick glucose and diagnose initially with a noncontrast head CT: ischemic areas appear hypodense; hemorrhagic areas appear hyperdense. Remember in an ischemic CVA a head CT may appear normal early on (<12 hours) as the damage progresses. However, diffusion weighted imaging can show damage within 15-30 minutes of the onset of an ischemic CVA. Angiography can be utilized for *diagnosis* and *treatment*. If signs of ICP or hemorrhage, refer immediately to neurosurgery. A hemorrhage must be ruled out in order to start thrombolytic therapy (start IV tPA within 3-4.5 hours of symptom onset for acute ischemic strokes). *Complications* include permanent neurologic deficits and death.

Review Video: Overview of Strokes
Visit mometrix.com/academy and enter code: 310572

Spontaneous Intracranial Hemorrhage and Cerebral Aneurysm

A **spontaneous intracranial hemorrhage** occurs with sudden bleeding from a blood vessel in the brain. It is usually due to HTN or when vascular lesions in the brain leak/rupture.

A **cerebral aneurysm** is a dilatation in the wall of a cerebral artery that is usually asymptomatic until it leaks or ruptures. It may be saccular ("berry") or fusiform (spindle-like) in shape. About 5% of the population has this and the risk of rupture is ~1%; however, mortality is >50% once it ruptures.

Signs & symptoms vary depending on the area/size of the intracranial hemorrhage, but some include a severe headache (often with activity) described as "the worst of their life," speech and memory issues, confusion, visual deficits, N/V, paresthesias or paralysis, other deficits, and LOC. AVMs may have less severe bleeding, therefore less severe symptoms, or may even be asymptomatic. If non-emergent, these can be diagnosed with MRI, MRI angiography (preferred over CTA), or definitively through angiography. If it ruptures follow emergency protocol (e.g., ABCs, fingerstick glucose, and noncontrast head CT) and immediately refer to neurosurgery. *Complications* from these include a subarachnoid hemorrhage (which is a medical emergency), chronic neurologic deficits, and death.

Disorders of Cerebral Function

Coma	A state of complete unconsciousness with no response to pain or any type of external or internal stimuli. A patient in a light coma may have some reflexive activity but no purposeful movement while a patient in a deep coma has no motor response. Coma may result from disease, injury, or drugs, such as induced coma.
Persistent vegetative state	A condition in which the patient has no cognitive function but retains some autonomic functions and may partially arouse. Criteria include remaining in this condition for at least 3 months after non-traumatic brain injury or 12 months after traumatic brain injury. A court order is generally required to terminate life support.
Brain death	A condition in which all brain functions are lost and life support is required. The patient does not respond to painful stimuli or exhibit reflex movements. Brain death is a legal definition of death. Legal requirements may vary, but requirements usually include failure of the apnea test, separate neurological confirmations by two physicians, and two isoelectric electroencephalograms 24 hours apart. Confirmatory tests, such as cerebral angiography, is a requirement for infants less than one year of age.

Aphasias

Aphasias are defined as the loss of the ability to produce or understand language, generally as the result of brain injury.

- **Broca's** aphasia is an expressive aphasia. Patients are unable to produce fluent, understandable language. Comprehension is intact.
- **Wernicke's** aphasia is a receptive aphasia. Patients are able to speak fluently; however, the content is often incorrect. Comprehension is poor.
- **Global** aphasia is a combination of both Broca's and Wernicke's aphasia, both language production and comprehension are impaired. It results from injury to both Broca's and Wernicke's areas of the cerebral lobe of the brain.

The diagnosis of aphasias is made clinically. Treatment is with speech therapy and supportive care.

Cavernous Sinus Thrombosis

The cavernous sinus is located at the base of the brain and comprises a cavity with networks of veins that drain deoxygenated blood from the brain and facial veins for transport back to the heart. **Cavernous sinus thrombosis** occurs when one or more of the veins becomes obstructed by a blood clot, usually as the result of bacterial rhinosinusitis. Most infections (70%) are caused by *Staphylococcus*. The mortality rate for the infection is about 30%, usually associated with CNS infection or sepsis. About 50% of survivors have residual deficits (visual, cranial nerve). Signs and symptoms include headaches, cranial nerve deficits, and history of sinusitis or furuncle of mid face. Diagnosis is per CBC (polymorphonuclear leukocytosis common), CT, and or MRI with contrast or

MR venogram (preferred). Lumbar puncture with examination of cerebrospinal fluid may aid in diagnosis. Treatment includes antibiotic therapy (typically a penicillinase-resistant penicillin and cephalosporin,3rd or 4th generation), usually administered IV for 3 to 4 weeks. Anticoagulation with heparin is also often used but there is not yet consensus as to value, and use of thrombolytics is experimental. Corticosteroids are used to reduce inflammation.

Concussion and Postconcussion Syndrome

Concussion is a mild traumatic **brain injury** that causes a disturbance in brain function. This commonly results from **sports injuries**. *Signs and symptoms* may include headache, dizziness, visual disturbances, light and noise sensitivities, confusion, amnesia (retrograde or antegrade), issues with concentration, LOC (only present in about 10%), emotional changes, N/V, and balance or coordination issues. Persistent vomiting may be a sign of increased intracranial pressure and should be investigated further. Athletes should be immediately removed from play and should not return until cleared medically. *Diagnose* clinically and possibly imaging to rule out other injuries. Order a CT if LOC, a focal neurologic deficit, signs or symptoms of ICP, or GCS <15.

Postconcussion syndrome involves continued symptoms from the **concussion** and may persist for days, weeks, or months after the injury. This usually resolves but may become permanent. *Signs and symptoms* include chronic headaches, continued light and noise sensitivities, sleep disturbances, fatigue, personality changes (being more emotional or irritable), concentration issues, and short-term memory deficits. *Diagnose* clinically and *treat* with supportive care. Patients with repeated concussions (especially boxers and football players) are at an increased risk of developing **chronic traumatic encephalopathy** which may not present until years after the last concussion. This causes progressive degenerative changes in the brain which may manifest as mood/behavior issues, dementia, and motor dysfunction.

Myasthenia Gravis

Myasthenia gravis (MG) is an **autoimmune neurologic disorder** that causes **skeletal muscle fatigue** with activity. **Autoantibodies** are produced that block the **postsynaptic acetylcholine receptor sites** at the neuromuscular junction leading to fewer nerve signals being sent to muscle cells, which results in weakness. There is no definite known cause of MG, but the **thymus gland** may play a role in producing the antibodies for the disease. It most commonly affects middle-aged men and women, but typically appears earlier in women (20-40 years old) vs. men (>50 years old). There are two main forms; **ocular** and **generalized**. Patients usually present with ptosis, diplopia, and fluctuating skeletal muscle weakness that worsens with activity and improves with rest. This can include difficulty breathing, chewing, swallowing, talking, performing exertive motions, or controlling eye movements. In a **myasthenia crisis**, normal respirations are affected, causing difficulty breathing, and may even require a respirator; but mortality due to a crisis has greatly decreased through the years. A **cholinergic crisis**, which presents similarly to a myasthenic crisis, may also occur in MG patients, but this is due to ingestion of too much acetylcholinesterase inhibitor (e.g., pyridostigmine). *Diagnose* with an AChR-Ab (anti-acetylcholine receptor antibody) test. A MuSK-Ab (muscle specific kinase) test may be used if the first is negative. Use a CXR or chest CT to rule out a thymoma. In patients with ptosis a bedside ice test may be used to see if symptoms improve (improves in MG). An IV edrophonium (Tensilon®) test will also show improvement in symptoms in MG (caution: may cause bradycardia so atropine should be readily available). *Treat* symptoms with the acetylcholinesterase inhibitor pyridostigmine. Also, over time, most patients improve after a thymectomy even if a thymoma is not present. Steroids and other immunosuppressants, plasmapheresis, and IVIG may also help reduce symptoms. The primary *complication* is respiratory failure.

Review Video: Myasthenia Gravis
Visit mometrix.com/academy and enter code: 162510

Tourette Syndrome

Tourette syndrome (**TS**) is a **neurological disorder** that manifests as repetitive, involuntary, nonrhythmic movements and vocalizations, referred to as **tics**. This is more common in males than females and there seems to be a genetic as well as an environmental component to this disease. These symptoms first appear in the preschool or early elementary school child, often becomes worse during puberty, and usually resolves gradually during adulthood. **Simple motor tics** might include eye movements, grimacing, shrugging, twitching, jerking; while **simple vocal tics** might include throat-clearing, coughing, grunting, or sniffing. **Complex tics** are created with combined, coordinated activities, full words, or phrases (e.g., kicking, jumping, animal sounds, yelling). **Coprolalia** (use of profanity or inappropriate words) and **copropraxia** (obscene gestures) only occur in a minority of patients.

Symptoms worsen with stress or times of excitement and do not go away during sleep. Comorbid conditions like ADHD, learning disabilities, OCD, and depression are often present. *Diagnose* clinically: rule out other causes, symptoms of both motor and vocal tics must be present for >1 year and must appear before 18 years old according to DSM-5-TR criteria. *Treatment* is not required unless the tics interfere with normal daily functioning. Dopamine-blocking neuroleptics and other medications (e.g., haloperidol, pimozide, clonidine, topiramate) may then be considered as a means of providing some control. Side effects of haloperidol and other neuroleptics include extrapyramidal symptoms (e.g., acute dystonic reactions, akathisia [feeling of restlessness], Parkinson-like symptoms, tardive dyskinesia) which may not be reversible with prolonged use of the medication(s).

Trigeminal Neuralgia

Trigeminal neuralgia is a **chronic disorder** that creates extreme pain, often described as stabbing or electric-shock-like, along one side of the **face** (follows the sensory distribution of CN 5, usually the maxillary and mandibular nerve branches). This condition is rare but usually affects women >50 years old. This is typically idiopathic. Underlying causes are more likely to be determined in patients younger than 40, generally multiple sclerosis or a swollen blood vessel or tumor providing pressure on the **trigeminal nerve**. The pain usually lasts seconds to 2 minutes and is typically sporadic at first but may increase in frequency and can be quite debilitating. The pain may cause a facial tic due to muscle spasms. Triggers of the pain may include sound, touch, vibration or stimulation of the area through brushing teeth, chewing, drinking, eating, or shaving. The neurologic exam is normal. *Diagnosis* is clinical but testing often includes magnetic resonance imaging (MRI). *Treatment* may include anticonvulsant medications (carbamazepine is usually first line), muscle relaxants (baclofen), or tricyclic antidepressants. More aggressive treatment entails referring to neurosurgery and cutting or destroying part of the trigeminal nerve (ablation), microcompression, tumor removal (if this secondary cause is found), or microvascular decompression.

Guillain-Barré Syndrome

Guillain-Barré syndrome (**acute inflammatory polyneuropathy**) is an acute condition in which inflammation occurs in the **peripheral nerves** throughout the body, resulting in **progressive muscle weakness and decreased reflexes**. This typically begins in the lower extremities and ascends, which may cause respiratory depression requiring mechanical ventilation. There is no definite known cause of this disease, but over one-half of the people who suffer from Guillain-Barré have a history of a respiratory or gastrointestinal illness (usually *Campylobacter jejuni* or CMV) 2-4 weeks before they develop symptoms, so it may be due to an autoimmune disorder. *Symptoms* can progress rapidly from hours to days and usually peak within 2-4 weeks. Depending on the type (demyelinating or axonal injury) it may take weeks to months to recover but may take years. Patients develop symmetric paresthesias and weakness (usually affects proximal muscles more) in the extremities (usually lower 1st) that gradually spread up the limbs and may cause paralysis. This may be accompanied with pain, hypotension, and bladder/bowel incontinence. *Diagnose* clinically and with nerve conduction studies, electromyography, and LP with CSF analysis (elevated protein but normal WBCs) to aid in the diagnosis process. Consult neurology, test for infectious cause and rule out other causes. Admit patients with suspected Guillain-Barré syndrome, monitor closely, and intubate as needed. *Treat* with IVIG or plasmapheresis. The disorder generally begins to resolve after approximately 1 month. Most people make a full recovery from Guillain-Barré with a small portion of patients having some degree of residual weakness. *Complications* include lasting sequelae, ARDS, and death.

ALS

Amyotrophic lateral sclerosis (Lou Gehrig's disease) is a progressive neurodegenerative disease that is generally fatal in 3 to 5 years. Amyotrophic lateral sclerosis causes degeneration of both upper and lower motor neurons. The cause is unknown and most cases are sporadic. Symptoms can be subtle at first. Patients may have weakness or clumsiness. Patients eventually develop difficulty speaking, swallowing, and breathing. The cause of death is usually respiratory failure. The diagnosis is made clinically based on the presence of both upper and lower motor neuron dysfunction. Electromyogram can be used to confirm the diagnosis. Riluzole is the only drug available for treating ALS and there is some evidence that it may slow the progression of the disease. Otherwise, treatment is supportive care with physical and occupational therapy, nutritional and psychosocial support.

Diseases of Muscle and Neuromuscular Function

Drug-Induced Myopathy

Drug-induced myopathy is characterized by muscle weakness and pain without the presence of muscle disease, caused by exposure to drugs or toxins. Muscle weakness derives from damage to muscle fibers. Severity may range from myalgia (pain and weakness) to myositis (pain and weakness with elevated CK, indicating muscle damage), to rhabdomyolysis (pain and weakness with elevated CK and myoglobinuria from severe damage to muscle tissue). Rhabdomyolysis can lead to compartment syndrome, renal failure, and death. Some reactions are inflammatory and others non-inflammatory. Common causative agents are statins and corticosteroids. Other agents may include fibrates, D-penicillamine, colchicine, vincristine, antimalarials, zidovudine, procainamide, illicit drugs (cocaine, heroin, and alcohol. Diagnosis is per symptoms and CK, test for myoglobinuria, and muscle biopsy (definitive). Treatment includes identifying and eliminating causative agent. Rhabdomyolysis may require IV fluids, electrolyte management, and dialysis.

Polymyositis and Dermatomyositis

Muscle disorder	Characteristics	Diagnosis and treatment
Polymyositis	Inflammatory condition or unknown origin resulting in muscle weakness, especially of proximal muscles of extremities and neck, most commonly affecting those in the 30s to 50s. Characteristics may include general muscle weakness dysphagia, aspiration pneumonia, and dyspnea. Often association with autoimmune disorders (SLE, RA, scleroderma, Sjogren's) as well as Raynaud's phenomenon, myocarditis, interstitial lung disease, and cancer.	Diagnosis includes tests for muscle enzymes and autoantibodies, EMG, MRI, and muscle biopsy. Treatment includes corticosteroids, azathioprine, methotrexate, rituximab, IVIG, PT and speech therapy.
Dermatomyositis	Inflammatory disease characterized by progressive muscle weakness and painful, pruritic violet/red rash on face and joints (knuckles, knees, elbows) and trunk. Associated conditions and characteristics are similar to those of polymyositis with the addition of the rash and calcinosis (calcium deposits in tissues). Calcinosis is more common in children.	Diagnosis and treatment are similar to polymyositis except for possible surgery to remove calcium deposits. Patients should wear sunscreen.

Primary Neurologic Disorders

Neurocutaneous Syndromes

Neurocutaneous syndromes are neurological disorders with cutaneous manifestations. Tumors may be present throughout the neurological system (brain, spinal cord), organs, skin, and/or bones. Diagnosis is per genetic tests, imaging, and hearing/vision/balance tests. The most common disorders include:

- **Tuberous sclerosis:** Sporadic or inherited (autosomal dominant) disease with seizures and psychomotor restriction in early childhood progressing to increasing mental deterioration. Cutaneous lesions (adenoma sebaceum) evident by 5-10 years on face and shagreen patches (leathery appearing) on trunk. Children may have retinal lesions/tumors and benign rhabdomyomas or organs, including the heart, lungs, and bones. Treatment is supportive.
- **Neurofibromatosis:** Sporadic or inherited (autosomal dominant) with multiple neurofibroma and many cutaneous lesions: (Type 1) AKA Recklinghausen disease includes multiple hyperpigmented macules and neurofibromas. (Type 2) Includes eighth nerve tumors as well as intracranial and intraspinal tumors and hearing impairment. Treatment of neurofibromatosis is supportive and may involve surgery to remove tumors and implantation of cochlear implants.
- **Sturge-Weber syndrome:** Sporadic congenital disorder with unilateral cutaneous capillary angioma (often disfiguring), leptomeningeal angiomatosis, and choroidal angioma. Seizures are common an may progress to hemiparesis, multiple eye problems, and hemisensory disturbance. Treatment is supportive, but surgical removal of tumors may be necessary.

Cerebellar Ataxias

Cerebellar ataxias may result from many different disorders (tumors, stroke, alcoholism, cerebral palsy, traumatic brain injury, multiple sclerosis and other autoimmune disorders, infections, metal poisoning, vitamin E, B12, or thiamine deficiency, and paraneoplastic syndromes) that impair functioning of the cerebellum because of damage or loss nerve cells. Additionally, some forms of ataxia are inherited as autosomal dominant diseases (spinocerebellar, episodic ataxia) or autosomal recessive disorders (Friedreich's, ataxia-telangiectasia, congenital cerebellar, and Wilson's disease). If involvement is of the cerebellar hemispheres, then ipsilateral symptoms occur, including incoordination, ataxia, and peripheral hypotonia. If the involvement is of the vermis cerebelli (controls pattern and timing of movements), then the trunk exhibits marked ataxia. Signs and symptoms may include incoordination, ataxic gait, fine motor deficits, dysphonia, dysphagia, and nystagmus. Diagnosis is per CT or MRI, spinal tap, and genetic testing. There is no specific treatment other than supportive, including assistive devices, PT, OT, and ST.

Pseudotumor Cerebri

Pseudotumor cerebri (AKA idiopathic intracranial hypertension) is a condition in which CSF is not properly reabsorbed and the increased volume of CSF results in increased intracranial pressure and symptoms similar to those caused by a tumor, including headaches (often worsening at night and early morning), double or blurred vision, nausea and vomiting, dizziness, neck stiffness, tinnitus, and changes in mentation or level of consciousness. The cause of pseudotumor cerebri is not clear, but risk factors include female gender, obesity, abnormal vasculature, sleep apnea, and some medications (steroids, lithium tetracyclines, and vitamin A derivatives). Diagnosis is per spinal tap, MRI or CT, and eye examinations. Treatment may vary depending on the cause and severity but may include dietary modifications (low sodium, restricted fluids), weight loss, and/or lumbar puncture and removal of spinal fluid to reduce pressure. Surgical treatments may include placement of shunt, stent, and/or decompression of fluid about optic nerve to protect vision.

Friedreich's Ataxia

Friedreich's ataxia is an autosomal recessive progressive spinocerebellar disorder. It is generally diagnosed in childhood. Patients generally present in childhood with difficulty walking. The disease progresses to involve the arms and trunk. Eventually speech is affected and scoliosis develops. Depressed knee and ankle tendon reflexes are seen on physical exam. Magnetic resonance imaging may show spinal cord and cerebellar atrophy. Echocardiogram may be significant for ventricular hypertrophy. There is no effective treatment for Friedreich's ataxia. Supportive care to treat symptoms should be offered. Patients generally die by the age of 35 years.

Huntington's Disease

Huntington's disease is an **autosomal dominant disorder** of the neurological system that causes **progressive destruction of brain cells** resulting in chorea, cognitive issues, and neuropsychiatric issues. Since it is an autosomal dominant disorder, only one parent needs to carry the gene for a child to develop the disease (50% probability). The disease results from a mutation on chromosome 4, and this primarily affects the caudate nucleus. There is no cure for Huntington's disease, it usually manifests around 30-50 years old, and patients have about a 10-30-year life expectancy after the onset of symptoms. Early *signs and symptoms* include personality changes, irritability, impaired concentration or memory issues, restlessness or clumsiness, and depression. Physical signs include imbalance, uncontrollable facial expressions, lack of coordination, and sudden spasm-like movements (chorea). These symptoms and dementia gradually progress to the point where patients are incapacitated and cannot care for themselves. *Diagnosis* is confirmed with genetic testing. 1st degree relatives should be offered genetic counseling and then genetic testing. Anticonvulsants, antipsychotics, and antidepressants can help with some of the symptoms. Physical therapy, occupational therapy, and kinesiotherapy can all help with range of motion, but will not be able to stop the progression of the disease.

SYNCOPE

Syncope is an abrupt **loss of consciousness and muscle tone** ("fainting spell") and the patient recovers from the episode on their own. There are numerous causes of syncope including a vasovagal response, hypoglycemia, dehydration, medications, orthostatic hypotension, arrhythmias, valvular or heart disease, MI, CVA/TIA, hyperventilation, breath-holding, and pregnancy. Anything that causes **decreased blood flow to the brain**, including decreased oxygen or glucose, may cause syncope. Those at increased risk include the elderly and those with cardiovascular disease. There may be presyncopal symptoms with a feeling of dizziness or light-headedness, weakness, sweating, blurry vision, or GI symptoms. Red flag *symptoms* include: palpitations, chest pain, syncope during exertion, syncope without a prodrome, severe headache or neurologic deficits, severe abdominal pain, and respiratory issues especially if accompanied with LE edema or calf pain. Workup includes a thorough history and PE, orthostatic BP (orthostatic hypotension is defined as: a sustained >20 mmHg decrease in systolic BP and a 10 mmHg decrease in diastolic BP within 3 minutes of standing from the supine position), and ECG. Also, a tilt table test, Valsalva maneuver, blood glucose, CBC, serum electrolytes, cardiac enzymes, and UA may be helpful in diagnosing. *Treatment* involves treating the underlying cause (e.g., vasovagal precautions/avoid triggers, orthostatic training/rise slowly, treat arrhythmias with meds or pacemaker, treat CHF with meds, stabilize blood glucose levels, rehydrate, etc.). If patient is at high risk admit for observation and further workup.

Disorders of the Eye

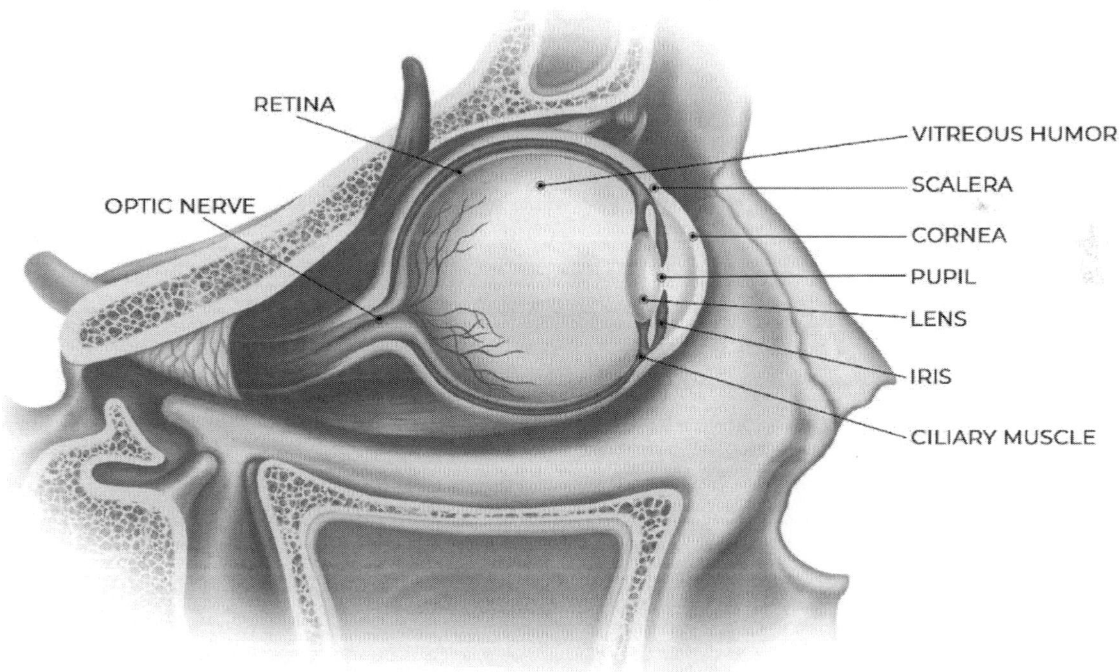

CORNEAL ABRASION

A **corneal abrasion** is caused by minor trauma to the surface of the eye, resulting in a scratching of the **cornea**. Patients will complain of pain and tearing of the eye, and may even complain of blurred vision. First rule out penetrating trauma, infection, and exclude the diagnosis of open globe before proceeding. To diagnose a corneal abrasion, topical anesthetics should be instilled in the eye. Fluorescein is then administered in the eye, and an UV light is used to examine the eye. The area of the cornea that is affected will brightly light up, indicating the area of abrasion. The eye should be gently irrigated to ensure there are no lingering foreign objects that can continue to cause damage. Topical antibiotics (most often ophthalmic fluoroquinolones (e.g., ofloxacin) OR trimethoprim/polymyxin B ophthalmic) are used until asymptomatic, as well as topical anesthetics. Anticholinergics (e.g., cyclopentolate HCl 1%) are used in large abrasions. This condition should heal within 2-3 of days of treatment. Recently patching has been called into question. Patching may not benefit patients and may delay healing time, however, is often used in patients with large abrasions. Do not patch if patient has a high risk of infection. Patients with contact lenses should be examined for corneal infiltrates or ulcers, and if found should be referred to ophthalmologist immediately. Contact wearers without infiltrate or ulcer should be treated with ofloxacin or ciprofloxacin drops 4 times a day for pseudomonas coverage. *Complications* include bacterial keratitis, corneal ulcer, and loss of vision.

Hyphema

Hyphema is blood in the **anterior chamber** of the eye. It is most frequently caused by blunt trauma to the eye, but can also occur following eye surgery or certain medical disorders, such as sickle cell anemia. A hyphema is very obvious because blood will be visible underneath the cornea and cause the iris to be blocked. There may also be conjunctival hemorrhages present. *Treatment* involves strict activity restrictions with avoidance of all strenuous activities. Aspirin and other anticoagulant medications should be avoided to decrease the risk of additional bleeding. If the hyphema is managed on an outpatient basis, patients should be re-evaluated every couple of days to assess for rebleeding. Bleeding can reoccur 3-6 days following the initial eye trauma and may be worse than the initial bleeding that caused the hyphema. Most hyphemas spontaneously resolve within 4 days. *Complications* include increased intraocular pressure, vision disturbances, and glaucoma, especially later in life.

Orbital Cellulitis

Orbital cellulitis is a soft-tissue infection posterior to the **orbital septum**; whereas, **preseptal cellulitis** (periorbital cellulitis) only involves the **preseptal structures**. Orbital cellulitis is a serious condition and must be managed urgently to prevent further complications. It is usually due to sinusitis caused by *Streptococcus, Staphylococcus,* or *Haemophilus influenzae* type B. Dental or other infections may also be the cause. Patients will have a painfully swollen, red eye/eyelid, sometimes severe enough to cause the eye to be swollen shut with drooping (ptosis). Patients may have blurred vision along with a fever and headache. Proptosis (bulging eye) and ophthalmoplegia (eye muscle paralysis) are hallmark signs of orbital cellulitis. On exam, the extraocular movements may also be restricted, depending on the amount of edema. A CT scan should be done to determine severity and to rule out the presence of a foreign body and to assess any damage to the optic nerve. Also order a CBC (complete blood count), blood cultures, and culture of a nasal swab. Patients should be hospitalized and *treated* with appropriate IV antibiotics. Immunocompromised patients may develop a fungal orbital cellulitis. Once the infection is controlled with IV antibiotics, patients can be discharged home on oral antibiotics for 2 to 3 more weeks with close follow-up. *Complications* include intracranial expansion, vision loss, and cavernous sinus thrombosis.

Blepharitis

Blepharitis is an inflammation or infection of the **eyelid and eyelashes**. There are two types: **Staphylococcal blepharitis** and **Seborrheic blepharitis**, with seborrheic being the most common. In addition to the eyelids and eyelashes, blepharitis can affect the eyebrows and scalp. Patients may complain of burning of the eyes and matting of the eyelashes. The eyes may be irritated with a gritty feeling. They can also appear red. Include questioning in the history regarding possibly allergens or use or retinoids. Note any history of eczema or acne. *Diagnosis* is made per clinical assessment, usually pink or reddened eyelid with crusting. Under otoscope, if a hard, crusty material is visible in eyelashes this most often indicates staphylococcal blepharitis, whereas if the material in the eyelashes looks likes oily flaky material, this is more compatible with seborrheic blepharitis. *Treating* blepharitis involves debriding the lid margin of the matted material, usually using a cotton applicator. Warm compresses may be helpful. Topical antibiotics may be given and should be applied in the morning and at bedtime to prevent blurred vision from interfering with activities. Antihistamine eye drops do not help to relieve the symptoms of blepharitis by either cause. However, if the irritation is allergic in origin, then the drops will have an immediate effect. Lubricating eye drops will not help. Patients, especially in unilateral cases, need to be evaluated for sebaceous cell malignancy.

Chalazion

A **chalazion** is caused by the inflammation of a **sebaceous gland** (meibomian glands) on the eyelid. It is not the same thing as a sty. A sty will also involve hair follicles and is more superficial appearing. It is commonly found in patients with rosacea or blepharitis. A chalazion usually occurs on the **upper eyelid**. There may be gradual swelling that increases over the course of a few days to a few weeks. The lesion may appear red and inflamed, and patients may complain of pain. Eventually, it becomes a painless nodular lesion. *Diagnosis* is made by clinical assessment. Warm compresses may help to relieve the pain and promote absorption of the oil that is trapped in the sebaceous gland. If a bacterial infection is superimposed on the chalazion, an ophthalmic antibiotic may be prescribed. If the chalazion is large and there is no sign of infection, an injection of triamcinolone (Kenalog®) directly into the mass may help to relieve the inflammation and promote healing. In rare cases, surgical incision of the mass may be necessary if it persists and is not resolving with more conservative treatments. If the patient experiences recurring chalazia, they should be assessed for carcinoma.

Ectropion and Entropion

An **ectropion** is a condition in which the **lower eyelid turns outward**. This usually occurs during the aging process due to laxity of the muscles within the eyelid. The ectropion causes dryness and irritation of the eye. A paralysis of the facial nerve can cause this to occur because of the loss of neuromuscular control of the facial muscles on the affected side. Scarring due to trauma or burns can also cause an ectropion. Repair of the ectropion is accomplished through surgery to tighten the muscles of the lower eyelid.

An **entropion** is a condition in which the **lower eyelid turns inward**. This is most commonly caused by the aging process due to muscle laxity causing the lower eyelid to involute. Facial nerve palsy and scarring can also cause this condition. Patients will complain of irritation of the eye with tearing and the sensation of a foreign body being in the eye due to the eyelashes rubbing on the sclera. *Treatment* is by surgical correction.

Hordeolum

A **hordeolum**, or "**stye**," is a condition in which an eyelash follicle becomes infected. Patients may complain of tenderness around the area. The small abscess will appear red and swollen. It will eventually come to a head and purulent discharge may be expressed from the small infection. *Treatment* of a hordeolum generally consists of frequent application of warm compresses to draw the abscess to a head so that the infectious material can be expressed. The hordeolum may not drain and can resolve on its own. If the condition becomes severe, if complicated by preseptal cellulitis, or if patients develop recurrent hordeola, oral antibiotics (e.g., cephalexin) may be given to eradicate the infection. Oral doxycycline may be used in adults if recurrent and/or multiple lesions, or if significant/chronic meibomitis (inflammation of the meibomian glands, which can lead to a chalazion). It is important to remember that children should not be given tetracycline antibiotics due to alterations that can occur in tooth or bone development, unless >8 years old and if a severe/life threatening infection. Tetracyclines should also not be given to females who are or may become pregnant (Category D) because of the risk of birth anomalies. *Complications* include lid deformity and progression to a chalazion.

Congenital and Senile Cataracts

Cataracts are a disease involving opacification of the **lens** and are the leading cause of **treatable blindness** in the world. They typically present as either congenital or senile cataracts.

- **Congenital cataracts** are usually due to intrauterine infections, metabolic disorders, or genetic factors. An irregular red reflex is the typical initial clinical finding. TORCH titers (toxoplasmosis, other infections, rubella, cytomegalovirus, herpes simplex virus) and a VRDL (Venereal Disease Research Lab) test for syphilis should be drawn. Surgical intervention before 17 weeks of age is recommended to prevent and minimize visual impairment, including irreversible amblyopia ("lazy eye") and sensory nystagmus (involuntary, rapid eye movements), which is especially seen in bilateral congenital cataracts.
- **Senile cataracts** involve a gradual thickening of the lens and present with gradual, progressive visual impairment (typically night vision and near vision issues). Patients often complain of a glare. *Treatment* involves unilateral or bilateral surgical lens extraction. The main *complication* is blindness.

Pterygium

A **pterygium** is a triangular-shaped raised lesion that grows on the **surface of the eye**. It most commonly occurs on the nasal side of the cornea and may appear red. Patients usually seek treatment for this because of cosmetic appearances, but it can grow to obstruct the visual fields. This occurs if it extends over the cornea. Occasionally, it can be irritating to the eye. *Diagnosis* is made by clinical assessment. Care should be made to differentiate it from any neoplastic conditions. *Treatment* involves surgical removal of the pterygium, though this is usually reserved for cases in which the lesion affects the visual fields or is irritating. Surgery may be necessary to replace a portion of the conjunctiva. An antimetabolite may also be applied during surgery to prevent recurrence of the lesion. Almost one-half of patients who develop a pterygium will go on to develop the lesion again. There are usually no long-term effects of decreased visual acuity following surgery if the lesion is not encroaching upon the cornea.

Macular Degeneration

Macular degeneration is the most common cause of **irreversible central blindness** in the Caucasian population. It is rare in other races. There are two types of macular degeneration: dry and wet.

- **Dry macular degeneration** is more common and occurs when drusen (yellow deposits) accumulate deep in the eye under the retina. It begins in middle age and progresses slowly, causing a loss of central vision eventually leading to blindness. It can, however, develop into wet macular degeneration.

- **Wet macular degeneration** occurs when capillaries break through the retina and grow behind the macula of the eye. This form of the disease progresses more rapidly to blindness (days to weeks). Any vision loss that occurs over a period of weeks or days requires urgent ophthalmic evaluation. Drusen may be seen under the retina on fundoscopic exam, even before there is any visual loss. Center vision deficits may be seen on visual field exam.

There is no definitive cure for macular degeneration. However, vitamin C, E, zinc, copper and beta-carotene may slow the process of dry macular degeneration. Medications (ranibizumab, aflibercept, or bevacizumab) and surgery may improve vision in wet macular degeneration. There is a genetic link with this disease and prevention is important. Eating leafy green vegetables high in carotenoids, quitting smoking, and protecting the eyes from UV light, can reduce risk. *Complication*: Dry macular degeneration can suddenly turn to wet macular degeneration, resulting in rapid vision loss.

RHEGMATOGENOUS RETINAL DETACHMENT

Rhegmatogenous is the most common form of **retinal detachment** and is a medical emergency. Refer to an ophthalmologist immediately. Rhegmatogenous retinal detachment occurs when there is a **tear in the retina**, allowing the vitreous humor to enter the space behind the retina and causing a detachment of the retina from the posterior eye. The most common cause of this type of retinal detachment is the aging process, which leads to shrinkage of the vitreous humor. This causes pulling on the retina, leading to a tear or hole in the retina. Patients will describe floaters and flashes of light with an associated decrease in vision. The loss of vision will occur in a curtain-type fashion, where the vision appears as a dark curtain descending over the visual field, usually starting at the upper periphery and marching downwards. This occurs as the torn retina flaps down. Patients complaining of floaters who present with mono decreased visual fields should be referred to an ophthalmologist immediately. This condition is a surgical emergency and needs to be *treated* immediately. Delay of even one day can result in some degree of permanent visual loss after surgical repair.

TRACTIONAL RETINAL DETACHMENT

A **tractional retinal detachment** occurs in conditions that cause scarring within the **vitreous humor**, such as diabetic retinopathy. This is the second most common type of **retinal detachment**. The fibrous strands that make up a scar cause traction to be applied to the retina. This traction results in separation of the retina from the posterior eye. Onset is usually gradual. Some patients may have floaters or flashes of light in their vision, along with the curtain-type vision loss, as seen with rhegmatogenous retinal detachment. More commonly, there will be visual loss with a description of blind spots in the vision. *Treatment* usually involves removing the vitreous humor, thereby removing the fibrous scar material. Gas or an oily substance may be injected into the eye to prevent recurrence of this condition. The best treatment is prevention by maintaining adequate control of blood sugar levels in diabetics to prevent the development of diabetic retinopathy. There is a chance of permanent visual loss with this condition, despite aggressive treatment.

EXUDATIVE RETINAL DETACHMENT

An **exudative retinal detachment** occurs when fluid builds up **behind the retina**. This can occur with multiple medical conditions, including various collagen-vascular diseases, posterior scleritis, neoplasms of the eye, infections, preeclampsia, and congenital abnormalities. This results in visual loss with patients complaining of experiencing blind spots in their vision. They may also experience floaters or flashes of light in their vision. Surgery is not always necessary to treat this condition. *Treatment* of the underlying condition is usually sufficient to prevent permanent visual loss. With chronic medical conditions that cause an exudative retinal detachment, achieving adequate medical control of the condition can result in reversal of the detachment as the fluid behind the retina dissipates. Urgent treatment of the cause of the retinal detachment is necessary to prevent permanent visual loss. Some patients may develop a chronic problem with this condition, and then surgery to prevent fluid accumulation behind the retina is necessary.

Diabetic Retinopathy

Diabetic retinopathy is the leading cause of **blindness** in the US in diabetics <65-years-old. It begins as tiny **microaneurysms in the retina**. Exudates form in the retina as these aneurysms rupture. Patients frequently have no visual loss at this stage. As retinopathy progresses, the exudates become larger and the rupturing aneurysms can lead to swelling of the **macula**. Patients may or may not have a decrease in visual acuity. Focal laser photocoagulation is done at this stage to decrease the **macular edema** by cauterizing the leaking microaneurysms. The final stages of diabetic retinopathy occur when new vessels are developed around the optic nerve. These vessels are very fragile and are easily ruptured, which leads to bleeding within the retina and vitreous humor. As scar tissue forms, the fibrous strands of the scar may cause a **tractional retinal detachment**. Focal laser photocoagulation can be performed to decrease the rupture of these new vessels, but visual loss is common with this condition, and blindness frequently occurs. Annual eye exams are critical to managing this disease.

Hypertensive Retinopathy and Malignant Hypertension

Uncontrolled blood pressure is the cause of **hypertensive retinopathy**. As pressure rises within the body's arteries, the small arteries in the eye are also affected. This results in narrowing of the **retinal arteries** and a decrease in blood flow to the structures of the eye. Patients may or may not notice a decrease in their visual acuity. On exam, possible changes include, narrowed retinal arteries, copper wiring from sclerosis of the vessels, arteriovenous nicking, cotton-wool spots (retinal ischemia), retinal hemorrhages, and possible optic disc swelling. A swollen optic disc (papilledema) can result with malignant hypertension, a hypertensive emergency in which the diastolic blood pressure is >120 mm Hg. *Treatment* of hypertensive retinopathy involves controlling the blood pressure with diet, exercise, and medications. **Malignant hypertension** is an emergency condition and should be treated immediately, but slowly over 24-48 hours. Visual loss that results from hypertensive retinopathy may be permanent, but control of the blood pressure can prevent additional damage. Hypertensive encephalopathy, stroke, and hemorrhage are additional possible *complications*.

Conjunctivitis

Conjunctivitis ("**pink eye**") is an inflammation or infection of the conjunctiva of one or both eyes. It can be caused by bacteria, virus, allergy, or an irritant. Patients will complain of a gritty, irritating, itching sensations in the eye, which is red from hemorrhage of small vessels. Vision is usually not affected. With **bacterial conjunctivitis**, there is a copious mucus discharge, and patients may have problems with the eye being matted closed in the morning. **Viral and allergic conjunctivitis** typically cause a watery discharge. This is a *diagnosis* of exclusion, based on clinical assessment. The following should be ruled out: stye, ulceration, or blepharitis. If bacterial conjunctivitis is suspected, *treatment* consists of erythromycin 5mg/g ointment ophthalmically applying a 1 cm ribbon 4-6 times per day for 5 to 7 days, or trimethoprim-polymyxin B ophthalmic 1 drop every 3 hours (max 6 drops/day) for 7 to 10 days, or other ophthalmic antibiotics. If no response to antibiotic drops the patient should be referred to ophthalmologist. Viral conjunctivitis only requires symptomatic relief. Patients should avoid rubbing the eye. Frequent hand washing can decrease transmission of the condition. Allergic conjunctivitis can be treated with ophthalmic antihistamines, but this condition may be chronic in patients who suffer from recurrent environmental allergies. Corneal injury may occur resulting in vision impairment.

Dacryocystitis and Dacryoadenitis

Dacryocystitis is a condition in which the **lacrimal sac** becomes inflamed. This inflammation can be due to a blockage at some point in the tear drainage system or a stone that has formed within the lacrimal sac. Patients will complain of pain along the inside corner of the eye. The area will appear red and swollen and may extend from the inner canthus of the eye to the upper nose or nasal bridge. If the dacryocystitis is chronic in nature, tearing is the most prevalent complaint. *Diagnosis* is made by clinical assessment. CBC may show elevated WBCs, and occasionally CT scans are ordered to show anatomy and surrounding areas of lacrimal sac. To *treat* this inflammation and infection, antibiotics can be given. Depending upon the severity, patients may require hospitalization for IV antibiotic therapy. If severe, incision and drainage may be necessary to treat an abscess. Once the inflammation and infection have resolved, surgery may be necessary to correct the blockage. If a stone is present within the lacrimal sac, this will need to be surgically removed to prevent future blockages leading to abscess formation. *Complications* include cellulitis, sepsis, meningitis, fistula, and abscess. **Dacryoadenitis** is the inflammatory enlargement of the lacrimal gland and presents as redness & swelling of the upper eyelid with a S-shaped ptosis (drooping of the upper eyelid).

Primary Open Angle Glaucoma

Primary open angle glaucoma is the most common form of **glaucoma**, is asymptomatic, progressive, irreversible, and causes optic nerve damage. It is more common in patients over 40, in African Americans, and in patients with a positive family history. Screening is vital since patients are asymptomatic; however, patients may notice peripheral visual field loss later in the disease. *Diagnose* by measuring intraocular pressure, corneal thickness, visual field testing, and ophthalmoscopy. Increased cupping of the optic disc and thinning of the neural rim may be seen on fundoscopic exam. *Treatment* begins with ophthalmic eye drops: Ophthalmic β-blockers (timolol), prostaglandin analogs (latanoprost), alpha-2 agonists (brimonidine), and carbonic anhydrase inhibitors (brinzolamide), and miotic agents (pilocarpine) that work on the muscarinic receptors of the eye to increase fluid flow may also be prescribed. Laser and traditional surgical treatments are usually reserved for when medical management fails to produce adequate results in decreasing the ocular pressure. Refer to an ophthalmologist for monitoring and chronic treatment. Permanent vision loss is the primary *complication*.

Angle Closure Glaucoma

Angle closure glaucoma affects approximately 10% of patients who have glaucoma. There are several types of **primary angle closure glaucoma**: subacute, acute (medical emergency), and chronic. The angle through which fluid drains from the eye is narrowed, resulting in an increase in ocular pressure. This is treated with surgery by creating an opening behind the iris through which the fluid can flow from the eye, resulting in a decrease in ocular pressure. In **subacute** and **chronic angle closure glaucoma**, the closure is usually gradual and can be asymptomatic unless there is an attack. **Acute angle closure glaucoma** results in the sudden onset of blurred vision with visual halos, pain/headache, red eye, and nausea and vomiting. This is a medical emergency and requires immediate treatment/referral to an ophthalmologist. The cornea may be edematous when examined, and ocular pressure readings are extremely elevated with this condition. Ophthalmic medications (e.g., pilocarpine, timolol, travoprost) can be given to reduce the corneal edema and intraocular pressure. Laser surgery (iridotomy) is necessary to open the angle so that fluid can flow from the eye to cause a decrease in the ocular pressure. *Complications* include optic nerve damage and vision loss.

Strabismus

Strabismus is a condition in which the **extraocular muscles** are weakened, leading to a gaze deviation in one eye. It differs from a "lazy eye," or amblyopia, because there is no loss of visual acuity associated with a strabismus. The condition is labeled by the direction in which the gaze is affected:

- **Hypertropia** occurs when the gaze is diverted upward.
- **Exotropia** when the gaze is deviated outward.
- **Esotropia** when the gaze is deviated inward ("cross-eyes").
- **Hypotropia** when the gaze is deviated downward.

A wide, flattened nose with a skin fold at the inner canthus can cause the appearance of esotropia and is called **pseudoesotropia**. This usually resolves with age. Eye muscle strengthening can be performed to help straighten the gaze in mild cases of strabismus. If this fails or if the strabismus is severe, surgery may be necessary to draw the affected muscles tighter in order to straighten the gaze.

Papilledema

Papilledema is **optic disc swelling**, typically bilateral, secondary to increased intracranial pressure. *Symptoms* may include headache, nausea/vomiting, pulsatile tinnitus, blurred, and double-vision. However, visual symptoms are often absent. Fundoscopic exam can show disc margin blurring, venous congestion with hemorrhages, exudates, and cotton-wool spots (indicates nerve fiber damage) around the disc. Initial findings typically present nasally. Test the visual field for enlargement of the blind spot. Order an urgent head CT or MRI with contrast to rule out a mass lesion. Once normal imaging is established, perform a lumbar puncture to assess opening pressure and to rule out neoplastic or infectious causes. Causes include brain tumor, head trauma/hemorrhage, meningitis, encephalitis, and idiopathic intracranial hypertension (pseudotumor cerebri). *Treat* the underlying cause. Blindness is the main *complication*.

Disorders of the Ear

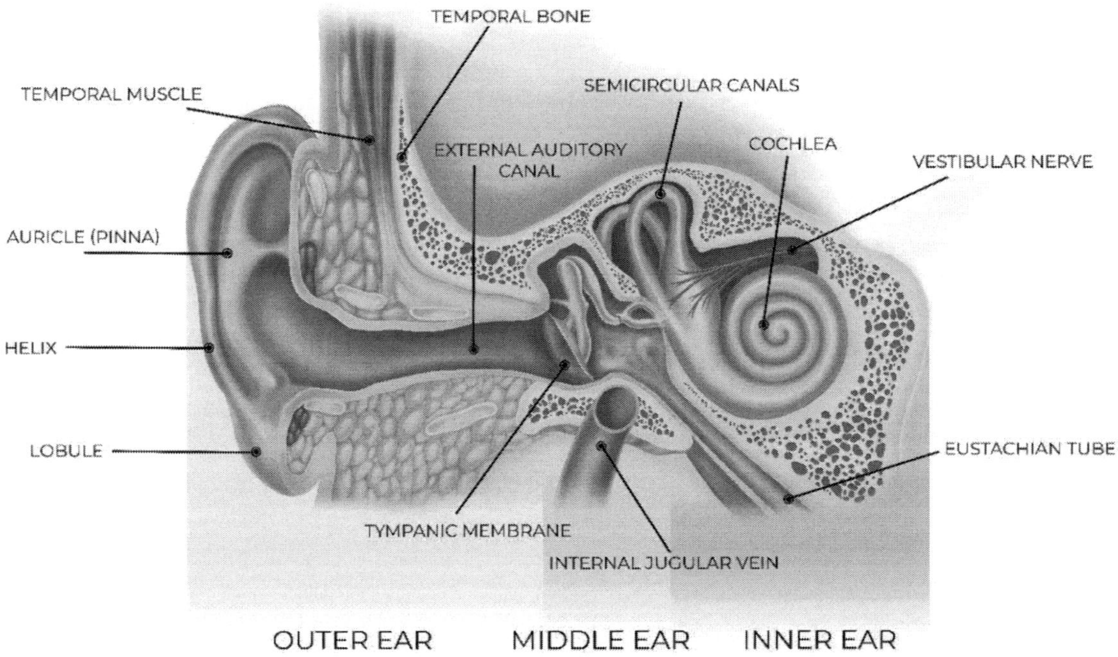

LABYRINTHITIS

Labyrinthitis is an inflammatory condition affecting the **labyrinth of the inner ear**. It usually occurs following a viral infection, such as a cold or the flu. Bacterial infections of the upper respiratory system, trauma to the head or ear, along with benign tumors of the ear may also cause this condition. Vertigo is the main *symptom* that patients will experience. This can be quite severe with nausea and vomiting, along with a complete loss of balance. Patients may have hearing loss, a headache, or tinnitus with this condition. The symptoms can be positional or may occur at rest. *Diagnosis* is made by clinical assessment, using imaging to rule out other disorders if needed. It is important to obtain an audiogram. Labyrinthitis is usually treated with bed rest, hydration, and anti-vertigo medications, such as meclizine. Viral labyrinthitis is also often treated with a tapering dose of corticosteroids, like prednisone. Antibiotics will be given if the condition is caused by a bacterial infection. For symptom relief, antihistamines, antiemetics, and benzodiazepines are commonly used, but should be used short term. *Complications* are not usually common, but include tinnitus and hearing loss (especially in cases of meningitis).

VERTIGO

Vertigo is the sense that the room is spinning. It can originate from a central (central nervous system, CNS) or peripheral cause.

- **CNS causes** include anemic or hemorrhagic episodes, tumors, trauma, or multiple sclerosis.
- **Peripheral causes** include labyrinthitis, Ménière's disease, vestibular neuronitis, and benign paroxysmal positional vertigo (BPPV).

In the US, vertigo is commonly caused by BPPV. It causes short-term positional vertigo accompanied with nystagmus (rhythmic movement of the eyes) and usually nausea. This is a clinical *diagnosis* which can be confirmed with an abnormal Dix-Hallpike maneuver (a test that elicits vertigo and nystagmus). Small stones (otoliths) within the labyrinth cause this condition, and the Epley maneuver can be used to change the position of the stones. Medications are not effective since they do not address the causative factor. *Complications* are rare after repositioning maneuvers, but include worsening vertigo and otoliths causing a canal jam.

OTITIS MEDIA

Otitis media (OM) is an infection of the **middle ear** and is the second most common childhood illness after upper respiratory infections (URI). It is most commonly bacterial or viral and affects children more often than adults because of the straight anatomic structure of the auditory canal and eustachian tube, which promotes the accumulation of fluid behind the tympanic membrane. The most common cause of otitis media in children is infection with *Streptococcus pneumoniae, Haemophilus influenza,* or *Moraxella (Branhamella) catarrhalis*. The incidence of infection with the first two organisms is on the decline, however, because of immunizations now available. *Signs and symptoms* include ear pain and fever and symptoms of an upper respiratory infection may also be present. On otoscopic exam, a bulging tympanic membrane with purulent effusion may be evident. There should be decreased movement of the membrane with insufflation. *Treat* with antibiotics if >6 months with severe otalgia, otalgia >48 hours, or temperature >39° C or if bilateral non-severe acute OM (AOM). Antibiotics may be started, but since many cases resolve on their own, a conservative approach can be taken if 6-23 months or older with a unilateral non-severe AOM. In this case, observe and start antibiotics if symptoms worsen or if there is no improvement within 48-72 hours of symptom onset. Amoxicillin is the drug of choice (unless used in the last 30 days) for uncomplicated OM without penicillin allergy. The most common dose is 500 mg every 12 hours (if >40kg). High dose Amoxicillin is an option in pediatrics (if >3 months and <40kg) of 80-90mg/kg/day ÷ every 12 hours. High dose Amoxicillin clavulanate is the antibiotic of choice for children in a daycare setting. Drug resistance varies across the US, so current guidelines for any specific area should be followed. *Complications* include mastoiditis, labyrinthitis, and hearing loss.

Mastoiditis

Mastoiditis is an infection of the **mastoid bone** of the skull and usually occurs following **otitis media**, especially in patients younger than 5 years old. It is typically due to *Streptococcus pneumoniae*. In the past, mastoiditis was relatively common and the leading common cause of death in children. Since the advent of antibiotics and prompt treatment of otitis media infections, the incidence of mastoiditis has greatly declined. Patients, if old enough, may complain of severe pain in the ear and behind the ear. There may be swelling and erythema in the area that causes the affected ear to stick out from the head. Patients may have a high fever and headache. A CT of the temporal bone will show an opacification of the mastoid air cells due to the infection. *Treatment* includes tympanocentesis with culture and sensitivity with aggressive IV antibiotics in order to penetrate the bone tissue and treat the infection. Once IV antibiotics are effective (afebrile for 48 hours), the patient will continue on oral antibiotics for 14 days to completely eradicate the infection. Myringotomy may be needed to remove fluid and ventilate the ear. If medical treatment is not effective, a mastoidectomy may be performed. *Complications* include hearing loss, facial nerve palsy (cranial nerve VII), brain abscess, and meningitis.

Cholesteatoma

A **cholesteatoma** is an abnormal growth of squamous epithelium in the **middle ear** which can cause permanent hearing loss. They can be congenital but is typically caused by **chronic tympanic membrane retractions** or from a **tympanic membrane perforation** (either traumatic or due to tympanostomy tubes). The patient with a history of ear infections, who presents with painless ear drainage (hallmark sign), hearing loss, and occasionally dizziness, should be evaluated for a cholesteatoma. *Diagnosis* is made on physical exam and by CT scan. Evaluation might include a hearing and balance test. Refer to an otolaryngologist since surgical removal is necessary, unless medically contraindicated. If left untreated, a cholesteatoma can lead to permanent hearing loss through bone deterioration, abscess formation, meningitis, and even death.

Otitis Externa

Otitis externa (OE) is an infection of the **external ear canal**. It is usually caused by *Pseudomonas* bacteria or *Staphylococcus aureus* infections. Occasionally, the infection can be due to a fungal infection. This is often referred to as "swimmer's ear" because of the prevalence in those who spend a lot of time in the water. Significant ear pain that is exacerbated with movement of the external ear is the main *symptom*. Patients may have enlargement of the preauricular lymph nodes. Exam of the ear canal will reveal edema, erythema of the ear canal, possibly with purulent discharge. *Diagnosis* is made by clinical assessment and history. The mainstays of *treatment* with OE involve cleaning the ear, treating the inflammation, controlling pain, and avoiding contributing factors. After cleaning the ear, the ear is treated with topical antibiotics with or without corticosteroids, antiseptics, or acidifying agents. For drops, tilt head towards opposite shoulder, pull superior part of auricle up and instill drops. The patient should side lie for 5 minutes or use a cotton ball in the ear. If swelling is severe, a wick is placed in the ear canal to facilitate installation of the solution. The wick may remain for 2-3 days. Aminoglycoside eardrops can also be used, but care should be taken to ensure the tympanic membrane is intact because of the risk of ototoxicity with these medications. *Complications* include necrotizing (malignant) external otitis, mastoiditis, and periauricular cellulitis.

Ménière's Disease

Ménière's disease (Idiopathic endolymphatic hydrops) is a condition affecting the **labyrinth of the ear**. The labyrinth is made up of bony and membranous portions. The membranous portion contains a fluid called **endolymph**. It is thought that Ménière's disease results when the membranous portion of the labyrinth ruptures, causing the endolymph to mix with **perilymph**, a fluid separating the membranous portion from the bony portion. *Signs and symptoms* include tinnitus, vertigo, and loss of hearing. Some patients experience a feeling of pressure within the affected ear(s). These symptoms are often not constant, but rather occur intermittently. *Diagnosis* is made by clinical assessment. Sensorineural hearing loss, tinnitus, and occasional episodes of vertigo as well as the occasional aural fullness are the usual qualifiers for a diagnosis. Other diagnoses should be ruled out. There is *no cure* of Ménière's disease. The symptoms can be decreased, though, with the dietary restriction of sodium, caffeine, and alcohol. Quitting smoking may help decrease the severity of symptoms. Gentamicin eardrops may help decrease the vertigo. With severe cases, the labyrinth can be surgically removed, but this will result in hearing loss in the ear. Benzodiazepines, antihistamines, and antiemetics are often used for acute episodes of symptoms. *Complications* include intractable vertigo and hearing loss.

Disorders of the Mouth, Nose, and Throat

Allergic Rhinitis

Allergic rhinitis affects the nose and eyes. It occurs in those individuals with allergies to **environmental irritants** such as pollen, animal dander, trees, and dust. *Symptoms* vary from minor allergic reactions to urticaria (hives) and throat constriction. The onset of symptoms can often be associated with exposure to an environmental irritant. Signs and symptoms include rhinorrhea (runny nose), itchy and watery eyes, mild cough, sneezing, facial itching, and sore throat. Patients may complain of a headache, possibly over the sinuses, with a feeling of pressure due to increased mucus production. Fatigue, irritability, reduced performance and possibly depression can be side effects. *Diagnosis* is made by clinical assessment, history, and findings. Allergic shiners, a nasal crease, boggy nasal turbinates, and cobblestoning of the posterior pharynx may be noted on physical exam. Allergy skin testing and allergen-specific serum IgE tests are useful. Treatment includes environmental controls to specific triggers, medication, and immunotherapy (subcutaneous or sublingual). Intranasal steroid sprays or antihistamines with decongestants are the most effective maintenance therapies. Antihistamines decrease the release of histamine and suppress the allergic symptoms; however, they have sedative side effects. Therefore, second generation antihistamines are usually preferred (loratadine, cetirizine, fexofenadine). *Complications* include sinusitis, otitis media, palatal changes, apnea, and asthma.

Acute and Chronic Sinusitis

Sinusitis (rhinosinusitis) is inflammation of the nasal passages and paranasal sinuses that is symptomatic. Mucus cannot drain because of the edematous sinuses, producing an excellent environment in which bacteria can thrive, leading to a sinus infection. It is classified as **acute sinusitis** if symptoms <30 days and **chronic** if >90 days. *Signs and symptoms* include a current or resolving upper respiratory infection (URI) and a headache (generally over the frontal, ethmoid, or maxillary sinuses). Complaints of positional increases in the headache, a fullness or pressure within the head, stuffy nose, fever, and aching in the teeth may also be present. *Diagnosis* is made per clinical assessment. It is important to attempt to distinguish bacterial from viral sinusitis. Sinusitis is likely **bacterial** if the patient presents with sinusitis symptoms for ≥10 days, especially if symptoms are severe with high fever, facial pain, and purulent nasal discharge. Since URI's typically last only 5-7 days, also consider when 7 days following a URI which was improving but suddenly presents with worsening symptoms. *Treatment* will be decided based on whether the sinusitis is of bacterial or viral origin. For both viral and bacterial sinusitis, symptoms can be improved with analgesia, mucolytics, decongestants, steroids, nasal irrigation, and antihistamines. First line treatment for acute bacterial sinusitis includes 14 days of high dose amoxicillin (80-90 mg/kg/day), clarithromycin, or azithromycin. Chronic sinusitis is typically treated with daily nasal irrigation, nasal steroids, and 3-6 weeks (or more) of antibiotics. Drug resistance varies across the US, so clinicians should be aware of local resistance trends. *Complications* include meningitis, cavernous sinus thrombosis, orbital cellulitis, and abscess.

Pharyngitis

Pharyngitis is an inflammation of the **pharynx**, causing a sore throat. It is most commonly caused by a **viral infection**. The most common bacterial cause of pharyngitis is **Group A Streptococci (GAS)**. Patients will complain of a very sore throat that may or may not be accompanied with other cold symptoms. Cold symptoms are usually present with viral forms of pharyngitis. A fever, headache, and soft palate petechiae may also be present. Children with GAS pharyngitis may also have nausea and vomiting. On exam, cervical and tonsillar lymph nodes will be enlarged, the oropharynx will appear edematous/erythematous, possibly with white exudates present. Centor criteria are symptoms that may be present and are used to guide the clinician: tonsillar exudates, absence of cough, fever (may be by history), and anterior cervical adenopathy. Patients with ≥4 have a 51-53% risk and are likely to have GAS. For patients that have 2 or more Centor criteria, use a rapid antigen detection test (RADT) to diagnosis GAS. Those with <2 Centor criteria, unless with a high risk for infection, are usually treated as viral pharyngitis. Culture confirms *diagnosis* (90-99% sensitive) but as RADT is very sensitive (70-90%), it is not often ordered. Viral pharyngitis is supportive with warm salt water, antipyretics, and analgesics. Penicillin is the drug of choice for GAS pharyngitis: e.g., penicillin VK, penicillin G benzathine (an IM form), and amoxicillin (preferred in children due to better taste tolerability). *Complications* include glomerulonephritis, rheumatic fever, scarlet fever, toxic shock syndrome, otitis media, sinusitis, cellulitis, and peritonsillar abscess.

Aphthous Ulcers

Aphthous ulcers, also known as **recurrent aphthous stomatitis (RAS)**, or **canker sores**, occur only within the soft tissues of the **oral cavity**. They can appear on the lips, oral mucosa, gums, or tongue. Canker sores are not contagious, typically start in childhood, and often resolve in the third decade of life. There is commonly a positive family history. However, they have no definite known cause, but irritants in the oral cavity, such as strongly acidic foods, may contribute to aphthous ulcers. Also, smoking cessation, stress, food allergies, and sodium lauryl sulphate, which is contained in many dental products, may contribute to RAS. Patients will complain of a painful area in the oral cavity with some local swelling. Exam will reveal a shallow, oval or round, yellowish or grayish ulcer that is well-demarcated with an erythematous halo. The ulcer is usually less than 2-4 mm in width and there is typically no bleeding present. *Diagnosis* is made per clinical assessment and history. *Treatment* involves topical corticosteroids and oral vitamin B-12 may help reduce RAS recurrences. Avoid predisposing factors and items that irritate the ulcer such as acidic foods and drinks, rough, hard foods. Over-the-counter topical numbing medications may be helpful in decreasing the pain. Aphthous ulcers generally resolve spontaneously within 7-10 days. Scarring is the main *complication*, but is uncommon.

Dental Abscess

A **dental abscess** is an infection that forms around the roots of a tooth, or teeth, or in the gum tissue. Infection within the **dental pulp** (periapical) is more common in children while an abscess in the **surrounding tissue** (periodontal) is more common in adults. Dental abscesses are polymicrobial. Patients will develop severe pain in an isolated area of the mouth. The cheek will be swollen and the gingiva will be warm and appear red and swollen. Also, the lymph nodes in the neck on the affected side may be enlarged. A fever and headache may be present. The abscess may rupture, but treatment is still necessary. *Diagnosis* is made per clinical assessment. *Treatment* includes antibiotics, usually amoxicillin/clavulanate, and drainage of the abscess. Antibiotic treatment is very important to prevent systemic spread of the infection. Refer to a dentist or an oral surgeon. *Complications* include deep tissue infections, osteomyelitis, sinusitis, Ludwig angina (a rapidly spreading cellulitis), and cavernous sinus thrombosis.

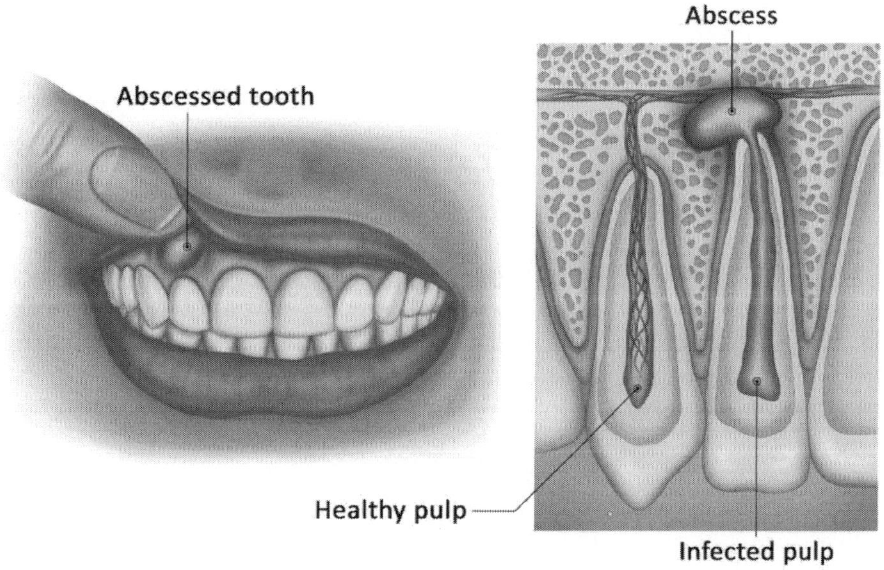

Oral Leukoplakia

Oral leukoplakia is a white patchy lesion found in the **oral cavity**. It can be caused by tobacco use (either smoking or chewing), alcohol use, chronic irritation, vitamin deficiency, candidiasis, or endocrine disturbances, and is considered a premalignant form of oral cancer. Another form of the condition is **hairy leukoplakia** (typically along the borders of the tongue), which is seen in HIV-positive patients or others with suppressed immune systems and is associated with the Epstein-Barr virus. Patients with oral leukoplakia will complain of a painless white patch in their mouths. This patch can be on the oral mucosa, the tongue, or gums. It is a slightly raised, rough patch that is white or grayish in color and cannot be rubbed off. There may occasionally be leukoplakia lesions or nodules that appear pink or red in color and these lesions have a strong potential for malignancy. *Diagnosis* is made by clinical assessment and confirmation by biopsy. *Treatment* involves surgical excision of the lesion. There is a chance that patients can develop these lesions again, especially if they continue to smoke or use smokeless tobacco. Quitting smoking and tobacco use is the best prevention of future lesions. Oral cancer is a possible *complication*.

Oral Candidiasis

Oral candidiasis, or **oral thrush**, is a fungal infection (typically *Candida albicans*) affecting the **oral mucosa**. It is usually not contagious and commonly occurs in those who wear dentures. It can also occur in newborns, diabetics, patients who take steroids (especially inhalation steroids), immunocompromised patients, and those undergoing head or neck radiation. It may also occur in those taking antibiotics due to alterations in the natural flora of the mouth. Patients will have white plaques over the oral mucosa which can be scraped off with a tongue depressor to reveal red, raw areas. The lesions may or may not be painful to patients. *Diagnosis* is most often made by clinical assessment, however if confirmation is needed, cultures can be taken. Topical or oral antifungals (e.g., nystatin, clotrimazole, fluconazole) are used to *treat* oral candidiasis. Resistance to the azole drugs is an increasing concern. Patients should be reminded to daily clean their dentures thoroughly. For patients using inhaled steroids, care should be taken to completely rinse their mouths after each treatment. There are usually no *complications* in the immunocompetent, but in the immunocompromised, candidiasis can spread to the blood stream, esophagus, heart valves, etc. Also, it can lead to malnutrition if eating becomes difficult.

Sialadenitis

Sialadenitis is an infection of the **salivary glands**. It differs from parotitis, or mumps, in that it involves a blockage of the flow of saliva, causing bacteria to grow within the **ducts**. This leads to a **bacterial infection**, usually caused by *Staphylococcus aureus*. The most common salivary glands affected are the parotid glands in the cheek and the submandibular glands under the chin. Patients will complain of pain in the affected area. Purulent drainage may flow into the mouth, causing a foul-smelling and foul-tasting sensation. Patients may have a fever and headache. *Diagnosis* is usually made by clinical assessment, but CT may be useful if stones are suspected but not palpable. *Treatment* is usually accomplished with appropriate antibiotic therapy and hydration. If infection is severe, the gland may need to be drained with culture and sensitivity testing performed on the extracted pus. If a stone is causing a blockage of the ductwork leading from the salivary gland, this will need to be surgically removed. *Complications* include abscess formation and patients may develop a chronic form of sialadenitis that causes recurrent flare-ups of the condition.

Peritonsillar Abscess

A **peritonsillar abscess** can occur as a complication of **bacterial tonsillitis**. The causative organism is usually group A beta-hemolytic streptococci. An abscess can develop in the soft tissue surrounding the **tonsil** and lead to a severe infection. Patients will have severe throat pain with enlarged lymph nodes on the affected side. *Signs and symptoms* include fever, headache, difficulty swallowing, muffled voice ("hot potato" voice), difficulty closing the mouth, drooling, neck swelling, ipsilateral ear pain, and trismus. Trismus can help distinguish an abscess from tonsillitis/cellulitis. *Diagnosis* is made by clinical assessment- deviation of the uvula and tonsil displacement. Immediately refer the patient to an otolaryngologist. Needle aspiration with culture of the fluid drained confirms the diagnosis. *Treatment* may be handled on an outpatient or inpatient basis. Treatment involves hydration, incision and drainage (with culture, if not previously performed), then appropriate antibiotics. High-dose IV penicillin, cephalosporins, and amoxicillin-clavulanate (if mononucleosis is ruled out) are good initial choices. As always, local patterns of susceptibility should be taken into consideration. If MRSA is common, use clindamycin or vancomycin or if severe or not responding. Patients may require future surgery to remove the tonsils and prevent recurrence of this infection. *Complications* include airway obstruction, sepsis, aspiration pneumonia, carotid artery pseudoaneurysm and rupture, thrombophlebitis (of the jugular vein), mediastinitis, and necrotizing fasciitis.

Skin and Subcutaneous Tissue

Skin Cancers

Basal Cell Carcinoma

Basal cell carcinoma (BCC) is the most common and slowest-growing form of skin cancer. It is an epithelial tumor of keratinocytes in the stratum basale (the deepest level of the epidermis) that is caused by excessive exposure to UV light. These usually appear on the head, face, and neck, and patients who develop BCC are likely to have more in the future. The lesions are usually pearly white to pink in color, may have a waxy appearance, and can be flat or scaly in appearance. These tend to recurrently bleed and crust over. There may be a depressed area in the center with surface telangiectases. *Diagnosis* is by a shave or punch biopsy and histology. *Treatment* of basal cell carcinoma involves removal of the lesion by a specialist. This can be surgically excised or removed with curettage and electrodessication, cryotherapy, or antineoplastic creams, such as 5-fluorouracil or imiquimod, or by using photodynamic therapy. Patients should be educated on the importance of protecting the skin from sun exposure. Sunscreen with a high SPF level should be used whenever patients are outside. *Complications* include increased risk for other types of skin cancer, disfigurement, and spreading of cancer (rare).

Squamous Cell Carcinoma

Squamous cell carcinoma (**SCC**) is the second most common type of **skin cancer** after BCC. It involves keratinocytes and invades the **dermis**. It is usually found on the head and neck (sun-exposed areas), can spread/metastasize, and can be fatal if left untreated. Though not as deadly as melanoma, SCC is more likely to cause serious complications when compared to basal cell carcinoma. SCC risk increases in patients with increased UV light exposure (especially fair-skinned), in men, in those with actinic keratosis, in the immunocompromised, and in those with a history of human papilloma virus (HPV). Patients often present describing a sore or ulcer that doesn't heal. SCC lesions can appear anywhere on the body and can be crusty or scaly, occasionally nodular, and may appear red or white when forming on mucous membranes. *Diagnosis* is made per histopathology. *Treatment* is similar to BCC and includes removal of the lesion with excision, curettage and electrodessication, Mohs microscopic surgery, or cryotherapy. For high risk lesions a more aggressive approach may be used including radiation for metastases. The skin should always be protected from sun by shielding or applying sunscreen with a high SPF rating. *Complications* include metastases to lymph nodes and organs, disfigurement, and death (uncommon).

Melanoma

Malignant melanoma is the most serious form of **skin cancer** and can be fatal. It develops in the **melanin cells** of the skin and can metastasize. It is more likely to occur in those who are fair skinned, have a high exposure to UV light, and those who have a positive family history of melanoma. Regular checks with a dermatologist and vigilant use of proper covering and sunscreen are necessary to help prevent melanoma. Melanoma can develop in a mole or may be a new lesion on the skin. Warning signs include changes to the shape, size, or color of a nevus or lesion. The skin may have asymmetry, irregular borders, uneven color, a diameter >6 mm, and be elevated. *Diagnosis* is made per histopathology from an excisional biopsy. The lesion is staged (Stage I-II= primary and localized; Stage III= regional metastasis; Stage IV= distant metastasis) and further categorized using the Clark levels and Breslow thickness classification. A sentinel lymph node biopsy may be needed to see if the cancer has spread to adjacent lymph nodes. Diagnostic studies should be done to ensure there have not been any metastases of the melanoma. *Treatment* consists of surgical excision to include a small amount of surrounding normal tissue (the margin size depends on the thickness of the lesion). Radiation and chemotherapy are used palliatively with advanced melanoma. *Complications* include metastases and death.

Dermatitis and Eczema

Contact Dermatitis

Contact dermatitis is an **inflammatory response** to an allergen or irritant. This can be caused by numerous agents such as lotions, soaps, nickel, poison ivy, or poison sumac. The skin rash associated with contact dermatitis often occurs quickly following exposure to an irritant and the rash is more painful than pruritic. Whereas, the rash associated with an allergen is a delayed hypersensitivity reaction, which, once sensitized, typically occurs within 1-2 days of exposure, and this rash is usually extremely pruritic. With contact dermatitis the skin becomes red and edematous with papules and vesicular lesions. In chronic exposure, the skin can become hyperpigmented with lichenification, plaques, fissures, and hyperkeratosis. *Diagnosis* is made mostly per history/physical. Finding and eliminating the possible trigger(s) can also be diagnostic. For cases that don't easily resolve, patch testing may be effective. *Treatment* consists of discontinuing exposure to the causative substance, cool compresses, topical corticosteroids, and antihistamines (e.g., hydroxyzine or diphenhydramine can be taken if the dermatitis is due to exposure to an allergen). If contact dermatitis is severe, oral steroids can be given to reduce the inflammation. *Complications* include neurodermatitis (lichen simplex chronicus-thick, leathery skin from chronic scratching) and infection.

Diaper Rash

Diaper rash is a form of **contact dermatitis** and commonly occurs in babies wearing diapers or in incontinent adults. It is caused by exposure of the skin to the moisture of urine and waste material. If severe, the rash can have an accompanying bacterial or fungal infection. The skin with prolonged moisture against it will become very inflamed, red, tender, and possibly broken or cracked. Often there is irritation in the convex surfaces of the infant's body. This irritation can be simple erythema, lesions, papules, or erosions. If a fungal infection develops because of the moisture, there may be small red papules, or satellite lesions, surrounding the inflamed area. *Diagnosis* is made clinically. The goal of *treating* diaper rash is to keep the skin clean and dry. Leaving the skin open to air and avoiding a wet diaper against the skin will help to relieve the rash. Barrier creams and ointment containing zinc oxide can help to prevent further irritation of the skin. An antifungal or antibacterial cream may be necessary if a secondary infection occurs. Persistent fungal diaper rashes can be a sign of an underlying immune condition or type 1 diabetes. *Complications* include candidal or bacterial infections.

Atopic Dermatitis

Atopic dermatitis, or eczema, is a **skin rash** that is more prevalent in children than adults though it can occur at any time in life. However, it usually presents before 5 years of age. The exact cause is unknown, but it is thought to be immune-mediated. It is frequently seen in families and along with asthma or hay fever. Patients have extremely pruritic, dry skin with reddish to dark-colored areas with scales, weeping, and lichenification. They may with have excoriations and papules that crust over after opening. The pruritus can be aggravated by temperature changes, hot showers or baths, or allergens (e.g., cigarette smoke). Atopic dermatitis most often occurs over the antecubital fossa and behind the knees, though it can occur anywhere on the body. *Diagnosis* consists of these essential features:

- Pruritus
- Eczema (either acute, subacute, or chronic)
- Typical distribution patterns (infants & children with facial, neck, or *extensor* involvement; h/o *flexural* lesions at any age; sparing of the groin and axilla)
- Chronic and relapsing nature

Treat with lubricating creams and oils immediately after bathing, topical corticosteroid creams or ointments, immunomodulators (e.g., tacrolimus), and avoid irritants and triggers to the outbreaks. *Complications* include neurodermatitis, skin infections, blepharitis, and sleep issues.

Nummular Eczema

Nummular eczema is a form of eczema that causes coin-shaped patches on the skin. Unlike atopic dermatitis, it is uncommon in children. It usually appears in males in the 6th-7th decade of life. There is no definitive cause, but it does tend to be aggravated by strong soaps and detergents, anything that dries the skin, and extremes in temperature. It begins as vesicles and papules that coalesce to form the characteristic erythematous, discoid plaque. They usually start on the legs, are very pruritic, often symmetric, and tend to be dry and scaly. The rash can resemble a fungal infection or ringworm, but tends to recur. *Diagnosis* is made per H&P. *Treat* with mid-to-strong corticosteroid creams or ointments and baths followed with immediate moisturizer use. With a severe outbreak, short-term oral steroids may be necessary as well as UVB phototherapy. Coal tar preparations can help with an outbreak, but they tend to stain clothes. Treat with appropriate antibiotics if a secondary skin infection develops. Avoid the triggers that cause flare-ups to help decrease the severity and frequency of outbreaks. *Complications* include skin infections and scars.

Dyshidrosis

Dyshidrosis, or dyshidrotic eczema, is a form of eczema that causes vesicular lesions to form on the **palms and soles**. This condition typically occurs between ages 10 and 40, and the exact cause is not known. It seems to occur more frequently during stressful times, and may be linked to exposure to metal salts. There is an increased incidence in those patients with atopy (a familial hypersensitivity to allergens). Dyshidrosis is a chronic condition with no known cure. *Signs and symptoms* include extremely pruritic vesicular lesions, that may form bullae, on the palms of the hands and soles of the feet. These can break open and crust over. As the lesions are resolving, the skin becomes very dry and cracked, which can be painful, and desquamation occurs. Secondary skin infections can also occur. *Diagnosis* is made upon clinical assessment: pruritus, reoccurrence, acute onset, deep seated bullae or vesicles on the soles and palms or the lateral finger. High-potency topical corticosteroid creams or ointments, cold compresses, antihistamines, antibiotics for secondary infections, UV light phototherapy, and immunosuppressants may *treat* symptoms and decrease the severity of the flare-ups. *Complications* include limited use of hands and feet, skin infections, and cellulitis.

Inflammatory Skin Disorders

Erythema Multiforme, Stevens-Johnson Syndrome, and Toxic Epidermal Necrolysis

Erythema Multiforme (EM) once thought to be a milder form of Stevens-Johnson syndrome, is actually an **inflammatory reaction**, usually due to a viral infection or sometimes a medication, that causes an acute, self-limited rash with characteristic target lesions that usually begin on the extremities and begins to resolve within 1 week. There are 2 forms: **EM minor** (localized eruption with little to no mucosal involvement) and **EM major** (mucosal involvement but <10% epidermal detachment).

Both **Stevens-Johnson syndrome (SJS)** and **toxic epidermal necrolysis (TEN)** are severe **hypersensitivity reactions** that usually occur due to a medication reaction (usually antibiotics, NSAIDs, or anticonvulsant meds) or sometimes an infection. Immunocompromised patients are more likely to develop this. Patients will have vague, flu-like *symptoms* for a few days followed by development of a progressing rash beginning on the face and trunk, usually with extensive mucosal involvement, and epidermal detachment (<10% for SJS and >30% for TEN). The following features are often present: acute onset of fever, a history of drug exposure often 1-4 wks before symptoms, diffuse erythema that progresses to vesicles and bullae, necrosis of the epidermis, positive Nikolsky sign (epidermal detachment when pressure is applied). Hospitalization is necessary to *treat* SJS or TEN with fluid replacement, wound care, and supportive therapy. If the syndrome is severe, treatment in a burn unit, IVIG, and skin grafting may be necessary. *Complications* include skin infections, skin issues (scarring, discoloring, and permanent hair loss), sepsis, ocular disease, organ damage, and death.

Folliculitis

Folliculitis is inflammation around the **hair follicle** due to an infection or non-infectious cause. The most common causes are frequent shaving, occlusion, hot/humid weather, and chronic inflammatory skin conditions. The most common causative organism is *Staphylococcus*. *Pseudomonas* is the most likely cause of hot tub folliculitis. Folliculitis can be superficial or deep, mild and self-limiting, or reoccurring. Patients will have pruritic or painful, small, erythematous pustules surrounding the hair. These pustules may break open and crust over. Deep lesions form nodules. Folliculitis can occasionally involve a large area and cause swelling and extreme pain. *Diagnosis* is made upon clinical evaluation. If folliculitis is chronic or resistant to treatment, further evaluation is needed including cultures, Gram stain, KOH preparations, or biopsy. Warm compresses can help relieve the symptoms, and folliculitis, if superficial, will usually resolve spontaneously without medical treatment after a few days with use of anti-bacterial soap and good hand-washing practices. Topical antibiotics (e.g., mupirocin, clindamycin 1%) can be used as first-line *treatment*. If severe, or caused by *Staphylococcus* or MRSA, oral antibiotics (e.g., cephalexin, dicloxacillin, clindamycin) are necessary to treat the condition. If available, always follow culture and sensitivity reports. *Complications* include cellulitis, skin damage (spots and scarring), and permanent hair loss.

Skin Infections

Onychomycosis and Paronychia

Onychomycosis or **tinea unguium** is a fungal infection of any part of the **fingernails or toenails**. This can cause pain and discomfort and can possibly lead to issues walking, especially in the elderly or those with diabetes. The nail appears thick (due to hyperkeratosis), deformed, white or yellow, and onycholysis (separation from the nailbed) may occur. *Diagnose* by direct microscopy with a KOH preparation. A fungal culture may be used if microscopy is unsuccessful. *Treatment* with topical agents is usually not very effective while newer oral agents (e.g., terbinafine, itraconazole) have better outcomes. *Complications* include cellulitis and ulcers, especially in diabetics.

Paronychia is a soft tissue infection of the **nail fold** and is the most common infection of the hand. Infection often occurs after trauma to the area by moisture, physical, or chemical damage. It can be acute (usually due to staphylococci) or chronic (usually fungal). The nail bed becomes red, swollen, painful, and yellow-green pus begins to collect and form an abscess. *Diagnose* clinically. *Treatment* includes warm soaks (if early infection), antibiotics, and incision and drainage if an abscess forms. If the infection reoccurs after treatment, suspect a fungal cause. *Complications* include this infection occasionally spreading beyond the nail fold.

Impetigo

Impetigo is a common **bacterial skin infection** caused by streptococci, staphylococci, or both that enter through a break in the skin. It is highly contagious and the most common bacterial infection in children. Impetigo can be nonbullous or bullous and appears as multiple vesicles or pustules filled with clear, yellow fluid that easily burst. These leave behind a red, raw area of irritation and a honey-colored crust. The rash is most common on the face and lips but may spread to other areas. Mupirocin ointment is recommended for *treatment*, but oral antibiotics (e.g., cephalexin, clindamycin) may be needed for severe cases or cases involving MRSA.

Erysipelas

Erysipelas is a **superficial skin infection** which is caused by streptococci, usually Group A streptococci. Patients may note a recent trauma or pharyngitis and may experience a prodrome of malaise, fever, and chills. Erysipelas appears as a well-circumscribed, painful area of marked erythema and inflammation. This is different from cellulitis as it is more raised and has definite borders. *Diagnose* clinically and treat with oral or IM penicillin or alternately, cephalexin or erythromycin if allergic to penicillin. *Complications* include abscess, scarring, sepsis, and gangrene.

Cellulitis

Cellulitis is an **acute bacterial infection** causing inflammation of the skin and subcutaneous tissues. It is commonly caused by staphylococci or streptococci that enter the skin through a portal of entry (e.g., cut, insect bite, wound). Patients complain of a spreading, painful area of erythema, inflammation, and warmth. *Diagnosis* can be made clinically; however, further investigation is warranted if systemic symptoms are present (e.g., fever, chills, tachycardia) or if signs of more serious infection are present (e.g., violaceous bullae, hemorrhage, gas in the tissue). *Treat* empirically with antibiotics and, as always, follow the antibiotic guidelines for your area. Abscesses, if present, should be incised and drained. Hospitalization and proper consultations (e.g., surgery) is needed for patients with signs of serious infection. *Complications* include abscesses, gangrenous cellulitis, necrotizing fasciitis, septic shock, or death.

Parasites and Bites

Lice and Scabies

Lice are parasites that live on humans either on the head, body (live on clothes), or pubic area. They can only crawl and have a lifespan of about 30 days. A female lays about 300 nits (eggs) in her lifetime. Nits hatch in 6-9 days and mature about 7 days after hatching. Itching is the main complaint. *Diagnose* through direct or microscopic observation. *Treatment* involves environmental controls (most important) and medicine (e.g., pyrethrin shampoos or creams, malathion) that must be repeated in 7-10 days. There is increasing resistance to lindane.

Scabies are mites (*Sarcoptes scabiei hominis*) that burrow under the skin usually seen in the webbed spaces, flexor surface of the wrist, belt-line, and pubic areas. *Diagnose* microscopically through a burrow scraping. *Treat* with topical permethrin cream, lindane lotion (not if <2 years-old), or oral ivermectin (2nd-line). It is important to treat close contacts simultaneously.

Clinically Significant Spider Bites

Clinically significant **spider bites** in the U.S. include bites from the black widow and brown recluse.

- **Black widow spiders** have a red, hourglass shape on the ventral abdomen. Their bites are neurotoxic and can cause immediate pain, diaphoresis, cramping, and in the worse cases, headache, HTN, nausea, and vomiting.
- **Brown recluse spiders** have a violin-shaped pattern on their cephalothorax. Their venom is cytotoxic and hemolytic causing pain hours after the bite, as well as inflammation and ischemia. Ulceration usually occurs 7-14 days after the bite.

Treatment of spider bites is supportive with wound care and pain meds. Antivenom is occasionally used for black widow bites, but reserved for severe cases. Cool compresses are helpful to impede the venom, which is temperature dependent, in brown recluse spider bites. Antibiotics and skin grafts may be necessary.

Drug Reactions/Eruptions

Drug reactions	Characteristics	Treatment
Toxic erythema	Maculopapular exanthematous reactions. Morbilliform is most common and caused by antibiotics (ampicillin, sulfonamides, TMP-SMZ), sulfonylureas, diuretics, and barbiturates. Usually begins within 7 to days and spreads from trunk to extremities, clearing in 3 to 5 days.	In most cases, identifying and stopping the drug will relieve symptoms, but severe cases may need an antihistamine and/or epinephrine. Topical or systemic steroids may be indicated.
Erythema nodosum	Inflammation and cutaneous nodules on extensor aspects of legs associated with oral contraceptives. Some may experience fever, arthralgia, and pain.	
Fixed eruptions	Single or multiple round, defined erythematous plaques, often hyperpigmented (which remains after healing). Results from antimicrobials, analgesics, barbiturates, heavy metals, antiparasitics, antihistamines, NSAIDs, and heart drugs.	
Urticaria	Raised, red, itching wheals, sometimes with angioedema. Caused by penicillins, NSAIDs, sulfonamides, opioids, salicylates, ACEIs and ARBs.	In most cases, identifying and stopping the drug will relieve symptoms, but severe cases may need an antihistamine and/or epinephrine. Topical or systemic steroids may be indicated.
Allergic vasculitis	Purpuric papular lesions and urticaria (>24 hours), usually on the legs. May include vesicles, bullae, or necrotic ulcers. Caused by phenytoin, propylthiouracil, and sulfonamides.	

Soft Tissue Conditions

Soft tissue conditions	Characteristics	Treatment
Gas gangrene	Life-threatening infection of muscle tissue usually caused by bacterial infection with *Clostridium perfringens* at a surgical or injury site, especially wounds contaminated with dirt or feces. The infection produces blisters and gas bubbles. The patient has tachycardia, tachypnea, putrid foul-smelling discharge, and severe pain. Some may have nausea and vomiting and develop jaundice.	Includes high dose antibiotics (usually both penicillin and clindamycin) and surgical debridement, which may necessitate amputation. Hyperbaric oxygen therapy is also utilized if available.
Necrotizing infections	Infection/Inflammation occurs in the subcutaneous tissue although cellulitis, myositis, and fasciitis may all be present. Patients may have severe pain even without external evidence. Skin may appear normal, erythematous, or gay-tinged. Edema and weeping of tissue may be evident. Patients may experience fever, tachycardia, and hypotension. The infection may spread rapidly to large areas. The most common areas affected are the extremities. The condition is life-threatening.	Immediate extensive debridement of affected tissue is critical. Antibiotics are indicated should not be used without surgery. Wounds are usually left open and multiple operations may be necessary.

Pigment Disorders

Pigment disorders	Characteristics	Diagnosis and treatment
Vitiligo	Long-term autoimmune disorder with absence of melanin pigment in patches on the skin (localized, generalized, or segmental), usually about orifices (such as the mouth) and on areas of light skin, such as on the hands, feet, neck, face, and body folds. Most common in dark-skinned individuals. Onset usually before age 20.	Diagnosis is by history and physical, skin biopsy, and laboratory testing to identify underlying autoimmune disorders. Treatment includes topical corticosteroids, calcineurin inhibitors, and/or psoralen and light therapy to restore pigmentation or depigmentation to remove remaining pigment (indicated for widespread disorder).
Melasma	Gray-brown discoloration of the skin, usually on the nose, cheeks, forehead, chin, and above the lips but may also occurs in areas exposed to the sun. More common in darker-skinned females (90%) and frequently occurs with pregnancy because of hormonal changes. The cause is not often clear.	Discoloration usually recedes after pregnancy, but treatment may include topical hydroquinone to lighten skin. Other treatments include topical corticosteroids, tretinoin, azelaic acid, kojic acids, microdermabrasion, laser treatment, and chemical peel. Patients should limit exposure to the sun and wear sun block.
Acanthosis nigricans	Dark and thickened velvety discoloration of the skin in areas of creases and folds, such as the neck, axillary regions, groin areas, genitals, stomach, under the breasts, palms, soles, and knuckles. The skin may be dry, rough, and itchy. The condition may result from insulin resistance (obesity, diabetes), changes in hormones, genetics, medications (birth control pills, corticosteroids, supplements, and niacin), and cancer (rare).	Diagnostic procedures include skin biopsy and various tests to determine the underlying cause. Treatment includes identifying and treating or avoiding the cause.
Xeroderma pigmentosa	This autosomal recessive genetic disorder is characterized by the decreased ability of the body to repair damage to DNA caused by ultraviolet light. XP affects the skin and the eyes. Any exposure to ultraviolet light can result in burning and blistering. Patients are at increased risk of developing skin cancer and other types of cancer. Patients often develop progressive neurological disorders as well.	Diagnosis is per genetic testing. Treatment is primarily preventive (using sunscreen, avoiding sun exposure, avoiding light fixtures with UV light, wearing protective clothing and face shields.)

Photosensitivity Dermatoses

Photosensitivity dermatoses	Characteristics	Diagnosis and treatment
Porphyria cutanea tarda	May be sporadic or hereditary. Characterized by non-inflammatory blisters on areas exposed to sun, particularly the hands (dorsal surface), and facial hypertrichosis. Associated with alcoholic liver disease, hemochromatosis, and hepatitis C. May be caused by some medications (estrogens, sulfonamides, oral contraceptives, barbiturates, anticonvulsants), smoking, or drinking alcohol.	Diagnosis per observation and laboratory tests: urine porphyrins, liver function tests, iron levels. Treatment can include avoiding trigger, phlebotomy, chloroquine, and/or hydroxychloroquine to reduce iron.
Photodermatitis	Reaction to exposure to light, results in painful or pruritic erythematous vesicular rash on sun-exposed areas of the face, neck hands, and chest as well as facial hypertrichosis. Classifications include primary (idiopathic, immunologic), drug- or chemically-induced, UV-associated, and genetic. Patients may experience nausea, vomiting, fever, GI symptoms, and malaise during acute episode.	Laboratory tests are usually not conclusive although eosinophilia may be present. Treatment includes avoiding sun exposure, using sunscreen, supportive care, and corticosteroids or azathioprine for severe reactions.

Miscellaneous Skin Disorders

Condyloma Acuminatum

Condyloma acuminatum is a sexually transmitted **genital wart** that is usually benign and involves human papilloma virus (HPV) type 6 or 11. There are about 40 HPV types that spread through sexual contact. HPV type 16 and 18 are responsible for the majority of cervical, anal, oropharyngeal, vaginal, and penile cancers. There is an HPV vaccine available against HPV 6, 11, 16,18, 31, 33, 45, 52, 58 which is a series of 2 injections at 0 and 6-12 months (recommended at 11-12 years old, but can be from 9 to <15 years old) or 3 injections at 0, 2, and 6 months if 15-26 years old. The lesions are pink or gray and can become pedunculated. Genital warts are *diagnosed* through histopathology and *treated* topically or through excision. *Complications* include disfigurement and cancerous transformation.

Verrucae and Molluscum Contagiosum

Verrucae (**warts**) are common, benign epidermal lesions caused by HPV (usually type 1-4, 27, 29) that can spontaneously regress in 1-2 years. They are usually asymptomatic, but can be painful, especially if a plantar wart. *Diagnose* clinically and treat topically (e.g., salicylic acid), through excision, cryosurgery (liquid nitrogen), or medication (e.g., cimetidine).

Molluscum contagiosum is due to a **poxvirus** and causes grouped, pink, dome-shaped **lesions** with central umbilication and a central plug. These are highly contagious by direct and indirect contact, but are benign and can spontaneously resolve in 1-2 years. This is common in children and young adults. *Diagnose* clinically and treat with cryosurgery, curettage, or topical agents.

Actinic Keratosis and Seborrheic Keratosis

Actinic keratosis is a slow-growing, **precancerous skin lesion** that is due to UV light exposure. It typically appears after the 4th decade of life, but may appear sooner if the patient is fair or lives in an area of intense UV exposure. It can progress to invasive squamous cell carcinoma about 10% of the time. Lesions are rough, keratotic, and pink, red, or brown. Confirm *diagnosis* with a skin biopsy. *Treatment* varies due to the number of lesions and includes surgery, cryosurgery (e.g., liquid nitrogen), resurfacing procedures, and medical treatment (e.g., topical 5-FU, imiquimod, photodynamic therapy). Prevention is key and the primary *complication* is progression to invasive squamous cell carcinoma.

Seborrheic keratosis is another common **skin lesion** in older patients, but it is completely **benign**. It is a slow-growing, wart-like epithelial lesion that appears stuck on the skin. They vary in color from white to black, but are usually tan to brown. They can be found on any skin area, except the palms and soles. *Diagnosis* is confirmed with a shave biopsy which can also be used to remove the lesion. No *treatment* is necessary, but these can be removed (e.g., cryotherapy, electrodesiccation, curettage) for cosmetic reasons. There are no *complications*.

Psoriasis

Psoriasis is a very common, chronic, inflammatory disease affecting 1% to 2% of the U. S. population. The cause is unknown, but current theories support an autoimmune origin and/or genetics. Psoriasis results from an **accelerated skin reproduction cycle** and **lymphocyte infiltration**. Lesions show parakeratotic cells, scales, and a thinned or absent stratum granulosum. It occurs most frequently on elbows, knees, scalp, intergluteal cleft, glans penis, and lumbosacral areas. Other triggers can include stress, skin irritation, sunlight, alcohol consumption, AIDS, chemotherapy, or other autoimmune conditions. There are a variety of forms of psoriasis including plaque-type, arthritic, nail, inverse, guttate, pustular, and erythrodermic psoriasis. Guttate psoriasis can be confused with *pityriasis rosea*, but pityriasis rosea, which is self-limited, begins with a herald patch and has a Christmas-tree distribution. The most common form of psoriasis is called **chronic plaque psoriasis**, which accounts for about 75% of cases. With chronic plaque psoriasis, there are erythemic, raised, sharply-defined plaques with thick, silvery scales. The lesions are usually symmetrically distributed and often on extensor surfaces. The plaques can be asymptomatic or pruritic. *Diagnosis* is made by history and clinical assessment. *Treatment* includes topical treatments (e.g., steroid creams and ointments, retinoids, salicylic acid, emollients, vitamin D_3 analogs), phototherapy, and systemic treatments (e.g., methotrexate, cyclosporine, adalimumab, etanercept, infliximab, ustekinumab). *Complications* include 2° infections, psoriatic arthritis, cardiovascular disease, metabolic syndrome, MI, lymphoma, depression, and kidney disease.

Lichen Planus

Lichen planus is a recurrent skin condition that appears to be immune-mediated. The exact cause is unknown, but it has been associated with hepatitis C and certain medications (e.g., penicillamine, NSAIDS, β-blockers). The appearance of the lesions is easily remembered with the **5 P's**: pruritic, purple, planar (flat-topped), polygonal papules and plaques that usually form in a row. It most commonly occurs around the flexural surfaces of the ankles or wrists. Oral lesions occur in about 50% of cases, can burn, and Wickham striae are usually noted (a fine network of lines on the surface of lichen planus lesions). Once the lesions fade, they may leave a darker pigmented area or scar. *Diagnosis* is made per clinical evaluation; however, a skin biopsy may be needed. On H&P, note mediations that may induce this disorder. Lichen planus usually resolves spontaneously within 1 year, but symptoms can be controlled with topical steroid creams or ointments, topical or oral retinoids, antihistamines, UV light therapy, or immunomodulating medications. If severe, oral or intralesional steroids may be necessary. *Complications* include infection, permanent alopecia, and increased risk of skin cancer.

Bullous Pemphigoid

Bullous pemphigoid is a chronic, auto-immune **blistering disease** that usually affects the elderly. The cause is unknown, but possible triggers include medications, trauma, radiation, and other diseases (e.g., psoriasis, lichen planus, DM, RA). Patients complain of a pruritic, blistering rash. Tense bullae appear on the trunk, flexural surfaces, and in intertriginous areas, but usually spare the mucous membranes. Nikolsky sign is negative. *Diagnosis* is made by skin biopsy and immunofluorescence studies. It is important to differentiate bullous pemphigoid from pemphigus vulgaris (flaccid bullae that usually involve the oral mucosa), which has a worse prognosis. *Treatment* includes topical or oral steroids. *Complications* include scarring and possible death in the elderly.

Lipomas and Epidermal Inclusion Cysts

Lipomas are benign, slow-growing fatty tumors and are the most common **soft tissue tumor**. They are usually found subcutaneously, are not fixed to fascia, and are soft and painless. *Diagnosis* is clinical; however, further investigation is necessary if the tumor grows rapidly or is fixed to fascia (rule out a liposarcoma). *Treat* with excision by fully removing the tumor, including the capsule, if symptomatic or large.

Epithelial or epidermal inclusion cysts form when epithelial tissue implants in the dermis and are typically found on the face, neck, and trunk. They are usually solitary, skin-colored to yellow, dome-shaped lesions with a central punctum, and they contain a foul-smelling, cheesy material. *Diagnose* clinically; however, a biopsy or fine-needle aspiration may be helpful in diagnosis. If not infected, treat with either watchful waiting or with complete excision including the capsule. If infected, *treat* with appropriate antibiotics (e.g., dicloxacillin, clindamycin).

Rosacea

Rosacea is an extremely common inflammatory disease of the skin. It is characterized by facial erythema, papular and pustular lesions. It generally affects adults over the age of 30 years. It is sometimes referred to as adult acne. Patients generally present with flushing, papules, pustules, and telangiectasia on the face. These symptoms are aggravated by alcohol, spicy food, hot beverages, exercise, and temperature extremes. The diagnosis is made clinically. *Treatment* includes avoiding exacerbation factors, oral antibiotics, topical metronidazole, and isotretinoin. Complications include rhinophyma, a buildup of tissue around the nose, and ocular rosacea. Ocular rosacea causes a burning, gritty sensation in the eyes.

Alopecia

Alopecia, a polygenic disorder, is the loss of hair, occurring when the hair follicles are attacked by the immune system. The triggering factor is not known. Different types of alopecia include:

- **Alopecia areata**: Hair loss is patchy. Hair may grow back, but loss may occur in other parts of the body.
- **Alopecia totalis**: Hair loss is restricted to the scalp.
- **Alopecia universalis**: All hair on the body, including eyebrows and eyelashes, is lost.

While treatment options are available, treatment is not successful for all patients. Most treatments utilized for alopecia are not FDA-approved for the condition. Treatment options for mild/moderate hair loss (less than 50% of scalp involved) include intralesional corticosteroid injection, topical corticosteroids, topical minoxidil, and anthralin cream or ointment. For severe hair loss (greater than 50% of scalp involved), additional therapies may include topical immunotherapy (diphencyprone, dinitrochlorobenzene, squaric acid dibutyl ester) and immunomodulators, such as tofacitinib and ruxolitinib. Some patients utilize scalp prostheses (wigs).

BURNS

Burns are damage to the skin or tissue due to thermal, chemical, radiation, or electrical causes. They are classified as first-, second-, or third-degree burns. They are also described according to the **total body surface area (TBSA)** that is affected. **First-degree burns** only affect the epidermis and appear red and are painful. **Second degree (partial thickness) burns** affect part of the dermis and can be superficial or deep with redness, blisters, and are very painful. **Third degree (full-thickness) burns** extend down into the subcutaneous tissue/fat, are whitish, blackened, and without sensation. Sometimes a designation of a **4th degree burn** is used when the burn involves deep fascia, muscles, and bones. When assessing a patient with burns, it is important to first stop the burning process and begin with the **ABC's** (airway, breathing, circulation). Assess for an inhalation injury and CO poisoning if there is soot or burns around the mouth or nose. By using the rule of nines, one can quickly determine the TBSA affected (see figure below). Also, for small burns, remember the patient's palm is 1% of the TBSA. Patients with TBSA >10% need IV fluids and if ≥20% will require IV fluid resuscitation. Patients should be referred to a burn center if the burn of any thickness is >20% TBSA, 2nd degree >10% TBSA, 3rd degree >5% TBSA, 2nd or 3rd degree burns of critical areas (e.g., joints, face, hands, feet, genitalia), electrical/lightning burns, chemical burns, or inhalation injury. Small burns may be *treated* with silver sulfadiazine.

RULE OF 9'S

The **Rule of 9's** is helpful when assessing burn patients to determine if IV fluids (needed if ≥10% TBSA) or transfer to a burn unit is necessary (needed if >20% TBSA, 2nd degree >10% TBSA, 3rd degree >5% TBSA).

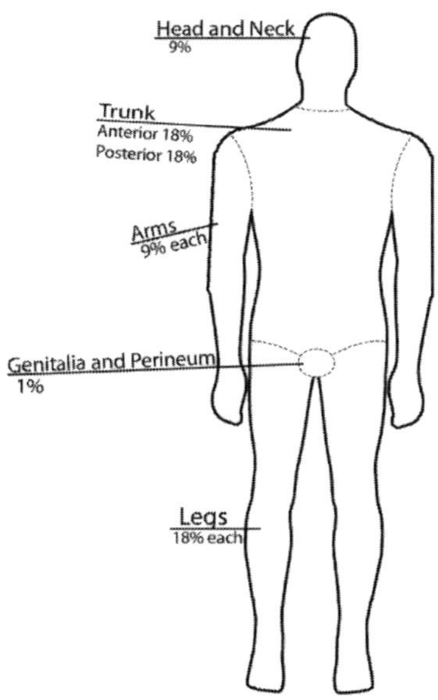

Pressure Ulcers

Risk Assessment

The **Braden scale** is a risk assessment tool that has been validated clinically as predictive of the risk of patient's developing pressure sores based on risk factors. It was developed in 1988 by Barbara Braden and Nancy Bergstrom. The scale scores 6 different areas with five areas scored 1-4 points, and one area 1-3. The lower the score, the greater the risk;

- 23:(Best score) excellent prognosis, very minimal risk.
- ≤ 16: Breakpoint for risk of pressure ulcer (will vary somewhat for different populations.
- 6: (Worst score) prognosis is very poor, strong likelihood of developing pressure sores.

Sensory perception	(1) Completely limited, (2) very limited, (3) slightly limited, (4) no impairment
Moisture	(1) Constantly moist, (2) very moist, (3) occasionally moist, (4) rarely moist
Activity	(1) Bed, (2) chair, (3) occasional walk, (4) frequent walk
Mobility	(1) Immobile, (2) limited, (3) slightly limited, (4) no limitations
Usual nutrition pattern	(1) Very poor, (2) inadequate, (3) adequate, (4) excellent
Friction & shear	(1) Problem (skin frequently slides down sheets and needs help to move), (2) potential problem (skin slides somewhat during moves, needs assistance, (3), no apparent problem.

Staging

Pressure ulcers result from pressure or pressure with shear and/or friction over bony prominences. The National Pressure Injury Advisory Panel (NPIAP) stages include:

- **Suspected deep tissue injury**: Skin discolored, intact or blood blister.
- **Stage I:** Intact skin with non-blanching reddened area.
- **Stage II:** Abrasion or blistered area without slough but with partial-thickness skin loss.
- **Stage III:** Deep ulcer with exposed subcutaneous tissue. Tunneling or undermining may be evident with or without slough.
- **Stage IV:** Deep ulcer, full thickness, with necrosis into muscle, bone, tendons, and/or joints.
- **Unstageable**: Eschar and/or slough prevents staging prior to debridement.

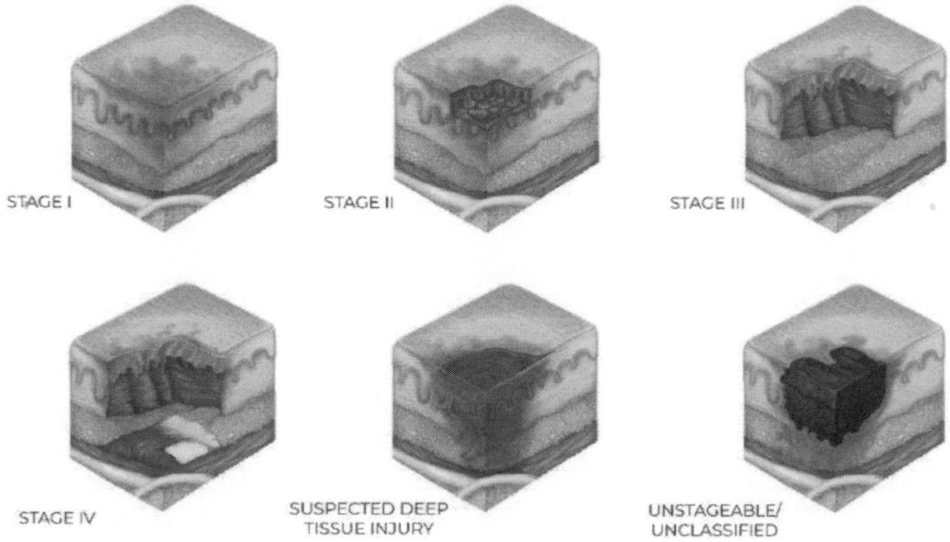

Patients should be placed on pressure reducing support surfaces and turned at least every two hours, avoiding the area(s) with a pressure ulcer. Wound care depends on the stage of the wound and the amount of drainage, but includes irrigation, debridement when necessary, antibiotics for infection, and appropriate dressing. Patients should be encouraged to have adequate protein and iron in their diets to promote healing and to maintain adequate hydration.

Preventative Measures and Treatment

Prevention	Treatment
Ensure adequate hydration and nutrition.	Continue preventive measures.
Inspect skin carefully and promptly treat breaks in skin or pressure areas.	Conduct nutritional assessment.
Reposition patients every 2 hours.	Cleanse wound or irrigate at 10 to 15 psi (pressure below 4 psi will not clean wound).
Cushion bony prominences.	Debride wound (autolysis, enzymes, maggots, sharp debridement, surgical debridement).
Use appropriate assistive devices.	Treat infection (broad-spectrum antibiotic and/or topical antibiotics).
Use pressure-relieving cushions on chairs/wheelchairs.	Utilize appropriate dressing to maintain a moist environment and absorb discharge.
Limit sitting to <2 hours at a time for those acutely ill.	Utilize compression therapy if indicated.
Position patient in 30° lateral position instead of 90° side-lying position.	Apply off-loading measures.
	Control pain.
	Monitor progress.

Musculoskeletal System

Joint

Septic Arthritis

Septic arthritis is an infection in a **joint**, most commonly the **knee** though other joints may be affected. It is important to diagnose quickly since joint destruction can occur within 48 hours of the start of the infection. This is usually due to bacteria that has spread to the joint, but it can also be caused by a virus or fungus. The most common **bacterial causes** are *Staphylococcus aureus* (most common in <2 and >55) or *Neisseria gonorrhea* (most common in younger, sexually active adults). Patients at increased risk of developing septic arthritis include those with chronic illnesses (e.g., rheumatoid arthritis, DM), prosthetic joints, IV drug users, and those at risk of STDs, Patients will complain of acute onset of significant pain in the affected joint, fever, reduced ROM, and the joint will appear red, swollen, hot, and very tender to the touch. Patients may or may not be aware of a recent bacterial infection elsewhere in their body. *Diagnose* with arthrocentesis; consult orthopedist. Arthrocentesis with culture and sensitivity, blood cultures x2, and STD testing should be performed before empiric antibiotics are started (follow local sensitivity patterns). Synovial fluid may show purulent discharge with elevated WBCs. *Treatment* is with IV antibiotics started at the time of diagnosis, followed by a course of oral antibiotics for a total of 2-4 weeks. Joint aspiration is usually necessary, and if the condition is severe, surgery rarely may be needed to drain and clean the joint. The primary *complications* are joint destruction and chronic arthritis.

Osteoarthritis

Osteoarthritis (OA) is a very common condition that occurs due to overuse of the joints. It is characterized by a wearing down of the cartilage and other structures within the joints and is a gradually progressive condition. It usually affects those >50 years old and commonly occurs in the hands (DIP, PIP, and joint at base of thumb) and large weight-bearing joints, such as the hips and knees; but it can affect any joint in the body. Patients may note a gradual onset of a deep aching pain in the affected joint, especially with activity; and may note joint stiffness in the morning or with inactivity that is relieved within 30 minutes with movement. There may be swelling in the joint and osteophytes may be noted: Heberden nodes in the DIP joints and Bouchard nodes in the PIP joints. On exam, crepitus can be felt with flexion and extension of the joint and reduced ROM may be observed.

X-rays (gold standard) may show joint space narrowing due to worn down cartilage, sclerosis, and marginal osteophytes. *Treatment* includes acetaminophen and rest of the affected joint, heat, or ice when it is painful; NSAIDs may be used if acetaminophen is not helpful. Exercise should still be performed but not to the point that pain occurs. Physical therapy may help with muscle strengthening, and exercises that decrease the stress on joints as well as weight loss can be helpful. When OA is severe, surgery may be necessary to clean up or replace the joint.

Rheumatoid Arthritis

Rheumatoid arthritis (RA) is a chronic, progressive autoimmune disease that affects the **synovial linings of the joints**. The body's **white blood cells** attack this synovial lining and destroy it, leading to deformity and destruction of the joint. It is usually diagnosed in middle age and is more likely to occur in females than males. Patients typically start with fever, malaise, weakness, morning stiffness, and arthralgias followed by a gradual progression of symmetric inflammation, erythema, and joint pain that generally starts in the small joints of the hands, wrists, and feet which eventually may spread to include the larger joints of the body. Swan-neck and Boutonnière deformities of the fingers, as well as subcutaneous nodules (a later finding) may be present. There is decreased movement/ROM as the disease progresses. *Diagnose* clinically (>6 weeks of typical symptoms; multiple joint involvement), with x-rays, elevated rheumatoid factor (RF), elevated anti-cyclic citrullinated peptide (anti-CCP), elevated ESR, and elevated CRP. There is no cure for rheumatoid arthritis, but the disease process can be slowed and pain symptoms can be managed. DMARDs (disease-modifying antirheumatic drugs) like methotrexate (first-line) or sulfasalazine are started at diagnosis to help slow the progress and damage caused by the disease. NSAIDs and steroids can help with pain relief as the patient waits for DMARDs to become effective. Some biologic DMARDs such as the immunomodulator abatacept (Orencia®), or the TNF-α inhibitor etanercept (Enbrel®), can help reduce damage, control symptoms, and increase function. In severe cases, joint replacement surgery may be necessary.

Juvenile Idiopathic Arthritis

Juvenile idiopathic arthritis (Juvenile rheumatoid arthritis) is a chronic arthritic disease affecting children <16 years old causing **joint inflammation and pain** for >6 weeks. JIA may be **pauciarticular** (≤4 joints), **polyarticular** (>4 joints), or **systemic** (spike fevers at predictable times, rash, HSM). It may affect large or small joints and may be asymmetric or symmetric. JIA also may be associated with uveitis or psoriasis. The cause is unknown, but there is a **genetic and autoimmune component**. Patients typically present with a limp with either an abrupt or insidious onset. Other *signs and symptoms* may include morning stiffness, joint inflammation and warmth, guarding, pain, reduced ROM, and possibly systemic symptoms (e.g., fever, lymphadenopathy, rash). *Diagnosis* is made with clinical criteria. X-rays or MRI, and RF (may be + or -), ANA (if positive rule out SLE), anti-CCP (may be + or -), and CBC tests may be used to help confirm JIA and rule out other disorders. Be careful to rule out acute lymphocytic leukemia, septic arthritis, and postinfectious arthritis as these may have similar presentations. Patients start *treatment* with a NSAID, which helps with the pain; intra-articular steroid injections also help treat the inflammation and pain in active disease. DMARDs (disease-modifying antirheumatic drugs; e.g., methotrexate) may be added to slow the progression of the disease; the goal is complete remission. Patient care involves a team approach.

Reactive Arthritis

Reactive arthritis (previously Reiter syndrome) is a collection of three conditions: **arthritis**, **conjunctivitis**, and **urinary tract symptoms** (urethritis); and is more common in young adult males. This condition is called reactive arthritis because it can occur in response to an **infection** (usually due to an STD or GI infection) somewhere in the body. The most common predisposing infection is *Chlamydia*; however, the bacteria *Salmonella, Shigella, and Campylobacter jejuni* may also cause reactive arthritis. *Symptoms* usually appear 1-4 weeks following the infection. Along with the triad of symptoms, patients may present with an acute onset of fever, fatigue, arthralgias, myalgias, skin lesions or ulcers, and may have sausage-shaped fingers or toes. Arthritis primarily affects the large joints in the lower extremities and spine (low back pain). Sacroiliitis and spondylitis of the spine are common. Conjunctivitis and uveitis also may occur. Patients may have complaints of dysuria, urinary frequency, discharge, and prostatitis in men. *Diagnose* clinically. *Treat* symptoms. NSAIDs and corticosteroid injections can be helpful. If there is an active infection, appropriate antibiotics should be given. Refer to or consult a rheumatologist, an ophthalmologist if uveitis is present, and cardiologist if the heart is affected. This becomes chronic in 30% of patients.

Gout

Gout occurs when there is increased **uric acid** in the blood, leading to urate crystals settling in a **joint**. Gout can be due to excess consumption of foods high in **purine** (e.g., asparagus, liver/kidneys, beer), reduced excretion by the kidneys, or elevated production of uric acid. It is more common in men and usually affects the big toe MP joint but can occur in other joints. Patients complain of a sudden onset of severe pain, swelling, and erythema in the affected joint; even light pressure causes significant pain. Sometimes fever and chills are present. *Diagnose* clinically and with serum uric acid (>6.8 mg/dL) and synovial fluid analysis. *Treat* acute attacks with NSAIDs (indomethacin), colchicine (if tolerated), and steroids. Allopurinol can be taken regularly for prevention of acute episodes and for chronic gout. Allopurinol reduces production of uric acid; the goal is a level <6 mg/dL). Patients should also be counseled on dietary changes to lower intake of purine-rich foods. *Complications* include gouty arthritis, tophi formation, and uric acid kidney stones.

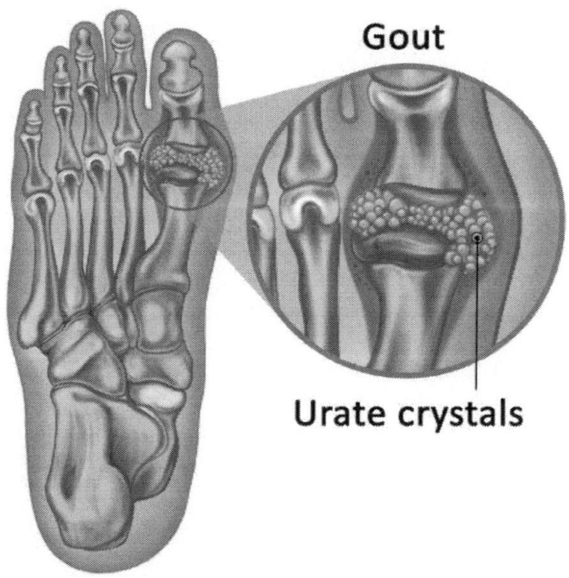

Pseudogout

Pseudogout is very similar to gout, except the causative agent is deposition of **calcium pyrophosphate dihydrate crystals (CPPD)** within a joint. It affects men and women equally, may be associated with OA, has a genetic component, and is self-limited (usually 10-14 days). The most common joints affected by pseudogout are the knees, but it can occur in other, often large, joints. Patients complain of an insidious onset of severe pain in the affected joint (takes days vs. hours) which appears red, swollen, and is extremely tender on PE; fever may be present. *Diagnose* by examining the synovial fluid and x-rays. *Treatment* includes NSAIDs, colchicine (may cause several GI side effects; may not be well tolerated), and steroids. Maintenance therapy with colchicine may help reduce the number of acute attacks of pseudogout. Aspiration of the joint fluid can be performed to relieve pressure on the joint and help to reduce pain.

Hydroxyapatite Deposition Disease

Hydroxyapatite deposition disease (HADD) is the deposition of calcium hydroxyapatite crystals (clumps of HA molecules) in or about the joint (especially in the tendons), typically the supraspinatus tendon and biceps tendon of the shoulder in middle-aged individuals although it can affect other tendons as well in other parts of the body. In some cases, the condition may progress to destruction of the joint. Some may develop the Milwaukee shoulder syndrome (typically females over 70 years) in which the rotator cuff is destroyed. The cause of calcific tendinitis is unknown although it may be associated with repeated trauma to the joint. Diagnosis is per x-ray, CT, MRI and/or high-resolution US and identification of crystals. Treatment may include ultrasound ablation, conservative treatment (rest, heat or cold, PT, NSAIDs), corticosteroid injection to joint (may lead to further calcification), or surgical removal of calcium deposits. Some patients may eventually require joint replacement.

Ganglion Cyst

Ganglion cysts, also referred to as **Bible cysts**, are soft-tissue cysts that are usually associated with **tendon sheaths and joint capsules**. It is more common in women (3:1) and is most often located on the **dorsal wrist**. It can also be found on the palmar (volar) side of the wrist, in the finger, knee, ankle, and toe joints. It may appear gradually or rapidly, is most often accompanied by pain that worsens with joint use, and the lump may grow more prominent when the joint is engaged. The average size is 1 to 3 cm which may fluctuate with time, and is usually a solitary mass. The mass is soft, movable, and will transilluminate. *Diagnose* clinically. Ultrasound can also be useful in determining the makeup of the cyst. If not painful or interfering with function, no *treatment* is necessary as they may resolve on their own. Thick, clear fluid can be aspirated from the cyst to help relieve symptoms. If the cyst is problematic, surgical excision may be needed for some, but recurrence is common.

Knee Injuries

The main knee injuries include anterior (ACL) and posterior cruciate ligament (PCL), collateral ligament, and meniscal injuries. All these are more common in athletes, especially in contact sports.

ACL injuries involve **hyperextension of the knee**, usually when stopping quickly and changing directions. Patients usually report hearing or feeling a "pop," pain, and instability of the joint. The Lachman (most sensitive), anterior drawer, or pivot shift test helps *diagnose*, and an MRI confirms the diagnosis. *Treatment* involves conservative management and if a candidate, surgical repair.

PCL injuries are less common since the PCL is the strongest ligament of the knee and involve hyperflexion injuries, posterior force with hyperextension, or trauma to a bent knee (e.g., falling). Patients may report instability or pain when weight bearing on a semi-flexed knee (e.g., walking down stairs). *Diagnose* clinically (posterior drawer test, posterior tibial sag sign), x-rays help rule out fractures, and may confirm with an MRI. *Treat* conservatively (R.I.C.E. & PT) or surgical repair.

Collateral ligament injuries involve the **medial collateral ligament (MCL)** when outward (varus) force is placed on the knee while **lateral collateral ligament injury (LCL)** involves inner (valgus) force. This can involve complete or partial tears or sprains of the ligament. Patients may present with pain, swelling, stiffness, and instability (if severe). *Diagnose* clinically (varus & valgus stress tests); x-rays or an MRI may be ordered. *Treat* with R.I.C.E., NSAIDs, and if severe, surgical repair.

Meniscal injuries involve the C-shaped **cartilage between the femur and tibia**. This is usually due to rotational force injuries and the medial meniscus is injured more often. *Symptoms* include pain, edema, and knee locking or buckling. *Diagnose* clinically (McMurray and Apley test); x-rays and MRI as needed. *Treat* with RICE and surgical repair, if needed, and PT.

Ankle Sprains

Ankle sprains involve the overstretching or tearing of a **ligament**, which connects 2 bones together (vs. strains—stretching or tearing of a tendon/muscle). Ankles are the most common sprain site in the body and are usually due to foot inversion and involve the anterior talofibular ligament. Assess stability, rule out fracture, and treat with R.I.C.E. (rest, ice, compression, elevation), NSAIDs, and protect with splints or braces. Casting may be necessary in severe sprains. For grade 3, refer to ortho.

Grades of sprains:

- Grade 1: microscopic tearing only
- Grade 2: partial tearing and moderate loss of function
- Grade 3: complete rupture, inability to bear weight, and significant instability of the joint

Degrees of strains:

- 1st degree: microscopic tearing
- 2nd degree: partial tearing
- 3rd degree: complete tear or rupture

Shoulder Bursitis

Shoulder bursitis involves inflammation of a **bursa**, which is a fluid-filled sac that helps reduce friction between tendons/muscles and bones. The bursa in the shoulder are: **subacromial bursa** (most common site of bursitis), **subdeltoid bursa**, and **subcoracoid bursa**. This can be caused by overuse, trauma, inflammatory arthritis (e.g., gout, RA), or infection. *Symptoms* may include pain, swelling, erythema, and reduced ROM, especially with abduction. *Diagnosis* is usually clinical but may need an ultrasound or MRI. Aspirate bursa and study fluid if infection, inflammatory arthritis, or hemorrhage is suspected. *Treat* primarily with rest, ice, and NSAIDs; occasionally steroid injections around the bursa or surgery is needed.

Rotator Cuff Tear

Rotator cuff tear involves an injury to one of the muscles that insert into the **shoulder (glenohumeral) joint** that help stabilize the humerus; it can be a partial or complete tear. The rotator cuff consists of the **supraspinatus** (most common tendon tear; used in abduction), **infraspinatus** (external rotation), **teres minor** (external rotation), and **subscapularis** (internal rotation) muscles. This may occur acutely, insidiously, or may be due to age (often affects those >40). *Symptoms* depend on the location of the tear and include pain (often at night), weakness, and reduced ROM. *Diagnose* clinically: Supraspinatus and infraspinatus— use Jobe or Neer test; Teres minor—use Hornblower's sign, this indicates a major rotator cuff tear; Subscapularis—use the lift-off test (patient places hand flat against back and tries to lift it away from their back). MRI (best) and ultrasound may be used to evaluate the tear and x-rays rule out changes in the bone (e.g., fracture, arthritis). Initially *treat* with conservatively with rest, ice, and NSAIDs. Then work on restoring ROM with stretching and strengthening exercises. Steroid injections and surgery may be needed.

Localized Joint Syndromes

Hip and Pelvic Pain

Hip and pelvic pain may result from a variety of different conditions:

- **Osteoarthritic changes** to the joint may result in increasing pain in the anterior or posterior hip and pelvic area as well as stiffness and reduced mobility. Pain increases on weight bearing.
- **Trochanteric bursitis** causes pain in the hip and lateral thigh, worsening with activity and weight bearing.
- **Hip dislocation** usually results from a traumatic injury. Typically, the pain is severe and the patient unable to bear weight or move the leg.

- **Snapping hip syndrome** results in snapping sound or sensation when the hip is extended because thickened connective tissue bands catch as they slide over the femoral head. This condition may be accompanied by bursitis.
- **Hip labral tear** is damage to the cartilage that lines the outside rim of the hip socket, resulting in pain in the hip or groin area. decreased mobility, stiffness, and clicking or catching of the joint.

Foot and Ankle Syndromes

Foot and ankle syndromes include:

- **Pes cavus**: High arch remains locked in place with weight bearing so foot loses flexibility and does not flatten. Often associated with CP and Charcot-Marie-Tooth and may result in callus formation and pain.
- **Pes planus**: Flat foot in which the medial arch is weak and cannot support weight, resulting in pain and deformity.
- **Ankle sprain**: Damage to a joint, with a partial rupture of the supporting ligaments, usually caused by wrenching or twisting that may occur with a fall. The rupture can damage blood vessels, resulting in edema, tenderness at the joint, and pain on movement with pain increasing over 2-3 hours after injury. Most sprains are inversion injuries with tearing of lateral ligaments.
- **Ankle strain**: Overstretching of a part of the musculature ("pulled muscle") that causes microscopic tears in the muscle or tendon, usually resulting from excess stress or overuse of the muscle. Strains may be caused by blunt trauma to a muscle or overstretching related to sports activities.
- **Ankle impingement**: Pain in bony or soft tissue structure at front of ankle during dorsiflexion caused by pinching of the joint capsule.

Raynaud Disease/Phenomenon

Raynaud's disease is a form of intermittent digital arteriolar vasoconstriction, especially in response to cold or stress. Primary RD occurs in 2-6% of the population, usually females, but RD can be secondary, primarily to rheumatic diseases. Secondary RD is usually more severe and may result in ulcerations or gangrene. **Raynaud's phenomenon** refers specifically to the vasoconstriction of arterioles of the hands and/or feet, resulting in pallor or cyanosis. A recovery phase results in hyperemia or rubor. Thus, symptoms are described as a progression from white to blue to red. The fingers are more often affected than the toes. Initially, just one or two fingertips are involved, but as the disease progresses, the entire fingers to the distal palm are affected. Symptoms are bilateral with primary RD but may be unilateral with secondary RD. Symptoms may be triggered by exposure to cold, vasoconstrictive medications, and cigarette smoking. Treatment involves avoiding triggers, calcium channel blockers (nifedipine), or sympathectomy (for severe cases).

Shoulder Dislocation

Shoulder dislocations occur when the **humeral head** separates from the **glenohumeral fossa**, usually anteriorly. This can occur due to a fall on an outstretched arm or other trauma. The acromion is prominent and the patient does not want to move the arm. If anteriorly dislocated, the arm is held slight abduction and external rotation. If posteriorly dislocated, the arm is held in an adducted and internally rotated position. Assess that nerves and blood vessels are intact. Order AP, axillary, and possibly Y-view x-rays. *Treat* with reduction then immobilization (sling & swathed) for 1-3 weeks.

Skeletal

Osteomyelitis

Osteomyelitis is inflammation and destruction of the **bone** caused by an **infection** (usually bacterial), and may be acute or chronic. The most common **pathogen** is *Staphylococcus aureus*; and the **lower extremities** are the most common site. This may occur due to trauma (especially open wounds), surgery, or may be bloodborne. Those at increased risk include those with DM, vascular insufficiency, or who are immunocompromised. Patients usually present with local pain, swelling, erythema, and may have a fever. *Diagnose* clinically and confirm with x-rays (takes about 2 weeks to be visible on x-ray; periosteal thickening, soft tissue swelling, and bone loss may be noted), MRI, or bone scan. Blood cultures and bone biopsy with culture and sensitivity may be performed before antibiotics are begun. *Treat* with IV and oral antibiotics for 4-6 weeks following local empiric antibiotic susceptibility trends, and then if necessary change to follow C & S results. Surgery may be performed to debride necrotic tissue and to remove areas of infection, including any fistulas or sinus tracts that may have formed in chronic cases.

Osteoporosis

Osteoporosis is a **metabolic bone disease** in which there is a decrease in the **bone mineral density (BMD)**. It may be classified as **primary** (postmenopausal, type I; or age-related/senile, type II) or **secondary osteoporosis** (e.g., due to cancer, hyperparathyroidism, steroid use, etc.). Type I involves mainly **trabecular bone loss** and type II involves mainly **cortical bone loss**. Osteoporosis is more common in Caucasians and in women than men; it is usually due to post-menopausal causes. **Estrogen** is thought to be bone-protective and, with the decrease in estrogen levels after menopause, the bones may begin to weaken. Other risk factors include smoking and alcohol use, medications, such as chronic steroid or heparin use, hormonal imbalance, such as hyperparathyroidism, reduced calcium intake, inactivity, and hypogonadal states. Patients may suffer an osteoporotic fracture, such as a compression fracture, as a result of little or no trauma. Patients are asymptomatic until a fracture occurs; therefore, screening is vital. Screen all women ≥65 years old and all men ≥70 years old; screen earlier if risk factors present. A DXA (dual-energy x-ray absorptiometry) bone mineral density scan of the hip or lumbar spine will show a bone density T-score of at least -2.5 standard deviations below the value of peak BMD. If a child, premenopausal, or a man <50 years old, use a Z-score ≤-2.0 SD below the BMD that is expected for their age and sex for diagnosis. The FRAX tool can help identify those at increased risk of developing osteoporosis. *Treatment* includes weight-bearing exercise, modifying risk factors, calcium and vitamin D supplementation. Also, bisphosphonates x 5 years (Fosamax®, Boniva®, Actonel®; first-line) and calcitonin that reduces bone reabsorption or other newer medications like denosumab may be used for osteoporosis.

Osteosarcoma

Osteosarcoma is a type of **bone cancer** that usually occurs in **metaphyseal region of long bones** as they are growing. It is most often found at the distal femur, proximal tibia, and proximal humerus. It commonly affects children and young adults from 10-20 years of age. Some hereditary diseases, such as hereditary retinoblastoma and bone dysplasia, may cause children to be more susceptible to developing osteosarcoma; and exposure of bone to high doses of radiation can also increase the risk of this disease. However, osteosarcoma will often occur without any known cause. Patients typically complain of bone pain that may have been present for months, may have nocturnal pain, there is usually swelling at the site of the cancer, and muscle atrophy may be present. This condition may be mistaken for an injury or growing pains. Systemic *symptoms* like fever and fatigue are uncommon. X-rays may show Codman triangle (a triangular area caused by the periosteum being lifted away), a sunburst lesion, or lytic lesions. This is followed by an MRI for staging and is then diagnosed with a bone biopsy. *Treatment* for osteosarcoma is surgery to remove the affected portion of the bone and chemotherapy (may also be given before surgery). In some cases, the cancer spreads to other organs of the body, especially the lungs. Refer to an orthopedic surgeon.

OSTEOCHONDRITIS DISSECANS

Osteochondritis dissecans is a disorder characterized by necrosis and ultimately separation of subchondral bone. It most commonly occurs on the medial femoral condyle and it is the most common cause of a loose body in the joint space in pediatric patients. It is usually due to repetitive stress to the bone. It typically presents in teenage athletes, who complain of the gradual onset of vague knee pain. Pain may worsen and swelling may develop following physical activity. The diagnosis is usually made by x-ray or MRI. Stable lesions may be managed conservatively by modifying activity. More advanced unstable lesions are managed with surgery.

Connective Tissue

SYSTEMIC LUPUS ERYTHEMATOSUS

Systemic lupus erythematosus (SLE) or lupus is a **chronic inflammatory condition** with periods of remittance and flares in which the body's **immune system** turns against itself and begins attacking organs and tissues. It is primarily known to affect the skin, joints, kidneys, heart, nerves, and blood cells. This affects young women much more than men, and in the U.S. appears more often in African Americans and Asians. There is no definite known cause of SLE, but genetic and environmental factors (e.g., sun exposure, medications) play a role in the development of this autoimmune disease. Patients may present with fever, fatigue, arthralgias, myalgias, a discoid rash, a photosensitive rash, or the typical malar rash (butterfly) across the nose and cheeks. Oral ulcers, serositis (e.g., pericarditis, pleuritis), Raynaud phenomenon, and renal (e.g., proteinuria) and neurologic disorders (e.g., depression) may also be present. *Diagnose* clinically and by confirming the presence of autoantibodies and other lab criteria (e.g., + ANA, anemia, proteinuria, + renal biopsy for lupus nephritis). Patients must meet 4 of the 11 ACR criteria or 4 of the 17 SLICC classification criteria to be diagnosed with SLE. There is no known cure for SLE, but the symptoms can usually be *controlled*. Start the antimalarial hydroxychloroquine in patients with SLE to help decrease flares and mortality. NSAIDs and corticosteroids can help to decrease inflammation during an acute flare-up. Immunosuppressant medications (e.g., cyclophosphamide, azathioprine) may also be helpful in decreasing the symptoms in severe disease. Consult or refer patients to specialists as needed.

SJÖGREN SYNDROME

Sjögren syndrome is a chronic autoimmune disorder causing **dry eyes and mouth**. It is often seen with other types of connective tissue disorders (e.g., SLE, RA) and is much more common in women >50 years old. It is not known what causes Sjögren syndrome though it is suspected that hereditary factors may play a part, and there may also be a link with viral infections being a trigger. Although the primary symptoms seen with Sjögren are dry eyes and a dry mouth, it may also affect almost any area of the body including the lungs, kidneys, liver, joints, nervous system, and skin. Patients may complain of dry eyes, dry mouth, dry nasal passages, dry skin and pruritus, vaginal dryness, parotid enlargement, a dry cough, difficulty swallowing, and arthralgias. Since it is commonly seen in conjunction with other connective tissue disorders, symptoms of those accompanying diseases may also be present. *Diagnose* clinically and may be supported with a + ANA, + anti-SSA/Ro, a + anti-SSB/La, or a + RF. Topical gels and artificial tears can help with the dry eyes and saliva production may be increased through chewing gum and/or using lozenges. Systemic medications to *treat* the symptoms include corticosteroids and immunosuppressants, especially if another connective tissue disorder is present. If dry eyes are severe, surgery can be performed to block small openings in the eyelids that drain tears from the eyes, thereby retaining moisture within the eyes. *Complications* include dental caries, eye infections, and an increased risk of lymphoma.

Scleroderma

Systemic sclerosis (Scleroderma) is a chronic condition in which **fibrosis** (hardening) of the skin and connective tissues occurs due to excessive **collagen deposits**. This can be localized, limited (CREST syndrome), or diffuse and may become progressively worse and lead to involvement of the organs, like the GI tract, heart, lungs, and kidneys. There is no definite known cause of systemic sclerosis, but it is an **autoimmune connective tissue disorder**. It is more common in women and in those 20-60 years old. Risk of developing systemic sclerosis is increased in those with silica or solvent/chemical exposure. Patients may complain of whitish fingers or toes with exposure to cold (Raynaud phenomenon), telangiectasias, puffy digits, and areas of tight, thickened, or hardened skin that will not go away, usually in the fingers, toes, or face. As the condition progresses, the skin becomes stiffer, range of motion (especially of the distal limbs/digits) decreases, and weakness develops. Scleroderma can even affect organs, such as the esophagus and stomach, leading to dysphagia and reduced gastric motility. If it affects the kidneys, it may result in renal failure. *Diagnose* clinically and support with presence of autoantibodies (e.g., +ANA, +RF). *Treatment* is symptomatic; d/c smoking. Topical medications and creams may help with the involved skin. NSAIDs and corticosteroids may help with pain as stiffness occurs. Medications to improve circulation (Ca^{++} channel blockers) can help as can immunosuppressants to decrease the symptoms and progression of this disease. *Complications* include contractures, distal ulcers, renal failure, and pulmonary HTN.

Ankylosing Spondylitis

Ankylosing spondylitis is a chronic systemic inflammatory form of **arthritis** involving where **ligaments and tendons** attach to bone (entheses), usually in the **vertebral column and the sacroiliac joints** (spondyloarthropathy). This inflammation causes **bony overgrowth**, especially in the spine, and may lead to fusion of the **vertebral bodies**. When it occurs at the joints of the ribs and spine, mobility of the rib cage can be affected, restricting respirations. Other systems that may be involved include the eyes, heart, lungs, kidneys, and GI tract. This has a genetic predisposition (HLA-B27) and is more common in men and in those in their late teens to 40 years old. Patients typically complain of fatigue and pain and stiffness in the affected joints (usually back and SI joints) that's worse in the morning and with inactivity. The pain may occur at night and improves with exercise but not with rest. Ankylosing spondylitis may lead to kyphosis and possibly depressed respirations. Uveitis (or iritis) and inflammatory bowel disease may also be seen with this. *Diagnose* clinically (see above: pain ≥3 months and onset ≤40 years old) and by documenting SI joint involvement (sacroiliitis) on x-ray. X-rays may also show erosions with sclerosis, narrowing, or bony fusion ("bamboo spine") in the vertebral column. Blood testing includes CRP, ESR, and CBC, but these are non-specific. *Treatment* includes anti-inflammatory drugs (NSAIDs are first-line) and steroid injections may be necessary to decrease inflammation. DMARDs and biologics are used second line and may help to decrease symptoms. PT is helpful and surgery may be needed to stabilize joints.

Spine

Cauda Equina Syndrome

Cauda equina syndrome is a condition in which there is severe compression of the **nerve roots** that exit the spinal cord below its termination at **L1** (resembles a horse's tail). This can cause permanent **neurologic disabilities** and is a medical emergency. It is usually caused by an **acute herniated nucleus pulposus** (herniated disk); or may be caused by compression from a **tumor**, or can occur due to **progressive degenerative changes** causing severe spinal stenosis in the lower lumbar spine. Patients usually have low back pain with pain radiating into one or both of the lower extremities. There will be saddle anesthesia present along with bowel and bladder retention or incontinence (all red flags). The lower extremities are numb and/or weak and have depressed or absent reflexes. *Diagnose* with an MRI and refer immediately to neurosurgery. *Treatment* of cauda equina syndrome is urgent surgical intervention within 24-48 hours of severe symptom onset. If treated promptly, there is a chance that patients' symptoms will be reversed. The longer the symptoms are present, however, the less likely patients will reach a full recovery. Steroids can be started to reduce the inflammation, but this is usually only until surgery is performed.

Spinal Stenosis

Spinal stenosis occurs when there is narrowing of the spinal canal or neural foramen causing compression of the **spinal cord or nerve roots**. This most often affects the **cervical and lumbar spine**. Spinal stenosis is most often degenerative in nature (e.g., osteoarthritis, bone spurs) and therefore usually affects those >50 years old; however, there is an increased risk of developing this if there is congenital narrowing of the spinal column, and may occur along with disk herniation or spondylolisthesis (slipping of the vertebrae). Patients typically complain of chronic pain in the affected portion of the spine and may have radiating pain, numbness, and/or weakness extending into the upper or lower extremities, depending on the stenosis location. With myelopathy (spinal cord injury), there will be profound weakness and hyperactive reflexes/spasticity. *Symptoms* of neurogenic claudication are due to lumbar spinal stenosis and include pain that is aggravated with walking (especially downhill) and standing, and is usually relieved with sitting and leaning forward. Severe lumbar spinal stenosis can cause cauda equina syndrome. *Diagnose* with an MRI (preferred) or CT/CT myelography which shows narrowing of the canal. Symptoms may be slightly relieved with NSAIDs (first-line), pain relievers, antispasmodics, and epidural steroid injections along with PT. Surgical correction in those with more severe symptoms (neurogenic claudication, radiculopathy, myelopathy) can be performed with a laminectomy or X-Stop procedure that relieves the pressure being applied to the spinal canal; refer to neurosurgery.

Herniated Nucleus Pulposus

A **herniated nucleus pulposus** (herniated disk) occurs when the softer interior of the **intervertebral fibrocartilage** herniates through the outer fibrous material that surrounds the **nucleus pulposus**. This can occur anywhere in the spinal column but is most often seen in the **lumbar spine**. The disk can bulge in one direction or may be central. If this occurs above the level of L1, there is a risk of **spinal cord compression**. Herniated disks are seen more often in those with heavy-lifting jobs and incidence increases as we age. Patients may be asymptomatic or complain of pain at the level of the spine where the herniation occurs, along with radicular pain following the dermatome of the affected nerve. For example, if the herniation occurs at L5-S1, patients may complain of sciatic-type pain. Patients may develop numbness or tingling in the affected dermatome, along with weakness of the affected limb. Assess strength, ROM, and thoroughly check for an intact neurologic system. *Diagnose* with MRI or CT. Patients may be managed conservatively with NSAIDs and pain relievers. Often, the symptoms will resolve with conservative *treatment*. Physical therapy to help with pain relief and stretching and strengthening can help. Steroids, either orally or per epidural injection, can help to reduce the inflammation. If neural deficits or signs of structural instability, refer to neurosurgery. Surgery may be performed with a microdiscectomy to remove the portion of the disk that has herniated.

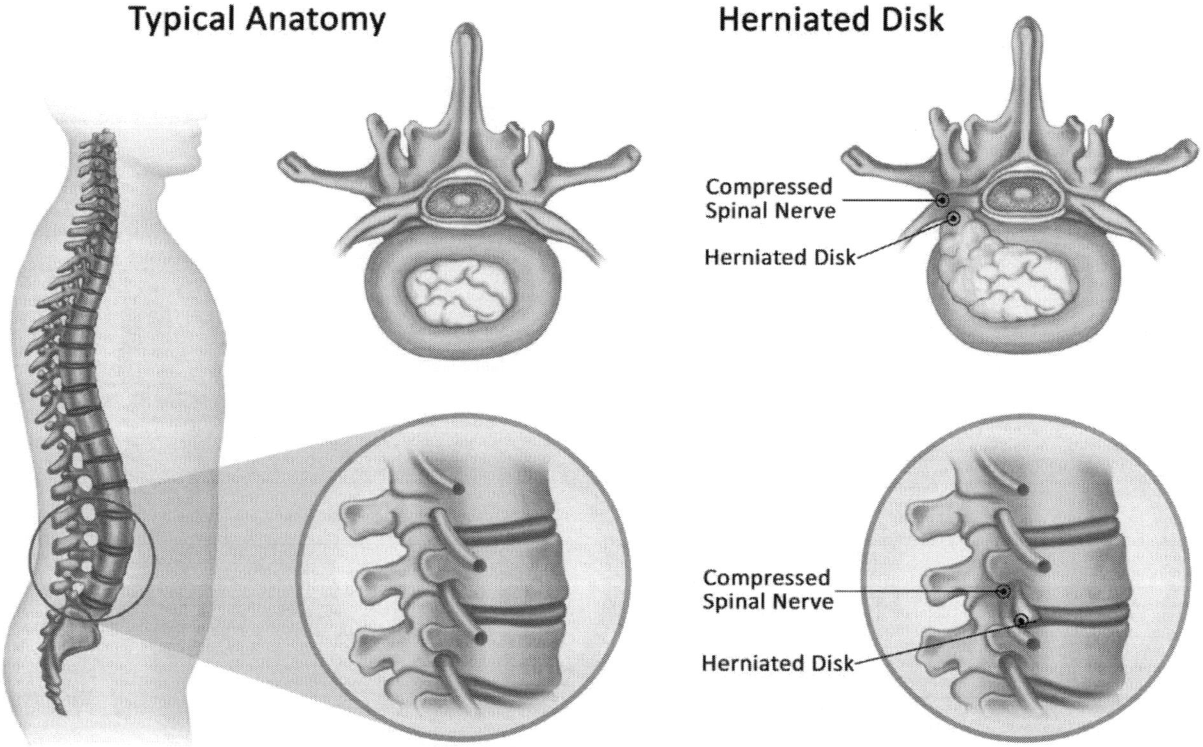

Low Back Sprains and Strains

Low back injuries and pain are a common presenting complaint of patients. A **sprain** is an injury to a **ligament** (connects bone to bone) and a **strain** is an injury to a **muscle or tendon** (connects muscle to bone). This often occurs due to sports and in those whose jobs require heavy lifting. The L4-L5 and L5-S1 are the most frequent locations of injury; however, injuries may occur anywhere along the back. **Back strains** are more common and this is often caused by overuse or a twisting motion while applying a force/muscle contraction (mechanical injuries). Patients usually present with a history of the injury event, localized muscle/tendon/ligament pain on palpation, increased pain with movement, may have some radiating pain, muscle spasm, and reduced ROM. Red flags that may indicate other issues include fever or other systemic symptoms, midline vertebral pain, a positive straight leg raise test (may indicate sciatica/nerve root compression or a herniated nucleus pulposus), significant muscle weakness or paresthesias, sensory deficits, saddle anesthesia, bladder and bowel retention or incontinence, nocturnal pain, and a history of osteoporosis or cancer. *Diagnose* clinically and reserve imaging studies for those with red flags or if it is chronic (most patients heal within 6 weeks). *Treat* symptoms with rest and ice (for 1st 2 days), NSAIDs, and possibly muscle relaxants. After the acute phase, begin ROM and strengthening exercises. Educate patients in proper back safety and lifting techniques, and lumbosacral muscle corsets may be recommended.

Scoliosis

Scoliosis is abnormal lateral curvature (≥10°) of the **spine** in a S or C shape. It can be classified as **infantile** (<3 years old), **juvenile** (3-10 years old), or **adolescent** (>10 years old). The cause is typically unknown but it may have a genetic component and is more common in girls. It usually has an insidious onset in late childhood or early teen years when **growth spurts** are common. This is often 1st noted on a routine physical or by a school nurse during screening (Adams forward bend test), but asymmetry of the shoulders (right is usually higher), protruding scapula, uneven ribs, or ill-fitting clothes may be noted by a caregiver. *Diagnose* with AP and lateral x-rays showing a Cobb angle measurement ≥10°. If the Cobb angle is 10-19° reevaluate every 6 months. Refer patients once it reaches ≥20° and braces may be used at this point. Surgery is not usually used until >40°.

Kyphosis

Kyphosis is an abnormal forward curvature of the **thoracic spine** (≥50°) causing a "hunchback" appearance. Kyphosis has many possible causes but is most common in older women due to **osteoporosis** (compression fractures). **Scheuermann's kyphosis** appears in adolescence and is slightly more common in boys. Patients may present with back pain, the curvature does not correct with hyperextension of the back, and patients may be cosmetically bothered by the curvature. *Diagnose* with PA and lateral x-rays of the spine showing a Cobb angle ≥50°. *Treat* symptoms as needed (NSAIDs), treat underlying osteoporosis, and PT and bracing may be helpful. Surgery is usually reserved for more severe cases where curvature is >65-75° or if neurologic deficits are present.

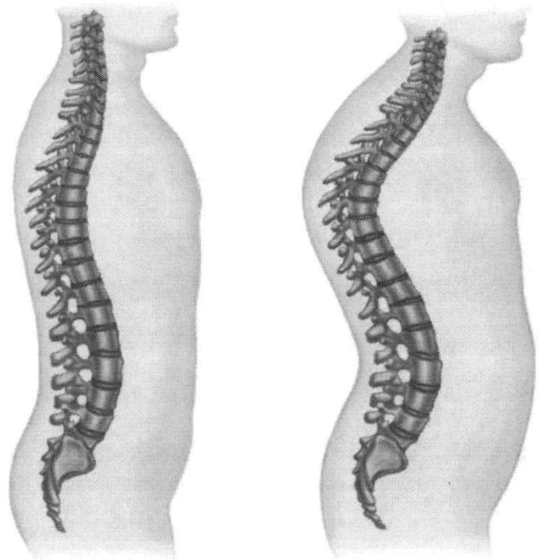

Muscle

Polymyositis

Polymyositis is an **inflammatory myopathy** in which chronic inflammation, degeneration, and weakness occurs in the **muscles**. It most commonly affects the muscles in the proximal large joints, such as shoulders and hips, and is gradually progressive. A definite cause is not known, but it may be due to an autoimmune reaction. This usually affects those >30 years old and is more common in women (2:1) and in the black population. Patients may complain of a slow progression of symmetric muscle weakness and sometimes pain. This is commonly present in the shoulders and arms, and patients will experience a sensation of fatigue after even light activity. Patients may have morning stiffness, arthralgias, progressive dysphagia, SOB, fever, and weight loss. Unlike dermatomyositis, polymyositis is not associated with a rash. *Diagnose* with a muscle biopsy and creatine kinase is typically elevated. First-line *treatment* for polymyositis involves corticosteroids (prednisone), along with physical therapy. There are medications available that work by suppressing the immune system, like azathioprine, methotrexate, and IVIG that can be used, especially in patients who don't respond to steroids. *Complications* of polymyositis include possible pneumonia due to decreased chest wall muscle expansion, aspiration pneumonia due to dysphagia; it is also associated with malignancy.

Pain

Polyarteritis Nodosa

Polyarteritis nodosa (PAN) is a systemic **vasculitis** in which necrotizing inflammation and damage occurs in the small and medium-sized **arteries**. This can occur anywhere within the body, but it most often affects the kidneys, intestines, skin, peripheral nerves, muscles, and joints; the lungs are usually not affected. It has no known definite cause, but it is often seen in patients who have been diagnosed with hepatitis B and sometimes hep C. Patients may present acutely or may have an insidious onset of and may affect one organ or many. Patients usually present with pain in the area that is affected by the arterial inflammation, fever, fatigue, weight loss, and weakness. If the damage is severe, there can be ischemia and infarcts of the bowel, kidney, or other affected organs. There can be asymmetric peripheral neuropathy if the PNS is affected, HTN if kidneys are affected, and if the skin is affected, ulcers, nodules, mottled skin, rashes, and purpura/cutaneous infarcts may be present. *Diagnose* with a tissue biopsy which shows necrotizing vasculitis and possibly with angiography. *Treatment* involves immunosuppression with corticosteroids (prednisone) and sometimes adding cyclophosphamide (not in hep B cases). If patients have hepatitis B, appropriate therapy should be started to treat this condition. If polyarteritis nodosa is severe and tissue death has occurred, surgery is performed to remove the damaged tissue and make repairs. Refer patients.

Polymyalgia Rheumatica

Polymyalgia rheumatica is a condition in which patients experience **proximal muscle stiffness** and severe pain usually in the shoulders, hips, and neck. It is more common in adults over the age of 50 and more prevalent in women (2:1). The cause is unknown but it may be an autoimmune disorder, it may have a trigger, and it is related to giant cell arteritis. It is self-limited but may last 3-5+ years.

Polymyalgia rheumatica can have an insidious onset or occur very quickly. As the disease progresses, it will affect both sides equally but may begin in a unilateral distribution. Patients typically complain of bilateral and symmetric muscle pain and stiffness in various proximal locations of the body (back, neck, shoulders, hips), especially first thing in the morning (may last ≥1 hour) and with inactivity. Patients may have bursitis and tenosynovitis. Patients may have a generalized feeling of malaise, fever, weight loss, and fatigue. Patients typically have normal muscle strength but a decreased ROM due to the pain. *Diagnose* clinically and ESR may be ≥40 mm/hr, elevated CRP, and anemia may be present on CBC; rule out other causes and rule out giant cell arteritis. *Treatment* is long-term corticosteroids and patients may require 1-2 years of treatment; taper slowly. Patients should be closely monitored and counseled on the risks of long-term steroid use; refer to a rheumatologist.

Complex Regional Pain Syndrome

Complex regional pain syndrome (**CRPS**) is a **chronic pain condition** that usually manifests after an injury. CRPS is the newer collective name for reflex sympathetic dystrophy and causalgia. CRPS includes **type I**, which is linked to an initial injury or insult, and **type II**, which is due to an injury to a nerve. This commonly occurs after a fracture, crush injury, limb immobilization/cast, surgery, or MI and the pain is disproportionate to the injury. CRPS involves autonomic dysfunction as well as sensory and motor issues and changes to the skin and possibly bone. This is more common in women and usually affects those in their 40's, although this may occur at any age. Patients usually describe a regional burning, aching, or throbbing pain that starts days to weeks after an injury (often to an extremity) with other *signs* including changes in: temperature (>1° C), color, edema , thinning skin, sweating, hair or nail growth changes, sensitivities to touch, muscle and joint stiffness, and decreased ROM. CRPS is a clinical *diagnosis* and requires 2-4 signs and 3-4 symptoms to be diagnosed as well as ruling out other causes. Sometimes x-rays are taken that may show osteopenia. Early *treatment* is important and involves a multidisciplinary approach with pain management, PT/OT, and psychological support. More research is needed, but medical treatment may include NSAIDs, opioids, corticosteroids, calcitonin/bisphosphonates, tricyclic antidepressants, gabapentin, clonidine, IVIG, and sympathetic ganglion blocks. Refer to neurology as needed.

Fibromyalgia

Fibromyalgia is a chronic **neurosensory disorder** in which patients feel fatigued, have pain "all over," have sleep disturbances, and have memory difficulties. This condition affects the muscles and tendons. The cause of fibromyalgia is not fully understood, but it is believed to be a condition in which the body's **central nervous system** becomes hypersensitive to **peripheral stimuli**. This typically affects women more than men and appears in their 20's-50's. Patients complain of chronic fatigue accompanied with tenderness or pain (must be continuous for >3 months) along with stiffness that is widespread. Signs of depression, difficulty sleeping, and concentration/memory problems may also be present. Many fibromyalgia patients also suffer from IBS and chronic headaches. Other disease processes like RA, SLE, hypothyroidism, and autoimmune disorders should be ruled out as the cause of the pain, but these diseases may be concomitant. Patients may be *diagnosed* with fibromyalgia if the Widespread Pain Index (WPI) is ≥7, the Symptom Severity scale (SS scale) is ≥5 [or the WPI 3-6 and SS scale ≥9], symptoms have been present for ≥3 months, and if another disorder doesn't explain the pain. Tender points may be assessed during the PE. *Treatment* consists of non-opioid analgesics (e.g., tramadol, acetaminophen), tricyclic antidepressants, anti-anxiety drugs, and anticonvulsants. Currently 3 drugs are approved for treating fibromyalgia: Lyrica® (pregabalin), an anti-seizure medication, Cymbalta® (duloxetine), a serotonin-norepinephrine uptake inhibitor (SNRI); and Savella® (milnacipran), an SNRI. Also, a healthy diet, exercise, stress management, sleep therapy, and psychotherapy can help.

Trauma

Blowout Fracture

A **blowout fracture** is a fracture of the **orbital floor** and involves the maxillary bone and the posterior medial floor of the orbit. It occurs due to **excessive facial trauma**. These patients will report trauma and complain of significant pain. Diplopia may be present because of restriction of the extraocular muscles. The eyelid may be edematous with crepitus present on palpation. A potential complication of a blowout fracture is possible entrapment of the orbital contents within the maxillary sinus. If this occurs, the eye may have a sunken appearance, or enophthalmos. *Diagnosis* is made per history and confirmed with imaging studies, usually CT scan. A blowout fracture will typically heal on its own with regular follow-up to ensure proper healing is occurring. Patients should be advised to avoid blowing their noses. Oral antibiotics may be given to decrease the risk of orbital infection. In some cases, such as with restrictive diplopia or enophthalmos, surgery may be necessary to repair the orbital wall. *Complications* include inferior rectus muscle entrapment leading to ischemia, nerve damage to the infraorbital nerve, and enophthalmos.

Fractures

Boxer's fracture occurs at the **distal end of the fifth metacarpal bone**. It earned its name because it is usually caused by force of a fist hitting a hard surface as with boxing. It usually heals within 3-4 weeks with splinting (ulnar gutter splint) and rest. Reduction and casting may or may not be necessary depending on the severity of the fracture. **Colles fracture** occurs at the **distal end of the radius with dorsal displacement** ("dinner fork" deformity); and is usually caused by breaking a fall with an outstretched (extended) hand. Depending on severity, surgery (open reduction) may be necessary, but often all that's needed is a closed reduction with a cast for 3-6 weeks until the fracture has healed. A **Smith fracture** is a fracture of the **distal radius with volar displacement** (opposite of a Colles and not as common). This usually occurs by falling on a flexed wrist. *Treatment* involves open or closed reduction with a cast for 6 weeks. For both Colles and Smith fractures assess for injury to the median nerve (palmar side of thumb, index, middle, and half of ring finger).

Scaphoid Fracture

Scaphoid fracture (navicular fracture) occurs from a fall on an outstretched hand and is the most common carpal fracture. This will cause tenderness in the anatomic snuffbox at the base of the thumb in the wrist. There is risk of interrupted blood supply to this small bone with this fracture, osteonecrosis may occur. *Treatment* is with a thumb spica cast or splint, sometimes up to 6-8 weeks, and surgery may be necessary. *Diagnose* the above fractures with AP and lateral x-rays. Add an oblique view for hand and carpal fractures. CT may be necessary; and sometimes an MRI may be necessary with suspected scaphoid fractures. Care must be taken to note involvement of the epiphyseal disk (growth plate) in children since an open reduction with fixation (ORIF) may be required. Patients should be referred to an orthopedist.

Slater-Harris Classification

The **Slater-Harris classification** of fractures is a method of classifying fractures in children that affect their growth plate. The classification helps determine the treatment and prognosis. The classification is as follows:

- **Type I** is through the physis. The growth plate is rarely disturbed and the prognosis is excellent.
- **Type II** is through the physis and metaphysis. These are the most common fractures. They carry a risk of growth disturbance.
- **Type III** is through the physis and epiphysis. These fractures involve the joint and orthopedic referral is indicated.
- **Type IV** fractures are through the metaphysis, physis, and epiphysis. These fractures can often cause chronic growth problems.
- **Type V** are crush injuries.
- **Type VI** are injuries to the perichondrium.

Mallet Finger, Jersey Finger, and Boutonniere Deformity

Mallet finger, or jammed finger, results when there is forced flexion of an extended distal interphalangeal (DIP) joint. The injury frequently occurs while playing basketball or baseball. The diagnosis is made clinically. An x-ray should be performed to rule out a fracture. Treatment is extension splinting.

Jersey finger is an injury to the distal interphalangeal joint often seen when a football player grabs the jersey of another player, leading to forced extension of the DIP joint. This causes an avulsion injury of the flexor digitorum profundus tendon. It is most often seen in the ring finger. Treatment is surgical repair.

Boutonniere deformity describes the abnormal position of hyperflexion of the PIP joint with hyperextension of the DIP joint. It can be caused by trauma or inflammatory conditions such as rheumatoid arthritis. Treatment is extension splinting.

Overuse Injuries

Nursemaid's Elbow

Nursemaid's elbow is a **subluxation of the radial head**. It usually occurs in children under 6-years-old. A pulling mechanism on the arm, such as when swinging a child, causes the **radial head** to pull out of the **annular ligament** in which it sits. This results in partial dislocation, or subluxation, of the arm. The child may initially experience pain, but then usually acts normally while refusing to use the affected arm; and will hold it in a slightly flexed, adducted, and pronated position. There is no visible deformity, swelling, or bruising of the arm; but the child will guard the arm and prevent any movement of it to prevent pain. *Diagnosis* is clinical; however, older children and adults may need an x-ray to rule out a fracture. A nursemaid's elbow is easily reduced using the supination-flexion technique (the child's pronated arm is held at a 90° ∠ with pressure applied to the radial head. Next, the hand is supinated and then the elbow flexed so the hand touches the shoulder) or the hyperpronation technique (the child's pronated arm is held at a 90° ∠ with pressure applied to the radial head; then the wrist is hyperpronated). A pop or click is usually felt if it has been reduced, and typically the child immediately begins to use their arm (some take ~30 mins.). If this does not reduce the subluxation, the arm may be placed in a sling and orthopedic evaluation obtained. The parents should be advised to avoid swinging or pulling the child, especially by 1 arm, to help prevent this from recurring (recurs in about 30%).

Gamekeeper's Thumb

Gamekeeper's thumb, or skier's thumb, is injury to the **ulnar collateral ligament** of the thumb. It is caused by a force that hyperextends the thumb away from the hand toward the body, as when falling on a ski pole. It earned its name from gamekeepers in Europe injuring the ligament while breaking rabbits' necks. It may also occur in sports (i.e. football, rugby), falls, and MVA while bracing for impact. Patients will have significant pain with this injury and, depending upon severity, it can be disabling. The pain is greatly exacerbated when trying to grasp or pinch anything (i.e. holding car keys). The area may be edematous, erythematous, or ecchymotic. Obtain AP, lateral, and oblique x-rays to rule out an avulsion fracture. Exam usually reveals ligament and first MCP joint instability by using a lateral stress test (local anesthetic is needed and this should not be performed if there is an avulsion fracture). *Treatment* consists of immobilization of the ligament with a thumb spica splint or cast for 4 weeks and NSAIDs. Surgery may be necessary if the ligament injury is not healing and is required for a complete tear or rupture. Prognosis improves when the patient seeks medical attention shortly after the injury; if required, surgery should be performed within 3 weeks. Chronic instability is the primary *complication*.

De Quervain Tenosynovitis

De Quervain tenosynovitis is a condition in which there is inflammation in the **abductor pollicis longus and extensor pollicis brevis tendons** in the thumb. They are held together in the thumb by the **extensor retinaculum**. If the tendons become inflamed and swollen, the retinaculum cannot expand to accommodate the inflammation, leading to tenosynovitis. This can be caused by overuse of the thumbs (i.e. mothers or day care workers picking up infants, carpenters), trauma, or arthritis which can cause edema in the tendons, leading to this condition. Hormonal changes of pregnancy and water retention may lead to constriction and pain of the tendons. Patients complain of pain with motion of the thumb and wrist, and there is usually thickening and pain on palpation at the radial styloid (1st dorsal compartment). *Diagnose* clinically and with the Finkelstein test (make a fist around the thumb and perform ulnar deviation; this elicits pain). *Treatment* consists of resting the thumb, splinting, and NSAIDs. If conservative treatments do not help, long-acting steroid injections into the sheath may reduce the inflammation. As a last resort, surgery can be done to release the extensor retinaculum.

Carpal Tunnel Syndrome

Carpal tunnel syndrome occurs when there is irritation and pressure applied to the **median nerve** within the carpal tunnel of the wrist. It can have no known cause, but most patients have experienced some type of repetitive movement of the hands that caused irritation within the carpal tunnel. *Signs and symptoms* are gradually progressive and include numbness or tingling of the palmar side of the thumb, index, and middle fingers (median nerve distribution). Patients may describe grip strength weakness and frequent dropping of objects at home. Symptoms may be worse at night and may wake patients. *Diagnose* clinically and may confirm with nerve conduction testing, EMG (electromyography), or ultrasound. Symptoms can be elicited by tapping on the volar surface of the wrist, over the carpal tunnel (Tinel's sign). Wrist splints in a neutral or slightly extended position should be tried at night for 3-4 weeks to help relieve pressure on the nerve. Anti-inflammatory drugs and resting the hands and wrists may help. If conservative *treatment* does not work, corticosteroid injections may help. If it is severe or these other treatments are not effective, surgery to release the transverse ligament over the carpal tunnel usually resolves the condition.

Lateral Epicondylitis

Lateral epicondylitis, or tennis elbow, is common and occurs due to overuse of the **extensor muscles** in the forearm. These muscles attach to a tendon that attaches to the **lateral epicondyle** of the elbow. With overuse, such as with playing tennis (backhand), painting, or computer keyboard use, microtears and inflammation in the tendon at its insertion can occur. Patients may complain of pain and tenderness over the lateral epicondyle that can radiate to the forearm which can be aggravated with extending the fingers and wrist. *Symptoms* will become worse while picking up an object or even shaking hands. *Diagnose* clinically. Testing involves having patients extend the wrist or fingers (especially the middle) against resistance or supination with resistance which produces pain. *Treatment* includes rest of the elbow and forearm, ice, NSAIDs, and splint or a counter force brace can be worn to help relieve pain. Stretching and exercises can also be done to help strengthen the extensor muscles of the forearm and decrease pain. Steroid injections can be performed around the tendon at the lateral epicondyle (not in the tendon because it will weaken and possibly rupture). Surgery may be needed if not improved in 9-12 months.

Medial Epicondylitis

Medial epicondylitis, or golfer's elbow, occurs due to overuse of the **flexor muscles** in the forearm. These muscles attach to a tendon that attaches to the medial epicondyle of the elbow. With overuse, such as with golfing, pitching, or typing, **microtears and inflammation** in the tendon insertion can occur. Patients will complain of pain and tenderness over the medial epicondyle, aggravated by flexing the fingers and wrist. Hand or wrist weakness may develop and *symptoms* can become worse while grasping an object. *Diagnose* clinically. Testing involves having a patient extend the palm and attempt to flex the wrist toward the forearm against resistance or pronating against resistance which should produce pain over the medial epicondyle. Use the Tinel sign (tapping on the ulnar nerve at the medial epicondyle) to check for ulnar neuropathy. *Treatment* includes rest of the elbow and forearm, ice, NSAIDs or acetaminophen, and a cock-up wrist splint or counterforce brace can be worn to help relieve pain. Steroid injections can be performed around the tendon at the medial epicondyle. Once pain is better, exercises can be done to help strengthen the flexor muscles of the forearm. Surgery is rare, but may be needed if the patient is not improved in 9-12 months.

Plantar Fasciitis and Morton Neuroma

Plantar fasciitis is pain in the **plantar fascia** which runs along the sole of the foot providing support in the **arch**. This is common in runners. Pain is usually more pronounced at the origin site at the medial calcaneal tuberosity, worse in the am, and later in the day. *Diagnose* clinically and treat with ice, NSAIDs, rest, arch/heel cushions, avoid high impact activities. May need steroids/night splints.

Morton neuroma involves the irritation and thickening of the **interdigital nerve** at the ball of the foot, usually between the **3rd and 4th metatarsals**. It is more common in women. This causes progressive paresthesias and intermittent sharp, burning pain. *Diagnose* clinically and may confirm with ultrasound or MRI. *Treat* by modifying footwear; or possibly steroid injections or surgery.

Bicipital Tendinitis

Bicipital tendinitis (biceps tendinitis) is inflammation of the long head of the **biceps** as it runs along the **bicipital groove of the humerus**. The biceps both flexes and supinates the arm. This is a common overuse issue especially in athletes (especially with throwing) and those who lift heavy objects and objects overhead. This is often associated with a rotator cuff tear or a SLAP lesion (superior labrum anterior to posterior tear). *Signs and symptoms* include anterior shoulder pain over the bicipital groove aggravated with flexion and supination; and, if unstable, may cause a "snap" during ROM exercises. *Diagnose* clinically (Speed test- pain with shoulder flexion against resistance, with the elbow extended and arm supinated; Yergason test- pain with forearm supination against resistance, with the elbow flexed and shoulder adducted) and x-rays, ultrasound, and MRI as needed. *Treat* initially with rest, ice (for 2 days), and NSAIDs for 3-4 weeks. Next, once pain free, PT may be used to stretch then strengthen the shoulder. Steroid injections may be used with careful attention not to inject into the tendon itself as that may cause atrophy and rupture of the tendon. Occasionally surgery may be necessary; refer to ortho. *Complications* include reinjury & biceps tendon rupture.

Shoulder Tendinitis

Shoulder tendinitis is inflammation of one of the **tendons** in the shoulder at its **insertion**. Common tendons affected by tendinitis include the **bicipital tendon** and **supraspinatus tendon**, which is often associated with an impingement issue since it runs under the acromion. Tendinitis typically occurs due to overuse from sports or work, especially with overhead and throwing motions. This results in pain (abduction & overhead motions), inflammation, and reduced ROM. *Diagnose* supraspinatus tendinitis clinically; pain at the greater tuberosity, Jobe test (pain or reduced strength when downward pressure, against resistance, is applied to an abducted and internally rotated arm), and Hawkins test (checks for impingement; pain with passive internal rotation of the shoulder, with both arm and shoulder flexed to 90°). X-rays help note bony changes (e.g., calcifications, sclerotic changes due to arthritis, and fracture); then obtain MRI for detailed information. *Treat* with rest, ice, NSAIDs, and as improves, use stretching and strengthening exercises. This should improve in 3-6 months.

Cardiovascular System

Cardiomyopathy

Cardiomyopathies are chronic conditions of involving a diseased heart muscle. There are three main types: dilated, hypertrophic, and restrictive.

- **Dilated cardiomyopathy** is the most common type of cardiomyopathy. It results in a reduction in strength of the ventricular contraction, which causes dilation of the left ventricle and a decreased ejection fraction. Most common *causes* are genetic, alcohol abuse, toxins and drugs, coronary heart disease (CHD), infections, and endocrinopathies (diabetes, thyroid disease), but it can also be due to an autoimmune or an idiopathic process. Infective myocarditis due to the coxsackievirus and other viruses can lead to dilated cardiomyopathy.
- **Hypertrophic cardiomyopathy** causes a significant hypertrophy of the left ventricle, especially the septum, which results in obstruction of the left ventricle. This is most often genetic in etiology (autosomal dominant) and may be first seen in young athletes as a sudden cardiac arrest. Hypertension may also contribute to development of this type of cardiomyopathy.
- **Restrictive cardiomyopathy** is rare and occurs due to some type of infiltrative process that results in decreased elasticity of the ventricles which causes diastolic dysfunction and heart failure. It can be idiopathic or due to conditions that result in endomyocardial fibrosis, such as sarcoidosis or amyloidosis.

Dilated Cardiomyopathy

Dilated cardiomyopathy will cause patients to feel short of breath, especially on exertion, and orthopnea and paroxysmal nocturnal dyspnea (PND) may be present, resulting in complaints of **fatigue**. Patients may also report edema and weight gain, especially around the abdomen. As the ejection fraction decreases, symptoms of CHF may present, such as rales, edema, S_3 gallop, and an increase in jugular venous distention (JVD). An echocardiogram will assess valvular function, flow, chamber sizes, and estimate the ejection fraction (EF). A cardiac catheterization can be done to determine the extent of CAD present and also ejection fraction. A myocardial biopsy may be done during a cardiac cath if an autoimmune or infiltrative process is suspected. Cardiac MRIs are increasingly being used in diagnosis. An ECG may show non-specific ST-T wave changes with left ventricular hypertrophy and possible conduction abnormalities. A chest x-ray may show cardiomegaly, pulmonary venous congestion, interstitial pulmonary edema (Kerley B lines), and pleural effusions. Lab work includes CBC, comprehensive metabolic panel, B-type natriuretic peptide assay (indicates fluid overload), cardiac biomarkers, and thyroid function tests. Finally, a urine or serum drug screen to identify presence of alcohol/illicit drug use. *Treatment* is aimed at reducing preload and afterload, diuresis, and airway support. ACE inhibitors are primarily used, but others include β-blockers, angiotensin II receptor blockers (ARBs), aldosterone antagonists, etc. to slow LV enlargement. Idiopathic dilated cardiomyopathy is highly familial, so when a new diagnosis is made, genetic screening should be done.

Hypertrophic Cardiomyopathy

Hypertrophic cardiomyopathy may not give any warning signs to patients and is frequently the cause of **sudden cardiac arrest** in the young athlete. If symptomatic, patients commonly complain of dyspnea on exertion (most common), episodes of syncope, angina, palpitations, or fatigue. A systolic crescendo-decrescendo murmur and S_4 can be heard with hypertrophic cardiomyopathy, but unlike the other types of cardiomyopathies, the intensity of the murmur will increase when patients are standing or performing the Valsalva maneuver, especially noted if it is obstructive. Also, a double carotid pulse and a jugular venous pulse with a prominent a wave may be noted. A 2-D echocardiogram is diagnostic and assesses diastolic function, valvular function, and EF. ECG changes seen with hypertrophic cardiomyopathy include ST-T wave changes, left ventricular hypertrophy, and deep Q waves. *Treatment* focuses on improving diastolic dysfunction by slowing the heart rate and decreasing the contractility of the heart, maintaining euvolemia, and controlling any arrhythmias. β-blockers and calcium channel blockers (verapamil) are used. Drugs that decrease preload should be avoided, e.g., ACE inhibitors, angiotensin II receptor blockers, nitrates. Also, because hypertrophic cardiomyopathy is primarily a genetic condition, patients' families should undergo a thorough cardiac evaluation. *Complications* include left ventricular outflow tract obstruction, CHF, endocarditis, thrombus, and sudden death.

Restrictive Cardiomyopathy

Restrictive cardiomyopathy is the rarest **cardiomyopathy** and marked by **diastolic dysfunction** due to noncompliant ventricular walls that resist diastolic filling which leads to pulmonary venous hypertension. It must be distinguished from constrictive pericarditis which has a similar clinical presentation. It may cause dyspnea on exertion, fatigue, orthopnea, paroxysmal nocturnal dyspnea, as well as peripheral edema and an increase in jugular venous distention. A heart murmur (AV valve regurgitation) may be auscultated, and patients may have chronic atrial fibrillation. This is a *diagnosis* of exclusion, as this physiology can be seen in many other disorders. Echo may show bilateral atrial enlargement and a restrictive pattern of filling. Though this can be idiopathic in etiology, a myocardial biopsy can be done to determine if an infiltrative process (sarcoidosis or amyloidosis) is present. Cardiac MRI is helpful in detecting pericardial thickening. *Treatment* is aimed at treating the underlying cause and symptoms, decreasing end-diastolic pressure, and correcting any arrhythmias. *Complications* include systemic emboli and a progressive decrease in cardiac function. Symptomatic restrictive cardiomyopathy has a poor prognosis.

Dysrhythmias

Atrial Fibrillation

Atrial fibrillation (**AFib**), also known as "holiday heart," is the most common **tachyarrhythmia** and results in an **irregularly irregular rhythm with no visible P waves on ECG**. The QRS complex is usually narrow, ≤0.12 seconds. The AHA classifies AFib as paroxysmal (terminates spontaneously or with intervention within 7 days of onset), persistent (does not terminate within 7 days), long-standing persistent (occurring >12 mo.), permanent, or nonvalvular (AFib without: rheumatic mitral stenosis, heart valve, or mitral valve repair). Common complaints include weakness, dizziness, dyspnea, and palpitations. However, some patients are asymptomatic. *Diagnosis* is confirmed through ECG. Assess causes (e.g., alcohol use or withdrawal), associated diseases, and perform a complete CV evaluation. Check TSH and T4. *Treatment* focuses on rate control, anticoagulation, and rhythm control (if AFib symptoms limit the patient). For rate control diltiazem, verapamil or β-blockers can be used. Digoxin may be used in patients with AFib due to HF, but is contraindicated in patients with preexcitation syndrome. Anticoagulation is based on stroke risk and includes aspirin, warfarin, heparin, and newer anticoagulants (dabigatran, rivaroxaban, etc.). Rhythm control options include cardioversion and ablation. Cardioversion is most effective when started within 48 hours of the onset of AFib. Cardioversion can be performed either chemically (ibutilide, dofetilide, flecainide, propafenone, or amiodarone) or electrically. For new onset AFib, effectively anticoagulate [>3 weeks with warfarin (INR of 2-3) or a new agent, or use a heparin bridge for a TEE cardioversion] and perform a TEE to assess for atrial thrombus before electrical cardioversion is performed. Continue anticoagulation for 4 weeks post-procedure. If >150 bpm and patients are unstable, immediate synchronized cardioversion should be done to normalize the rate. *Complications* include reduced cardiac output, thrombus formation, CVA, and heart failure.

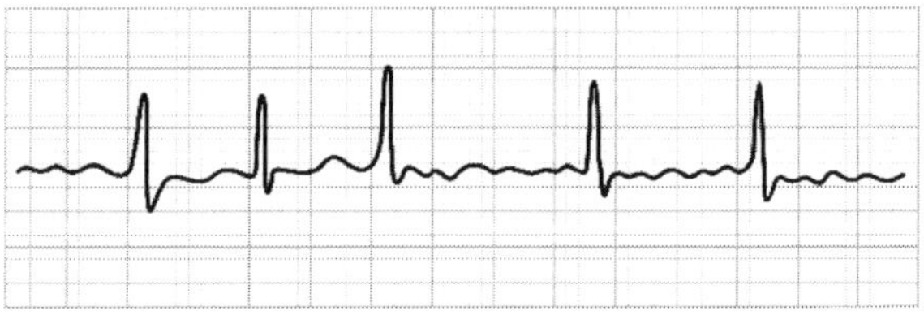

ATRIAL FLUTTER

Atrial flutter, the second most common **tachyarrhythmia**, results in a **regular rhythm on ECG** with an atrial rate between **240-360 bpm**. The P waves will follow a "sawtooth" pattern (most obvious in leads II, III, and aVF) two or more times followed by a narrow QRS. This is a macro reentrant arrhythmia with the reentry point just above the AV node. Commonly occurs when the atrial focus is irritated (e.g., atrial enlargement), resulting in multiple firings. The AV node will block some of these impulses from being sent to the ventricles which can cause an abnormal ventricular rhythm. Signs and *symptoms* include palpitations, fatigue, and presyncope. The heart rate is typically about 150 bpm due to the AV node block. *Diagnose* with ECG, and vagal maneuvers or adenosine may help unmask atrial flutter waves if not visualized clearly on ECG. Evaluate with a TTE. If the patient is unstable, the initial treatment of choice is immediate synchronized cardioversion. IV amiodarone is another option. If stable, the acute patient should undergo synchronized cardioversion or use oral dofetilide, IV ibutilide, and/or rapid atrial pacing for rhythm control or use IV β-blockers, IV diltiazem, or IV verapamil for rate control. Amiodarone may also be considered. In patients with ongoing atrial flutter, radiofrequency catheter ablation is the treatment of choice for rhythm control or may use β-blockers, diltiazem, or verapamil for rate control. For patients with >48 hours (or unknown length) of atrial flutter, check TEE for thrombus and give anticoagulation before and for a minimum of 4 weeks after cardioversion. If recurrent or chronic atrial flutter, continued use of anticoagulants is necessary and based on current stroke risk guidelines. *Complications* include syncope, CHF, and embolism.

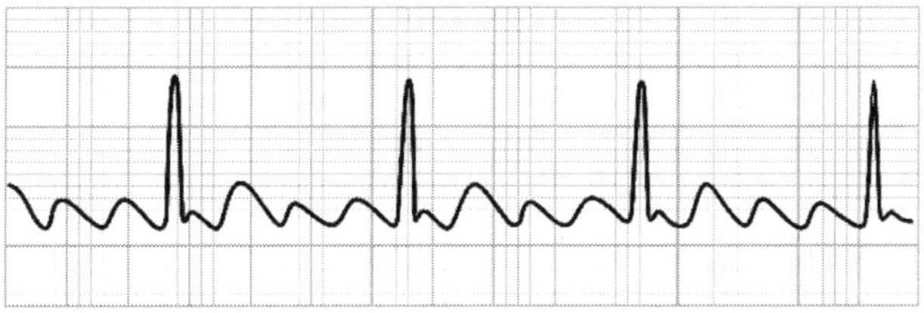

PREMATURE ATRIAL CONTRACTIONS

With a **premature atrial contraction** (**PAC**), also known as an **atrial premature beat (APB)**, there is an area within the atria that is irritated and is triggering delivery of sporadic impulses. This results in the atria contracting at a time out of sync with the regular rhythm of the atria. PACs are typically benign and found in both the young and elderly, and in those with and without heart disease. There are some known PAC *precipitants*—smoking, caffeine, stress, and alcohol. PACs are generally asymptomatic and not considered dangerous. Some patients may feel a palpitation or "skipped" beat. *Diagnosis* is made by ECG with an abnormally shaped P wave (but extra P waves may be hidden within the QRS complex or T waves) with a normal or narrow QRS. A Holter monitor may be worn to assess the frequency of PACs. *Treatment* is not required unless there is an underlying problem that needs to be managed (usually found in patients with frequent PACs). Avoid or minimize precipitants. If the patient has ongoing, symptomatic PACs, β-blockers can be used. Typically, there are no complications. However, PACs may trigger other dysrhythmias, especially AFib or atrial flutter.

Paroxysmal Supraventricular Tachycardia

Paroxysmal supraventricular tachycardia (PSVT) is an **elevated heart rate**, which begins and ends abruptly, that originates within the **atria** due to a reentry mechanism. The rate (usually >150 bpm and regular) is so fast that the underlying rhythm cannot be diagnosed. PSVTs can be seen in healthy patients or those with underlying heart or lung disease, as well as in digoxin toxicity and alcohol intoxication. *Signs and symptoms* vary depending on rate, but can include dizziness, syncope, shortness of breath, diaphoresis, chest pain, and palpitations. *Diagnose* clinically and on ECG. P waves are usually not present, or they are buried behind the QRS complex. The PR interval cannot be determined because of the absence of P wave, and QRS complex is usually very narrow. Screen for Wolff-Parkinson-White syndrome (due to increased risk of sudden death). If patients have a heart rate >150 and are clinically stable, vagal maneuvers may help convert the rate to a sinus rhythm. If this does not work, the next step for acute cases with a narrow QRS complex, IV adenosine should be given, or alternatively, IV verapamil or IV diltiazem. Avoid these AV node blockers if QRS is wide. Instead use synchronized cardioversion, procainamide, or amiodarone. If a patient has a HR of >150 bpm and is unstable, immediate electrical synchronized cardioversion is necessary to attempt to return to sinus rhythm. Long-term care options include radiofrequency ablation (first line) or calcium channel blockers, β-blockers, or digoxin. *Complications* are rare, but may include MI, CHF, and cardiac arrest.

Sick Sinus Syndrome

Sick sinus syndrome or sinus node dysfunction is a group of arrhythmias where the **sinoatrial (SA) node** doesn't function properly causing **bradycardia**; this is most common in patients >50 years old and tends to be progressive. It is represented by a pattern of irregular sinus bradycardia with possible long pauses (sinus pause; temporary disappearance of P waves) in conduction. There can even be sinus arrest (failure to generate an electrical impulse). There may also be an accelerated atrial rate or a pattern of bradycardia–tachycardia as the heart tries to correct its rhythm. Patients are often asymptomatic early on and there are often no clear symptoms, but vague complaints that could mimic other disorders. *Signs and symptoms* include a feeling of fluttering or "wrongness" in the chest, dizziness, fatigue, presyncope, syncope, dyspnea on exertion, a change in mental status, and altered consciousness. *Diagnosis* is made by ECG (possibly with a Holter monitor). If the patient is asymptomatic no treatment is necessary. If possible, stop medications causing bradycardia. Permanent *treatment* is provided by an internal pacemaker, and the associated surgical risks should be discussed with the patient. *Complications* of sinus node dysfunction include syncope, CHF, AFib or flutter, AV block, tachycardia-bradycardia syndrome, thrombi, emboli, stroke, and sudden death.

1st-Degree AV Block

First-degree AV block occurs when there is a delay in the transmission of the electrical impulse in the heart somewhere along the path from the SA node and through the AV node/His-Purkinje system. The most likely cause is a problem in the AV node itself, and incidence increases with age. This can also be caused by drugs (e.g., β-blockers, amiodarone, calcium channel blockers, digoxin) or can be found in well-trained athletes or those with increased vagal tone. 1st-degree AV block typically does not cause symptoms in patients. *Diagnosis* is made by ECG. Usually no change in the heart rate, but the ECG will exhibit a lengthened **PR interval** of >0.2 seconds. There are regular P waves followed by a QRS complex (all P waves conduct to the ventricles, therefore there are no missed beats). The rest of the ECG should be normal. No *treatment* is necessary. If patients have an underlying condition that could be contributing to the 1st-degree AV block, such as hypoxia, MI,

Lyme disease, collagen vascular disease, or dehydration, then treat those conditions appropriately. There are usually no *complications* from 1st degree AV block, but a few patients will progress to 2nd degree AV block.

2ND-DEGREE AV BLOCK

In **second-degree AV block,** not all atrial beats are conducted to the ventricles. This can be categorized as **Mobitz type I** or **Mobitz type II**. It may occur after a MI and can be transient and asymptomatic or due to digoxin, β-blockers, or calcium channel blockers. It must be determined if a 2:1 AV block is type I or type II as treatment varies.

- **Type I 2nd-degree AV block** occurs when the time it takes for the electrical impulse to travel from the SA node to the AV node increases in length until a **ventricular beat** is finally skipped. On the ECG, this will look like a gradually increasing PR interval until a QRS is dropped. If it results in symptomatic bradycardia, it can be *treated* with atropine and transcutaneous pacing can help normalize the rate. Further workup will determine if additional intervention is necessary.
- **Type II 2nd-degree AV block** occurs when the electrical impulse signal travels from the SA node to the AV node, but the signal does not always continue onto the ventricles to cause a **contraction**. On ECG, this results in a normal PR interval and a QRS that is usually dropped in the 3rd (3:1) or 4th (4:1) cycle. These patients are more likely to experience symptoms of dizziness, light-headedness, or syncope. This is *treated* with pacing, and transcutaneous pacing is necessary even in asymptomatic patients. Reversible causes should be investigated, and if none are found, patients should get a permanent pacemaker, as they have a high likelihood of progressing to complete heart block.

3RD-DEGREE AV BLOCK

Third degree AV block is considered **complete heart block**. The SA node continues to send its electrical impulse to the AV node, but the AV node is not transmitting this signal on to the ventricles. The ventricles are contracting, but this contraction is due to stimulation of the ventricular fibers, so the heart rate is usually decreased to <40 bpm. Some *causes* include idiopathic conduction disease, drugs that depress AV conduction, increased vagal tone and myocardial infarction. Myocardial infarction, resulting in cardiac hypoxia, can cause a disruption in the electrical system of the heart by damaging the AV node so the impulse cannot be transmitted from the SA node to the ventricles. *Signs and symptoms* include dizziness, angina, syncope, and exacerbation of HF symptoms. *Diagnosed* by ECG, this results in regularly-occurring P waves and regularly-occurring QRS complexes that are completely independently of each other. The atrial rate is normal at 60-100 bpm, but the ventricular rate will be bradycardic. The QRS complexes may appear wide indicating an infranodal block with escape rhythms coming from the His/or both bundle branches usually resulting in a hemodynamically unstable patient who doesn't respond to atropine. *Treatment* of this condition requires transcutaneous pacing until permanent pacing can be established. Patients should be closely monitored for a change in symptoms. *Complications* include asystole, VFib/V-tach, and death.

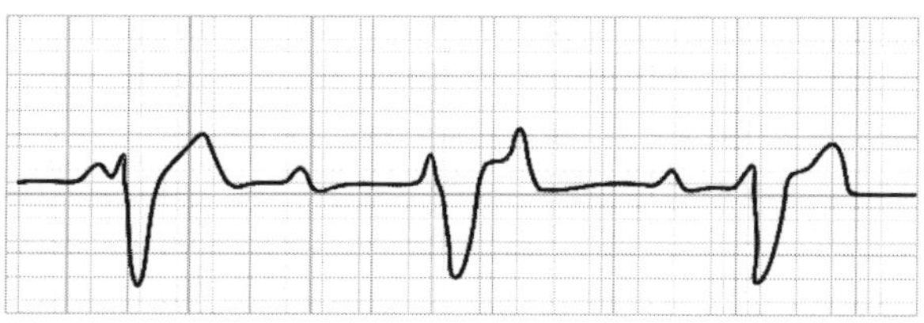

Bundle Branch Block

A **bundle branch block** (**BBB**) can occur within the left or right ventricle. It is usually due to an area of **muscle damage**. As the electrical impulse travels from the atria to the ventricles, the undamaged ventricle will transmit the signal normally. The damaged ventricle, however, will be delayed in transmitting the signal and this will result in **two QRS complexes** on ECG. Patients are most often asymptomatic and will have a normal heart rate and rhythm. The patient presenting with new onset BBB should have a complete cardiac workup. A quick way to *diagnose* a patient with a bundle branch block is to look at the V1, V2, V5, and V6 leads. With a RBBB (right BBB), the V1 and V2 leads will exhibit an abnormal, wide QRS complex with a "rabbit ears" appearance with an upward deflection of the QRS complex in V1. With a LBBB (left BBB), leads V5 and V6 will exhibit a widened QRS complex with a notched appearance with a downward deflected QRS in V1. Ventricular rhythms, Brugada syndrome (a genetic disease with increased risk of sudden cardiac death), and ventricular pacing should be ruled out. It is important to remember, that a patient with clinical symptoms representing an acute MI cannot be diagnosed with an MI by ECG alone if a LBBB is present. Sgarbossa criteria as well as other diagnostic labs will helpful in this situation. Typically, BBB does not require *treatment*. However, a pacemaker would be indicated with syncope (more often seen in LBBB). Prognosis of BBB is tied to underlying heart disease (e.g., a RBBB associated with a MI is associated with increased mortality).

Premature Ventricular Contractions

Premature ventricular contractions (PVCs) occur when there is an area of irritability within a ventricle, causing it to **contract early**. The cause of PVCs is often unknown, but can be due to electrolyte imbalance, medications (e.g., digitalis), alcohol/drugs, adrenaline (caffeine, anxiety, etc.), or myocardial injury (ischemia, acute MI). Most patients are asymptomatic, but some experience palpitations. The heart rate can vary and will depend upon the underlying rhythm. PVCs generally cause an irregular heart rate, but there can be regularity if bigeminy is present (occurs when a PVC is present after every regular ventricular beat). Trigeminy occurs when a PVC occurs during every third ventricular beat. On ECG, P waves are not present before a widened and unusually long QRS, usually followed by a fully compensatory pause. A pattern of bigeminy or trigeminy may be present. Check electrolytes and perform a cardiac workup if indicated. *Treat* the underlying cause, if it can be identified (e.g., oxygen if hypoxia is present). Often no treatment is necessary. β-blockers suppress PVCs in patients with ischemia and excess catecholamines. Antiarrhythmic medications (Lidocaine, amiodarone, etc.) may be necessary if the PVCs are complex and patient is symptomatic, especially in the setting of an MI. It is important to consider amiodarone in the peri-MI period to reduce the risk of ventricular tachycardia or ventricular fibrillation. *Complications* include increased risk of other arrhythmias and cardiomyopathy.

Ventricular Tachycardia

Ventricular tachycardia is a fast (>100 bpm) but regular rhythm with ≥3 **irregular beats** in a row that occurs when the ventricles repeatedly contract without coordinated atrial contractions. It can be **sustained** (>30 secs.) or **non-sustained** (<30 secs.) This can be a deadly arrhythmia and is considered a cardiac emergency. *Signs and symptoms* include syncope, palpitations, chest pain, SOB, anxiety, and dizziness. The rate is usually regular at around 150 up to 250 bpm. *Diagnosis* is on ECG with widened QRS complexes and typically no P waves are present. If the patient is unconscious or unstable, diagnosis is only made by physical findings and rhythm strip. If the patient does not have a pulse, ACLS protocol should be started, making sure to defibrillate the patient as quickly as possible. If the patient does have a pulse, assess if the patient is otherwise hemodynamically stable or unstable. If stable, antiarrhythmics, such as amiodarone, sotalol, or procainamide should be given to convert to sinus rhythm. If the patient is unstable, cardioversion is indicated (sedate if able). If the patient loses their pulse, defibrillation is indicated. In patients with monomorphic V-tach, with structurally normal hearts, catheter ablation or medication is the usual management. In patients with more complicated issues, an ICD should be placed, especially if there is a history of heart disease, to decrease risk of SCD. Correct electrolyte disturbances. *Complications* include sudden death.

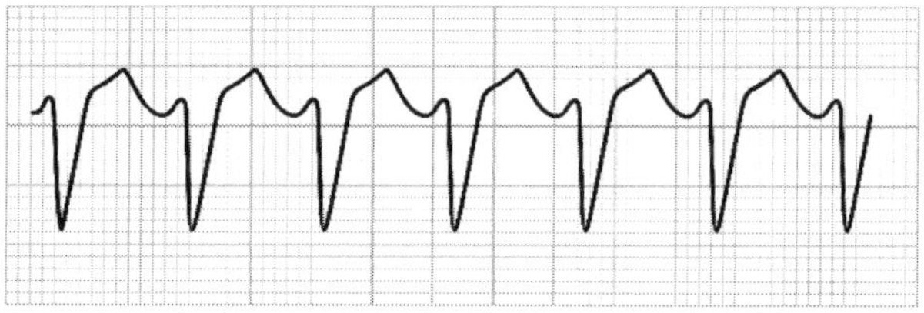

Ventricular Flutter and Torsades De Pointes

Three **types of ventricular tachycardia** include ventricular flutter, torsades de pointes, and repetitive monomorphic ventricular tachycardia. **Ventricular flutter** is a type of **rapid monomorphic ventricular tachycardia** that can degenerate into ventricular fibrillation. The rate is often about 300 bpm. The ventricles will spasm without any discernible pattern of organized activity. On ECG, there will be a monomorphic sine wave that looks the same even when the ECG is turned upside down. Ventricular flutter can resemble artifact, so the leads must be placed correctly on patients, and patient pulse checked. A magnesium or potassium deficiency can cause a form of polymorphic ventricular tachycardia called **torsades de pointes**. It is associated with a congenital or acquired (medication/electrolyte disturbance) prolonged QT interval. The name means "twisting of points" because of the changing axis of this rhythm. This rhythm will appear as a series of **widened QRS complexes** that vary in height in a wave pattern. This can also degenerate into ventricular fibrillation. Magnesium sulfate (usually 1-2 gm over 1-2 mins.) should be given. **Repetitive monomorphic ventricular tachycardia** is a recurring, monomorphic tachycardia. It is the most common type of idiopathic V tach. It occurs in those without cardiac structural disease. On ECG, it may appear as prolific ventricular ectopy or alternating nonsustained V tach with sinus rhythm.

Ventricular Fibrillation

Ventricular fibrillation (**VF**) occurs when the ventricles are in a state of uncontrolled **spasm** (quivering) without being able to complete a forceful contraction. This causes cardiac arrest and is a true emergency with death occurring within minutes of the arrhythmia. On ECG, the heart rate will not be able to be determined because of the irregularity. There are no discernible P waves, QRS complexes, or T waves. The rhythm can appear to be coarse or fine. VF can resemble artifact so the leads must be placed correctly on patients, and pulse checked. ACLS protocol should be followed for treatment of VF, including, high quality CPR, immediate defibrillation, epinephrine 1 mg every 3-5 minutes, amiodarone 300 mg bolus and possible 150 mg second dose. Patients should be well oxygenated and intubated if necessary. Look for *causes*, such as the 5 H's & 5 T's: Hypovolemia, Hypoxia, Hydrogen ions (acidosis), Hypo/Hyperkalemia, Hypothermia, Tension pneumo, Tamponade, Toxins, Thrombosis (cardiac), Thrombosis (pulmonary). Prognosis is often related to time of onset of VF and medical treatment. Anoxic encephalopathy and death may follow, even after initial successful resuscitation.

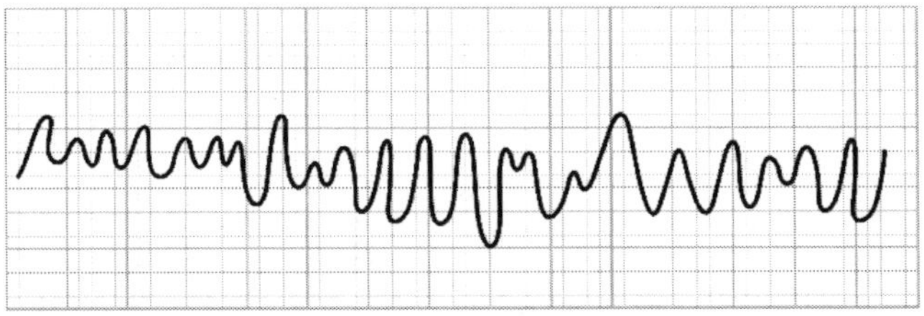

Symptomatic Bradycardia

Bradycardia (<60 bpm) may be benign in some patients but needs immediate intervention if the patient has serious symptoms related to the slow heart rate (after other causes are ruled out). Causes include sick sinus syndrome, myocarditis, hypothyroidism, electrolyte imbalance, congenital heart defect, heart damage, hypoglycemia, sleep apnea, hypothermia, and medications (such as beta blockers). Symptoms may include hypotension, pulmonary edema, chest pain, dyspnea, heart failure, fatigue, weakness, dizziness, altered mental status, and shock. The patient's perfusion should be assessed and, if adequate, the patient can be monitored, but if perfusion is inadequate, immediate interventions are needed, according to ACLS guidelines:

- Begin transcutaneous pacing if IV access is not yet available.
- If IV access available, begin with atropine 0.5 mg, repeated every 3-5 minutes to maximum 3 mg/6 doses while preparing for pacing.
- If bradycardia does not convert with atropine, begin transcutaneous pacing.
- If transcutaneous pacing is not effective (or while awaiting pacing instead of atropine in some cases), administer epinephrine 2-10 mcg/min or dopamine 2-20 mcg/kg/min.

Interventions should be carried out in rapid succession to prevent cardiac arrest.

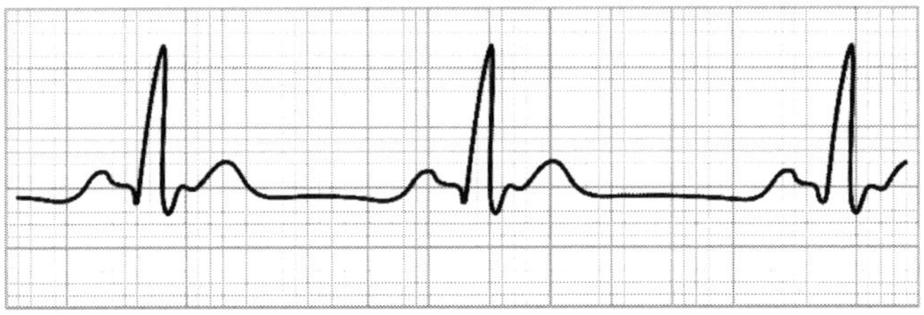

Congestive Heart Failure

Congestive heart failure (CHF) is defined as a condition in which the heart is unable to pump sufficient blood in order to meet the needs of all the body organs. Congestive heart failure is a common disorder that affects an estimated five million people in the United States. The prevalence is highest in older individuals. Causes of CHF include previous heart attack, hypertension, coronary artery disease, cardiomyopathy, congenital heart defects, valvular disease, cardiotoxic drugs, myocarditis, and endocarditis. The four stages of CHF include:

- **Stage A** – Individuals at risk for developing CHF.
- **Stage B** – Structural heart disease present without symptoms.
- **Stage C** – Structural heart disease present with symptoms.
- **Stage D** – Advanced symptoms often not responsive to medical treatment.

Heart Failure

Heart Failure with Preserved Ejection Fraction

Heart failure with preserved ejection fraction (HFpEF) is characterized by stiffening of the ventricular tissue with or without enlargement, resulting in a heart that is unable to fill normally. Filling of the left ventricle depends on increased pressure in the left atrium because the stiffness of the LV prevents the normal passive filling. Most patients have systemic hypertension and pulmonary hypertension, which leads to increased RV afterload and dysfunction, often resulting in atrial fibrillation. Systolic function is usually preserved although some abnormalities may be present, exacerbated by exercise. Typical symptoms include dyspnea on exertion and when lying flat, peripheral edema, and fatigue. Ejection fraction is preserved to at least 50%, but filling pressures are elevated at rest. Diagnosis include echocardiogram showing diastolic dysfunction and elevated brain natriuretic peptide (BNP) level Some patients may exhibit hemodynamic compromise only during exercise. Risk factors include hypertension, diabetes, coronary artery disease, CKD, COPD, OBA, obesity, anemia, and anemia. Treatment recommendations are not clear but usually begin with controlling hypertension and relieving symptoms, such as through diuretics.

Congestive Heart Failure

Clinical symptoms consistent with a CHF diagnosis include shortness of breath at rest or with exertion, chronic fatigue, and edema. Physical exam findings may show crackles present in the lungs, dependent edema, and elevated jugular venous pressure (JVP). Cardiac exam may be significant for the presence of an S3. Further work up should include chest x-ray, EKG, and echocardiogram. Chest x-ray may show evidence of an enlarged heart. Echocardiogram may show a decreased ejection fraction. Useful laboratory tests include the brain natriuretic peptide (BNP) test. Natriuretic peptide is a protein released by myocardial cells in response to stretch. It is a useful marker for the presence of CHF. Other laboratory exams that should be obtained include: CBC, electrolytes, BUN/creatinine, fasting glucose, LFTs, and thyroid function tests.

Heart Murmur

Heart murmurs are commonly heard in children during routine physical exams and many are innocent or functional murmurs. Signs that a murmur may be pathologic include the presence of cyanosis, shortness of breath, failure to thrive, chest pain, and edema. When a heart murmur is evaluated, it should be described by location, intensity, radiation, timing during the cardiac cycle, quality, and any variation with change of position of the patient. Murmurs that are grade III or louder, or occur during diastole, are more likely to be pathologic. Patients with suspicious murmurs should have an EKG, chest x-ray, and echocardiogram. All patients with pathologic murmurs should be referred to a cardiologist.

Congenital Disorders

Coarctation of the Aorta

Coarctation of the aorta is a non-cyanotic, congenital heart defect (which may present later in life) in which there is **narrowing of the aorta** usually distal to the left subclavian artery. This results in the development of **collateral circulation** through the intercostal arteries and the branches of the subclavian artery. It is most common in male children and is often associated with Turner's syndrome in females. Clinically, the patient may exhibit hypertension with blood pressure and pulse discrepancies between the upper and lower extremities. Symptoms of congestive heart failure may be present along with weak or absent femoral pulses. A systolic murmur will be heard predominantly over the back. Coarctation of the aorta is *diagnosed* using a chest x-ray and ECG. X-ray shows a "3" sign in the left upper mediastinal shadow and also rib notching will be evident due to the development of collateral vessels trying to pass over the coarctation. An ECG usually shows right ventricular hypertrophy in infants and left ventricular hypertrophy in adults. Echocardiogram may also be done; and helps measure peak pressure gradients. Diagnosis can be confirmed using a cardiac catheterization/angiogram. *Treat* symptomatic neonates with prostaglandin E1 to open the ductus arteriosus. Treatments include balloon angioplasty and possible stent placement to widen the aorta, resection, left subclavian flap aortoplasty, or patch aortoplasty. Post-op endocarditis prophylaxis treatment is required 6 months after the repair. Lifelong follow-up is necessary. *Complications* include hypertension, CHF, stroke, aortic dissection/rupture, cerebral aneurysm, coronary artery disease, and organ failure.

Atrial Septal Defect

An **atrial septal defect** (**ASD**) is a non-cyanotic, congenital heart defect in which there is an **opening between the left and right atrium** causing a left-to-right shunt. This can result in failure to thrive in the infant, but it is often not diagnosed until adulthood due to minimal symptoms that can be present in the first few decades of life. Although typically asymptomatic, the infant may exhibit dyspnea and excessive fatigue. On exam, a systolic murmur and a widely split and fixed S_2 will be heard. An atrial septal defect is *diagnosed* initially through a combination of exam findings, ECG changes, and chest x-ray. ECG findings may include right or left-axis deviation (depending on the position of the defect), an rSR' pattern in V1, or a right bundle branch block. An echocardiogram and an angiogram can be done to confirm the diagnosis. This is not diagnosed in utero because of the presence of the patent foramen ovale. It is usually detected within a couple of days of birth if the defect is large or in the 2nd-3rd decade of life. *Treatment* includes observation or closure if the defect is significant. Repair using cardiac catheterization techniques to patch the defect is preferred when possible or through surgical repair. Post-op endocarditis prophylaxis treatment is required 6 months after the repair. A small ASD, especially if central, may close during childhood and never cause an issue. *Complications* are often related to the size and can include heart failure, arrhythmias, stroke, and pulmonary hypertension.

Ventricular Septal Defect

A **ventricular septal defect** (**VSD**) is a non-cyanotic, congenital heart defect in which there is an **opening between the left and right ventricles**. This condition can be associated with Eisenmenger's syndrome (a VSD with cyanosis and pulmonary hypertension). Clinically, the infant may exhibit signs of pulmonary hypertension and congestive heart failure. Very rapid respirations may be present with sweating and pallor. The infant may have great difficulty eating because of the difficulty breathing, resulting in failure to thrive. On exam, a harsh, holosystolic murmur (with or without a thrill) can be heard at the LLSB. A VSD is suggested with exam findings and chest x-ray, but *diagnosed* with an echocardiogram. An ECG usually shows left ventricular hypertrophy, but if the defect is large, may show combined ventricular hypertrophy or right ventricular hypertrophy. Small VSDs may not need treatment. *Treat* heart failure with diuretics, digoxin, and ACE inhibitors. Closure of the ventricular septal defect can be attempted using cardiac catheterization techniques, but open surgery may be necessary or preferred. Post-op endocarditis prophylaxis treatment is required 6 months after the repair. *Complications* include arrhythmias, endocarditis, pulmonary hypertension.

Patent Ductus Arteriosus

Patent ductus arteriosus (**PDA**) is a non-cyanotic, congenital heart defect in which the **ductus arteriosus** fails to close after birth, causing a left-to-right shunt. The ductus arteriosus is an opening, present in utero, that serves as a shunt between the left pulmonary artery and the aorta. After birth, it normally closes within 10-18 hours of life. However, this opening can fail to close due to a rubella infection while in utero or other causes (e.g., prematurity, maternal phenytoin or amphetamine use). If the PDA closes spontaneously after this time, it typically occurs by 3 months of age. Clinically, the infant may be asymptomatic or exhibit pulmonary hypertension, difficulty feeding, and a failure to thrive. On exam, there will be a continuous machinery murmur heard at the LUSB. The apical impulse is displaced laterally, a thrill may be palpated, and a widened pulse pressure may also be present. PDA is *diagnosed* through a combination of exam findings, ECG, and chest x-ray, but is confirmed by echocardiogram. Closure of the PDA may be achieved using IV COX inhibitors (indomethacin) or IV ibuprofen. Other options include less invasive cardiac catheterization techniques or surgery may be necessary. *Complications* include pulmonary hypertension, heart failure, and endocarditis.

TETRALOGY OF FALLOT

Tetralogy of Fallot (**TOF**) is a cyanotic, congenital heart defect that comprises four conditions: a ventricular septal defect, right ventricular hypertrophy, right ventricular outflow obstruction (pulmonary stenosis), and overriding of the aorta. This is the most common **cyanotic infant heart disease**. Genetic factors, maternal rubella/other viruses, and some medications that are associated with the development of this condition. Clinically, the infant will be cyanotic with dyspnea, poor feeding/poor weight gain, and eventually clubbing. "Tet" spells, or severe cyanotic spells, may occur when feeding or crying. A holosystolic murmur can be heard on exam as well as a prominent right ventricular impulse and thrill noted at the LSB. TOF can be *diagnosed* using PE findings, CXR, ECG, and echocardiogram. A CBC will show polycythemia (elevated RBCs, elevated Hgb/Hct). Surgery is necessary, and usually done in the first year of life. Patients will always require endocarditis prophylaxis before all dental procedures and other invasive procedures throughout their lifetimes. *Complications* include endocarditis, emboli, and CHF. If untreated, this defect leads to disability and death by adulthood.

Hypertension

STANDARD CLASSIFICATIONS

Standard **classifications of hypertension** in adults, according to JNC 7 and based on 2 or more readings are below. (The more recently updated JNC 8 does not explicitly outline these ranges, therefore the JNC 7 ranges are listed.)

Classification	Systolic BP mm Hg	Diastolic BP mm Hgb
Normal	<120	And <80
Pre-hypertension	120 – 139	Or 80 – 89
Stage 1 hypertension	140-159	Or 90 – 99
Stage 2 hypertension	≥160	Or ≥100

* Guidelines from American College of Cardiology and American Heart Association in 2017 lower these:

Normal = <120/80; **Elevated** = 120-129 AND <80; **Stage 1** = 130-139 OR 80-89; **Stage 2** = ≥140 OR ≥90.

Hypertensive crises = BP >180/120

1. **Hypertensive urgency**: severe hypertension without target-organ damage found.
2. **Hypertensive emergency**: severe hypertension with acute target-organ damage.

Severe hypertensive retinopathy (malignant hypertension) is severe hypertension with papilledema and flame-shaped retinal hemorrhages and exudates. Hypertensive encephalopathy may be present as well.

Primary, Secondary, and Malignant Hypertension

Primary (essential) hypertension is the most common form of hypertension accounting for 90-95% of cases. The cause of this type of hypertension is unknown, but genetic and environmental factors play a role. Most patients are also unaware that they are suffering from this type of hypertension. It is diagnosed after patients have three separate episodes of blood pressure 140/90 or higher, not found to be due to some type of medical condition.

Secondary hypertension only affects about 2-10% of the population of patients who have been diagnosed with hypertension. It is due to another medical condition, such as renal disease (most common), renal artery stenosis, primary aldosteronism, or pheochromocytoma.

Malignant hypertension (hypertensive emergencies) is uncontrolled severe hypertension that causes end-organ damage and can be life-threatening. It can be due to secondary causes (e.g., renal artery stenosis, abrupt clonidine withdrawal) or the cause may be unknown. The goal is to provide immediate treatment by decreasing the mean arterial BP slowly, no more than 15-25% over the first minutes to 1-2 hours, and further titration based on symptoms. After the patient is stabilized, gradually reduce BP over 24-48 hours. Nitroprusside, clevidipine, nicardipine, labetalol, and fenoldopam are the most common IV medications used to initially treat this condition.

Treatment Options

Beta-Blockers

Beta-blockers (β-blockers) help to lower blood pressure by decreasing the heart rate and the force that is exerted by the ventricles with each heartbeat. Beta-blockers work on **beta-receptors**, though not all beta-blockers are created to work just on cardiac beta-receptors. Some of these medications, especially the older medications, work on all the beta-receptors in the body. Beta-blockers are now thought to be helpful in patients with known CAD, those who have had an MI, and those patients with known CHF. Although β-blockers are a routine part of therapy for those with heart failure, in patients with acute decompensated heart failure, they may exacerbate acute heart failure symptoms. Because β-blockers reduce the heart rate, there is a risk that they can cause the bradycardia and hypotension. This can result in dizziness, confusion, and possibly even syncope. The most commonly reported side effects of β-blockers are sexual dysfunction, depression, and fatigue. β-blockers are associated with increased airway resistance in patients that already have lung disease. β-blockers are *contraindicated* in those with 2nd and 3rd degree AV block, symptomatic bradycardia associated with sick sinus syndrome, asthma, and severe COPD. Sudden withdrawal from β-blockers can cause ischemic symptoms, especially those with coronary artery disease. Therefore, slowly reduce over several weeks. Some examples of β-blockers include metoprolol (Lopressor®), atenolol (Tenormin®), carvedilol (Coreg®), and acebutolol (Sectral®).

ACE Inhibitors

ACE inhibitors work on the **arteries** to cause dilation, which decreases the total peripheral vascular resistance (resistance of blood flow thorough the systemic blood vessels) and leads to a decrease in blood pressure. They work through inhibiting the **renin-angiotensin-aldosterone system**. Their effects help decrease morbidity and mortality in patients with heart failure, recent MI, renal disease, and proteinuria. Their anti-hypertensive effects are additive when used with thiazide diuretics. ACE inhibitors are not used as first-line treatment in African patients due to a possible increase risk of stroke. Because ACE inhibitors cause arterial dilation, they can, in rare cases, cause angioedema resulting in excessive dilation in the arteries of the lips, face, and larynx. Though rare, this type of allergic reaction is a medical emergency. A common potential *side effect* of ACE inhibitors is a chronic, nonproductive cough (5-20% of patients), which can be a reason for noncompliance in patients. Hypotension, pruritus, and rash are other related side effects. ACE inhibitors may cause the kidneys to decrease excretion of potassium, so patients should be monitored for hyperkalemia (especially patients taking K supplements or K-sparing diuretics). ACE inhibitors are *contraindicated* in pregnancy and patients with bilateral renal artery stenosis. Some examples of ACE inhibitors include captopril (Capoten®), enalapril (Vasotec®), and quinapril (Accupril®).

Angiotensin-Receptor Blockers

Angiotensin-receptor blockers (ARBs) work similarly to ACE inhibitors by working on the **renin-angiotensin system**. However, they block the effects of angiotensin II by binding to angiotensin type I receptors causing the arteries to dilate, which decreases the pressure within the arteries, and leads to a decrease in BP. Their effects also help patients with CHF by decreasing the risk of stroke and decreasing the risk of a future MI. ARBs are usually used when ACE inhibitors are not well tolerated. Both ARBs and ACE inhibitors are helpful in patients with DM (especially white, non-African patients), chronic kidney disease, and stroke. However, ACE inhibitors and ARBs should not be used in combination with each other. The reason that an ARB may be prescribed instead of an ACE inhibitor is due to a lower incidence of chronic cough and angioedema. Shared *side effects* between the two drugs include: hyperkalemia, renal dysfunction, and syncope due to hypotension. ARBs do have a higher rate of hypotensive symptoms than ACE inhibitors. They are *contraindicated* in pregnancy and in diabetic patients on aliskiren. Examples of ARBs include losartan (Cozaar®), telmisartan (Micardis®), and valsartan (Diovan®).

Diuretics

Diuretic classes include thiazide, potassium-sparing, and loop diuretics. **Thiazide diuretics** are used as first-line therapy in most patients and can be used alone or in combination (e.g., with a β-blocker or ACE inhibitor). Thiazides are particularly helpful in African patients with or without DM. **Potassium-sparing diuretics** work better in combination with other anti-hypertensive drugs. **Loop diuretics** can be used in patients with a decreased glomerular filtration rate or CHF. Diuretics work on the kidneys to increase the amount of water and sodium that are excreted from the body through the urine. This helps to reduce the actual fluid volume in the body, thus decreasing the amount of pressure within the arteries and resulting in a lowered blood pressure. Because diuretics work on the kidneys, they may not be appropriate for all patients, especially those with renal disease. Along with the water and sodium that is increasingly excreted from the body, potassium is also depleted with some of the diuretics. This can result in hypokalemia, so a potassium supplement is often prescribed along with the diuretic. Eating foods high in K^+ may also help patients prevent a decrease in potassium levels. An increase in urinary frequency is frequently seen, so patients should take diuretics in the morning to prevent having to get up frequently during the night. Examples of some diuretics include *Thiazide*: hydrochlorothiazide (HCTZ), chlorthalidone (Thalitone®); *Potassium-sparing*: spironolactone (Aldactone®), triamterene (Dyrenium®). *Loop-diuretics*: furosemide (Lasix®), and torsemide (Demadex®).

Calcium Channel Blockers Work to Control Hypertension

Calcium channel blockers are particularly helpful in African patients with or without DM. There are 2 categories of Ca^{++} channel blockers (CCBs): dihydropyridines and non-dihydropyridines. The **dihydropyridines** bind Ca^{++} channels in vascular smooth muscle to dilate the arteries, resulting in a decrease in BP. The **non-dihydropyridines** bind Ca^{++} channels in the SA and AV nodes and also have cardiac and some vascular effects, therefore decreasing the heart rate and the force of ventricular contractions. The newer CCBs, the dihydropyridines, only work to cause peripheral arterial dilation and may sometimes cause reflex tachycardia. They should be used cautiously in patients with CHF. The non-dihydropyridines, which cause a decrease in ventricular force, may worsen CHF and are *contraindicated* in severe LV dysfunction, moderate to severe CHF, and in patients with 2nd and 3rd degree heart block. Nifedipine is associated with an increase in mortality in the acute period after MI. Possible *side effects* while taking CCBs: headaches, flushing, dizziness, and edema. Constipation and gingival hyperplasia are specific adverse effects of the CCB verapamil. Dihydropyridines ("-pines") include amlodipine (Norvasc®), nifedipine (Procardia®), and felodipine (Plendil®). The non-dihydropyridines are diltiazem (Cardizem®) and verapamil (Calan®).

Orthostatic Hypotension

Orthostatic hypotension is a sudden drop in **blood pressure** that is symptomatic and affects approximately 20% of the elderly. It usually occurs when a patient stands up quickly or is rising from a lying to sitting or standing position. It is typically caused by autonomic dysfunction or hypovolemia. Medications are also a common cause of orthostatic hypotension, including antihypertensives, antidepressants (especially tricyclic), vasodilators (e.g., nitrates), and diuretics. Excessive alcohol use, prolonged bedrest, and adrenal insufficiency are other causes. Patients will describe a sudden dizziness or light-headed sensation, syncope, or near syncope when getting up too quickly. Other *symptoms* are leg buckling, blurry vision, confusion, and weakness/fatigue. Some patients may also experience these symptoms after eating. *Diagnosis* is based on a sustained >20 mmHg decrease in systolic pressure, a 10 mmHg decrease in diastolic pressure, or both that is noted within 3 minutes of standing after a 5-minute time of resting in the supine position. If there is not a corresponding increase in the heart rate, consider autonomic dysfunction. Whereas, a corresponding increase in heart rate by >30 bpm suggests hypovolemia or POTS (postural orthostatic tachycardia syndrome). *Treatment* includes discontinuing medications, if able, that could be responsible, correct hypovolemia, increase sodium intake, use elastic stockings, and exercise. Advise patients to rise slowly from a seated or lying position. If severe symptoms remain after nonpharmacologic intervention, consider fludrocortisone or midodrine. *Complications* include falls, strokes, and cardiovascular disease.

Vascular Disease

Peripheral Arterial Disease

Peripheral arterial disease (PAD) occurs when there is **obstruction or narrowing of an artery** that interferes with blood flow, typically in the lower extremities. This can be due to atherosclerosis, trauma, or inflammation. Patients will frequently complain of pain, achiness, or tiredness in their legs or calves after walking a short distance which is relieved with rest (intermittent claudication). Patients may also state they have burning, numbing, and tingling sensations in their extremities. Some male patients may complain about erectile dysfunction. Clinically, there may be obvious signs of obstructed blood flow, such as pallor, atrophic skin, and hair loss. Dependent rubor may be noted and pain may become worse when legs are elevated. Peripheral pulses may be decreased or absent if occlusion is present. In severe cases, arterial ulcers may be present with development of gangrene. An ankle-brachial index (ABI) of <0.9 (either a resting or exercise ABI) is used to *diagnose* PAD. Doppler ultrasound will identify decreased blood flow through the arteries. Angiography confirms the diagnosis and provides visualization of the narrowed vessels before surgery. Patients should also be assessed for CAD. *Treatment* includes risk factor modification (e.g., quitting smoking), exercise, cholesterol control medications, antihypertensives, antiplatelet medications, and blood glucose control. Cilostazol and pentoxifylline help treat symptoms of claudication. Endovascular therapy (e.g., stents, balloons) or open bypass surgery may be indicated. Critical limb ischemia is a possible *complication*, which can lead to infections/amputations.

ARTERIAL AND VENOUS THROMBOSIS AND EMBOLISM

An **arterial thrombosis** is a blood clot located within an **artery**. A **venous thrombosis** is a blood clot located within a **vein**. This is a stationary clot that can grow large enough to cause occlusion of the vessel. An **embolism** is the term used for the thrombus once it breaks free and begins moving through the **vascular system**. This embolism will eventually travel to an artery or vein that is too small to accommodate its size, resulting in an occlusion of the artery or vein with possible life-threatening results. *Treatment* is centered on prevention for high risk patients (e.g., arteriosclerosis, hypercoagulable state, immobility) such as risk modification, exercise, and wearing compression stockings (e.g., for venous insufficiency, varicose veins). Daily aspirin therapy (81 mg), or other anticoagulants, can provide antiplatelet activity that prevents platelets from forming a clot. Suspect a **deep venous thrombosis (DVT)** if patient presents with pain, swelling, redness in the calf with a positive Homans sign. Treat with heparin (LMWH, UFH, or fondaparinux) and oral warfarin to prevent a PE. Heparin can be D/C after therapeutic INR is reached for 24 hours (usually 4-5 days). If a thrombus does form and becomes an embolism, emergency treatment is necessary. For example, an arterial embolism can be fatal, but "clot buster" thrombolytic medications or even surgery to remove the clot may improve the patient's prognosis. Vena cava filters can be used in patients with a high risk for emboli. *Complications* depend on where the clot is located and include angina, MI, stroke, ischemia to limbs, pulmonary embolism, and postphlebitic syndrome.

PHLEBITIS AND THROMBOPHLEBITIS

Phlebitis is inflammation that is present in a vein and is usually superficial. It is gradual in onset and develops into a reddened, often streaky area that follows the path of a vein. It often occurs at an IV site and the area may be painful, swollen, indurated, and warm. If the phlebitis is superficial, warm compresses, elevation of the affected limb, and compression can help to resolve the problem. If recurrent phlebitis is occurring in the deeper vessels, an anticoagulant may be prescribed to prevent formation of a blood clot. **Thrombophlebitis** occurs when a **blood clot** forms within the inflamed vein. Patients complain of pain that may be gradual or sudden in onset, and the affected area may be red, swollen, or indurated. It is seen most often in more sedentary patients and in patients with a component of Virchow's triad (intimal injury, stasis or turbulent blood flow, and a hypercoagulable state). A hypercoagulable state may be seen with some malignancies. A superficial thrombophlebitis may extend and become a deep vein thrombosis (DVT). For both phlebitis and superficial thrombophlebitis, anticoagulants are typically not required and can be treated with NSAIDs, elevation, and hot/wet compresses. Compression stockings are particularly helpful in cases involving the lower extremity. If more severe, treatment consists of anticoagulants (e.g., low molecular weight heparin, fondaparinux) to prevent extension, recurrence, and to decrease the risk of embolism. *Prevention* is crucial in treatment with compression stockings, leg elevation, and decreasing the amount of time spent immobile.

ANTITHROMBOTIC THERAPY

Antithrombotic therapy is indicated for those with valvular heart disease, prosthetic heart valves, MI, unstable angina, and atrial fibrillation to prevent clots from forming and to reduce the risk of DVT, pulmonary embolism, heart attacks, and strokes. Antithrombotic therapy is also utilized with cardiac surgery. The two types of antithrombotic therapy include:

- **Anticoagulants:** These slow down the clotting process by reducing the formation of fibrin so that clots cannot form:
    - Warfarin: Blocks utilization of vitamin K, decreasing production of clotting factors.

- Heparin: Increases the activity of antithrombin III.
- Low molecular weight heparins (dalteparin, enoxaparin, bemiparin, tinzaparin, nadroparin, parnaparin, certoparin, reviparin): Increase activity of antithrombin III.
- Synthetic anticoagulants (bivalirudin, lepirudin and fondaparinux): Directly inhibit thrombin.
- **Antiplatelets:** These interfere with the function of the plasma membrane to prevent the clumping of platelets, thereby preventing the formation of clots. Antiplatelets include aspirin (the mildest) and newer drugs, such as clopidogrel, ticagrelor, dipyridamole, dipyridamole/aspirin, eptifibatide, prasugrel, and ticlopidine. These agents are ineffective to treat clots already present but prevent further formation.

Varicose Veins and Chronic Venous Insufficiency

Varicose veins occur due to faulty valves within the **distal veins**, leading to distention and stretching of the veins. Because the valves are not functioning properly, blood tends to pool in the extremities and cause further distention of the veins. Patients will complain of aching pain or heaviness in the legs that worsens after standing or sitting for extended periods of time. They may also experience pruritus and burning sensations around the veins, cramps, and restless legs. The veins will be visibly distended, bulging, and contorted. This may lead to **chronic venous insufficiency** (impaired venous return) causing the skin to be reddish and darkly pigmented with edema, and ulcers may form due to venous stasis. *Symptoms* are similar to varicose veins with pain that is worse when legs are dependent. The best *treatment* of varicose veins is prevention. This includes avoiding standing for prolonged periods of time, exercising regularly to keep weight under control, and wearing compression stockings or maintaining leg elevation to promote venous return from the lower extremities. Medical treatments include sclerotherapy, laser vein ablation, vein stripping, or, in severe case, complete removal of the varicose veins(phlebectomy). Surgery is typically ineffective for chronic venous insufficiency and treatment is centered around lifestyle modification, compression, elevation, and topical would care.

Giant Cell Arteritis

Giant cell arteritis, or **temporal arteritis**, is an inflammatory process that affects the **vessels**, most commonly the temporal artery, but may also involve other medium-sized arteries of the head and neck. It typically affects those >50 years old and is more prevalent among females. This condition can lead to occlusion of the temporal artery, resulting in blindness, so diagnosis and treatment should be started quickly. The most common *symptom* is a severe headache. This can be accompanied with a fever, malaise, fatigue, or weight loss. Approximately 50% of patients who are diagnosed with giant cell arteritis will also have a diagnosis of polymyalgia rheumatica. *Diagnosis* consists of erythrocyte sedimentation rate, C-reactive protein, biopsy (this is the standard), MRI, PET, and Doppler. Because of the nature of the illness, treatment is started before the biopsy results are available. *Treatment* consists of high-dose prednisone, usually 40-60 mg per day. Follow up with the patient 3 days after starting prednisone as the headache should improve within that time. Continue prednisone for at least 1 month and then taper. If symptoms return as the dose of prednisone is tapered, the dosage can be increased. Most patients require steroid treatment for about 2 years to monitor and protect the patient from the long-term effects of steroids. Low dose aspirin is usually given to reduce chance of blindness, TIA, and stroke. Chest x-rays or other imaging studies are done annually to assess for aortic aneurysm as a significant number of patients develop aortic aneurysm. *Complications* include blindness, stroke, peripheral vascular disease, and an increased risk of aortic aneurysm.

Aortic Stenosis

Aortic stenosis (**AS**) is a very common valve disease. Most patients are asymptomatic until they reach middle age. Aortic calcifications (aortic sclerosis) are frequently seen in those >55-years-old. Aortic stenosis can be due to a **congenital disorder of the valve** (e.g., bicuspid valve) or **rheumatic fever**. When AS patients become symptomatic or severe, the classic *symptoms* of syncopal episodes, chest pain, and heart failure may be present. They may complain of chest pain, fatigue, and shortness of breath with activity. Symptoms of CHF (SOB, DOE, orthopnea, and PND) can be present when the disease is advanced and prognosis is usually poor by the time these symptoms are present especially if the patient does not respond to meds. On exam, a systolic ejection murmur that is crescendo/decrescendo in nature during the middle to late portion of the cardiac cycle can be heard. This murmur will radiate superiorly to the carotid arteries and is best heard when the patient is sitting upright and leaning forward. There may also be an early systolic ejection click. *Pulsus parvus,* or a weakened pulse, may be palpated. *Diagnosis* consists of echocardiogram for initial diagnosis, and sometimes a transesophageal echo is needed. Medications can't reverse aortic stenosis, but they can decrease symptoms. Common meds used include antihypertensive meds, diuretics, meds to help with heart rate control, and β-blockers for angina. To correct AS, aortic valve replacement is needed. If the patient is not a good candidate for surgery, percutaneous valve replacement or percutaneous balloon valvuloplasty are options. Balloon or surgical valvotomy is used to repair congenital AS. *Complications* include arrhythmias, angina, syncope, heart failure, embolization, and cardiac arrest.

Aortic Regurgitation

Aortic regurgitation (**AR**), aka **aortic insufficiency**, occurs when blood flows back into the left ventricle during diastole due to the insufficiency of the aortic valve to close tightly. It can be an acute or chronic condition and can have many causes, including endocarditis, hypertension, rheumatic heart disease, syphilis, Marfan's syndrome, and congenital causes. If **acute**, patients will complain of sudden, severe SOB, possible chest pain, and signs of heart failure. If **chronic**, there is an asymptomatic time followed by progressive fatigue, SOB with activity, and palpitations. On exam, a high-pitched, decrescendo diastolic murmur will be heard, increasing when patients are seated and leaning forward and in full expiration. A widened pulse pressure will also be detected. Corrigan's sign, a water hammer pulse, may be present. Quincke's pulse, an alternating erythema and paleness in the nail beds with each heartbeat, may also be seen. De Musset's sign, patients visibly nodding the head with each heartbeat, may be evident. An Austin Flint murmur may be present which is a mid-diastolic, low-pitched rumbling over the cardiac apex due to the mitral valve leaflets vibrating. Patients may have all or only a few of these findings. *Diagnosis* is made by echo, which can help classify the regurgitation as mild, moderate, or severe. *Treatment* includes vasodilators, other meds, or valve repair/replacement. *Complications* include heart failure, cardiogenic shock, and death.

Mitral Stenosis

Mitral stenosis is characterized by blood flow being obstructed through the left atrium to ventricle by way of the damaged **mitral valve**. It is fairly common and most cases are female. The typical etiology is rheumatic fever presenting in the 3rd-4th decade of life; however, it can be congenital. Patients may complain of a cough, hemoptysis, or hoarseness that will not go away because of recurrent pressure being applied to the laryngeal nerve or bronchi due to an enlarged left atrium. On exam, findings include an opening snap, loud S_1 (unless stenosis is severe), and a low-pitch, diastolic rumble that is best heard at the apex when the patient in the left lateral position. The murmur increases with exercise and decreases with the Valsalva maneuver (which decreases preload). *Symptoms* of CHF may be present with dyspnea on exertion, crackles, and rales heard in the lungs as well as fatigue. Symptoms are worse during pregnancy because of the increased blood volume and the strain this puts on the mitral valve. *Diagnosis* includes echocardiography, TEE, or occasionally cardiac catheterization. Atrial fibrillation may be detected on ECG. Treatment can include diuretics, β-blockers, and Ca^{++} channel blockers. Secondary rheumatic fever prophylaxis is needed (follow current guidelines), and endocarditis prophylaxis is required in some (e.g., prosthetic valve, previous infective endocarditis). Anticoagulation should be used in patients who have had an embolus or AFib. Mitral valve surgery is indicated in symptomatic patients or patients with severe stenosis (mitral valve area <1.5 cm^2). Options include surgical or percutaneous valvotomy, or mitral valve replacement. *Complications* include AFib, thrombus/embolus, heart failure, pulmonary hypertension, pulmonary edema, and infective endocarditis.

Mitral Regurgitation

Mitral regurgitation (**MR**), aka **mitral insufficiency**, occurs when the mitral valve begins to degenerate. It can be due to rheumatic fever, myxomatous degeneration (MVP), congenital disorders, endocarditis, or dilatation of the left ventricle. Dysfunction of the papillary muscles, coronary artery disease, MI, and ischemia can also lead to MR. The *symptoms* of MR may be acute or chronic. Patients may complain of SOB with activity, orthopnea, fatigue, and weakness. A holosystolic high-pitched, blowing murmur can be heard over the cardiac apex, radiating into the left axilla, and is best heard in the left lateral position. An S_3 may also be heard. Patients may exhibit signs of pulmonary edema with rales, crackles, and dyspnea. *Diagnosis* is made by echo. Cardiac catheterization may be used to evaluate certain echo findings before surgery. A chest x-ray may show pulmonary edema, left ventricular hypertrophy, and left atrial enlargement. An ECG may show AFib and left atrial/ventricular enlargement. Treatment includes vasodilators, diuretics, and β-blockers for symptomatic patients. Anticoagulation is needed for patients with AFib or mitral annular calcifications. Surgical mitral valve repair or replacement is necessary if acute MR or if chronic MR symptoms progress or worsen. If due to papillary muscle dysfunction, patients may present in cardiogenic shock if a papillary muscle has ruptured. This is a life-threatening emergency with a very poor prognosis. *Complications* include infective endocarditis, arrhythmias, thrombus/embolus, and stroke.

Mitral Valve Prolapse

Mitral valve prolapse (**MVP**) is more common in females and is a condition in which the **mitral valve leaflets** are bulging into the atrium during systole. It is usually due to myxomatous degeneration of the leaflets or chordae tendineae which is typically idiopathic or can be congenital in nature with inherited connective tissue disorders (e.g., Marfan syndrome) or by autosomal dominant inheritance. It is frequently seen in multiple members of a family. Most patients are asymptomatic, but patients may complain of chest pain, SOB with activity, fatigue, or palpitations. On exam, a mid to late systolic ejection click can be heard possibly with a high-pitched, mid to late systolic murmur. This is best heard at the apex and with the patient in the left lateral position. The murmur is accentuated with the Valsalva maneuver or with standing. Confirm the *diagnosis* with an echo (2D TTE). Diagnostic echo findings are leaflet displacement ≥2 mm and leaflet thickness of ≥5 mm. Typically, no *treatment* is needed since most patients are asymptomatic. However, symptoms may be treated with β-blockers. Endocarditis prophylaxis is no longer recommended for MVP. If the patient is asymptomatic, reevaluate every 3-5 years with PE and echo. *Complications* include mitral valve regurgitation, arrhythmias, and endocarditis.

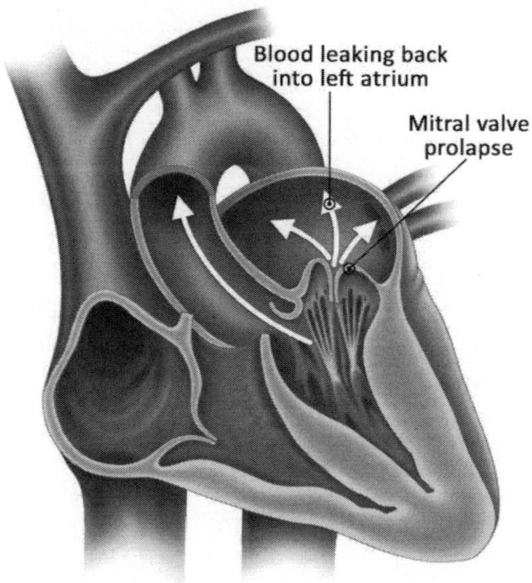

Tricuspid Stenosis

Tricuspid stenosis is not very common and involves narrowing of the **tricuspid valve opening** causing blood flow obstruction between the right atrium and right ventricle. Stenosis is usually due to rheumatic fever, and therefore, usually involves the aortic and mitral valves also. Other less common etiologies include carcinoid tumors, SLE, or endocarditis. Patients with tricuspid stenosis may be fatigued and frequently feel cold. They may notice a fluttering sensation in the neck or palpitations. If the condition is advanced, they may feel abdominal pain and bloating due to hepatomegaly. On exam, other symptoms of right-sided CHF may be seen (e.g., pitting edema), and a bounding pulse may be palpated in the neck over the carotid arteries. An opening snap may be auscultated with a mid-diastolic rumble. The murmur is louder and longer with leg raising and inspiration (maneuvers that increase venous return), and therefore softer with Valsalva and standing (maneuvers that decrease venous return). *Diagnosis* is confirmed with an echo (TTE) which can measure the amount of blood flow and determine the severity of the stenosis. Chest x-ray and ECG may show right atrial enlargement. *Treatment* includes antiarrhythmics, diuretics, and salt restriction, but requires surgery to repair or replace the valve if right heart failure or low cardiac output is present. Right atrial enlargement and arrhythmias are complications.

Tricuspid Regurgitation

Tricuspid regurgitation, aka **insufficiency**, is more common than tricuspid stenosis. Each time the right ventricle contracts, there is blood flow backward through the **tricuspid valve** into the right atrium during systole. It can be **primary** (organic valve problems) or **secondary** (normal valve, but problems occur due to right ventricular enlargement). Tricuspid regurgitation is typically due to secondary causes (e.g., pulmonary hypertension, mitral or pulmonary stenosis). Etiologies include endocarditis, rheumatic fever, MI, right ventricular overload/dilatation, and congenital anomalies. Ebstein's anomaly, a congenital condition, can result in an abnormally formed tricuspid valve, resulting in enlargement of the right atrium and CHF. Patients may complain of fatigue, SOB with activity, abdominal bloating, and swelling in their extremities that is not completely relieved with elevation. On exam, the symptoms of right-sided CHF may be observed (e.g., ascites, peripheral edema, jugular venous distention). A harsh, high-pitched, pansystolic murmur can be auscultated at the LLSB, and the murmur increases upon inspiration. While chest x-ray and ECG may show ventricular enlargement, echo is the *diagnostic* tool of choice. It also helps to evaluate severity. *Treatment* includes diuretics to remove fluid, digoxin, ACE inhibitors, and, if severe, annuloplasty or valve repair/replacement. *Complications* include ascites, heart failure, and thrombus/embolus.

Pulmonary Stenosis

Pulmonary stenosis is narrowing of the **pulmonary outflow tract** that causes blood flow obstruction between the right ventricle and the pulmonary artery during systole. It is most often due to congenital abnormalities and usually remain asymptomatic until the patient is an adult. It may be seen along with other cardiac abnormalities (e.g., Tetralogy of Fallot). Infants may exhibit failure to thrive and poor weight gain. It rarely occurs as a result of rheumatic fever or carcinoid. Patients may complain of fatigue, SOB with activity, chest pain, and syncope. Cyanosis may exist if a right-to-left shunt is also present. A normal S_1 followed by a systolic click and a mid-systolic murmur will be present, and the murmur tends to increase with deep inspiration. A wide split S_2 can be present with a right ventricular heave. *Diagnosis* is made per Doppler echo to assess the valve's anatomy, determine the location of the stenosis, and to check the right ventricle. Chest x-ray may show a prominent main pulmonary artery. Surgery is sometimes necessary to repair the valve. Balloon valvuloplasty is the treatment of choice and involves stretching the valve with a balloon in order to widen the opening. *Complications* include endocarditis, arrhythmias, and heart failure.

Pulmonary Regurgitation

Pulmonary regurgitation (**PR**), aka **insufficiency**, is when blood flows backwards from the **pulmonary artery** to the right ventricle. It most commonly occurs in patients with pulmonary hypertension. Occasionally it is due to endocarditis, congenital abnormalities, rheumatic heart disease, or carcinoid syndrome. There are usually no *symptoms* with this condition unless it becomes advanced. If right-sided heart failure does occur, patients may complain of SOB with activity (most common), fatigue, light-headedness, palpitations, chest pain, and syncope. On exam, a low-pitched murmur, which may increase with breathing, may be heard. When PR is due to pulmonary hypertension, pressure rises in the pulmonary artery, and a Graham-Steele murmur can be heard. This murmur is a high-pitched blowing decrescendo murmur and is best heard at the LUSB. There can be a split S_2, and a right-sided S_3 or S_4 may be heard and is accentuated during inspiration. If pulmonary HTN is not present, there will be a low-pitched crescendo-decrescendo murmur. *Diagnosis* is made per echo. Right axis deviation may be noted on ECG due to right ventricular hypertrophy/dilatation as well as a RBBB. Usually the symptoms are not severe enough to warrant treatment with replacement of the pulmonary valve, but surgery can be done if patients are extremely symptomatic. Most *treatment* will focus on correcting the underlying problem, such as pulmonary hypertension. Right-sided heart failure is rare, but is a *complication* of PR.

PROSTHETIC HEART VALVES

Prosthetic heart valves	Risks	Benefits
Mechanical valves (Types include caged ball, tilting disc, and bileaflet.) Recommended for patients over 65.	Increased risk of blood clots and emboli (heart attack, stroke) so patients must take anticoagulants. Thrombus formation may occur as well as hemolysis. Cavitation (formation of bubbles) can erode the valves.	Can last indefinitely.
Human donor valve (homograft) Recommended if life expectancy is under 15 years.	Few are available so the patient may have an extended wait for a valve. Surgical procedure is more complex than with other types of valves. Lasts only 10 to 20 years. Calcification of aortic wall may occur.	Does not require anticoagulants. Carries low risk of infection after surgery and low risk of thrombo-embolism. Good hemodynamics.
Biologic valves (xenografts) (derived from valves of pigs or bovine or equine tissue attached to metal frame or stent to form valve). Recommended for patients younger than 65.	Usually lasts only about 10 to 15 years, so best suited for those over 55. May be more susceptible to calcification than human valves.	The donor tissue is chemically treated to neutralize. Does not require anticoagulation.

Infections

BACTERIAL ENDOCARDITIS

Bacterial endocarditis can be classified as **subacute** (insidious onset) or **acute** (rapid onset). A further distinction can be made as to whether it is present in a **native valve** or **prosthetic valve**, or due to IV drug abuse. A patient with heart disease affecting the valves is at risk for developing endocarditis which includes those with congenital heart disease or valvular disease and those who have prosthetic valves. IV drug abusers, those with invasive procedures/surgery, and those who have had prior endocarditis are also at risk. Almost all patients with endocarditis will have a new, regurgitant-type murmur. Splinter hemorrhages may be evident in the nail beds with Osler nodes (tender nodules in finger/toe pads) and Janeway lesions (nontender lesions on palms/soles). Roth spots (retinal hemorrhages) may be evident on funduscopic exam and patients may show other signs of emboli being present, such as hematuria and renal dysfunction. After blood cultures are drawn, empiric antibiotic therapy is started for acutely ill patients, and IV Vancomycin 15-20 mg/kg every 8-12 hours is typically used. Nafcillin and gentamicin are used empirically in IV drug users. Appropriate antibiotics are started once culture and sensitivity results are in and continued for 2-8 weeks. These patients require prophylactic antibiotics for future dental or invasive procedures or surgery that involve the gingiva, respiratory tract, or infected skin or musculoskeletal tissue. Prophylaxis is given one hour before the procedure and oral options include: amoxicillin 2 g, or if allergic to penicillin, clindamycin 600 mg or azithromycin 500 mg. *Complications* include MI, heart failure, emboli, stroke, or organ damage.

Modified Duke Criteria to Diagnose Endocarditis

The **modified Duke criteria** for endocarditis states a patient must have 2 major criteria, 1 major and 3 minor criteria, or 5 minor criteria in order to have a definite diagnosis of endocarditis.

- The **major criteria** are: two positive blood cultures (BC) with typical endocarditis organisms, 2 positive BC taken 12 hours apart, 3 or more positive BC taken 1 hour apart, a single positive BC for *Coxiella burnetii*, evidence of endocardial involvement on an echocardiogram (e.g., vegetation), myocardial abscess, partial dehiscence of a prosthetic valve, or the presence of new valvular regurgitation.
- The **minor criteria** are predisposing risk factors (e.g., heart disease, IV drug use), a fever >100.4°F, vascular features (e.g., emboli, hemorrhage, Janeway lesions), immunologic features (e.g., glomerulonephritis, Osler nodes, Roth spots, rheumatoid factor), or a positive blood culture that does not meet major criteria. The blood cultures should be drawn three times 1 hour apart with the samples taken at different sites. The most likely organisms to cause endocarditis are *Staphylococcus aureus*, streptococci (e.g., *Streptococcus viridians*), and enterococci. The transthoracic echocardiogram (TTE) is typically used first, but a transesophageal echo may be necessary for accurate visualization of the valves.

Acute Rheumatic Fever

Acute rheumatic fever (**ARF**) can occur approximately 2-3 weeks following a group A streptococcal (GAS) infection. It usually affects children 5 to 15 years old, and is no longer as common in the United States. Approximately 60% of cases with carditis affect the mitral valve, followed by a combined aortic and mitral valve involvement. Patients usually first complain of a migratory polyarthralgia of the large joints and have a fever. For diagnosis of initial ARF, 2 of the major Jones criteria must be present *or* 1 major and 2 minor:

- **Major**: carditis, erythema marginatum, subcutaneous nodules, chorea, or migratory arthritis of the large joints;
- **Minor**: polyarthralgia, ESR >60mm/h or CRP >3.0 mg/dL, fever ≥101.3 °F, or prolonged PR interval on ECG.

Evidence of prior GAS infection includes a rising antibody titer (e.g., antistreptolysin O or anti-DNase B), a positive throat culture, or positive rapid antigen test. *Treatment* includes bed rest, penicillin or amoxicillin, aspirin (ASA) or other NSAID, and steroids (instead of ASA for moderate to severe carditis). Steroids are continued for 2-3 weeks and then tapered. ASA can be started as prednisone is tapered, and continued for 2-4 weeks after steroids are discontinued. Haldol may be given to control the movements of chorea. Rheumatic fever can be deadly and lead to permanent heart disease, CHF, and arrhythmias. The risk for recurring ARF is greatest in the first 5 years; therefore, antibiotic prophylaxis is recommended for 5 years or until the patient reaches 18 years of age. *Complications* include valvular regurgitation, stenosis (usually mitral or aortic), and heart dysfunction.

Myocarditis

Myocarditis is inflammation of the cardiac myocardium (muscle tissue), usually triggered by a viral infection, such as the Influenza virus, Coxsackie virus, and HIV. Myocarditis can also be caused by bacteria, fungi, or parasites or an allergic response to medications. Myocarditis can result in dilation of the heart, development of thrombi on the heart walls (known as mural thrombi), and infiltration of blood cells around the coronary vessels and between muscle fibers, causing further degeneration of the muscle tissue. The heart may become enlarged and weak, as the ability to pump blood is impaired, leading to congestive heart failure. Symptoms depend upon the extent of damage but may include fatigue, dyspnea, pressure and discomfort in chest or epigastric area, and palpitations. Diagnostic studies may include chest x-ray, ECG, echocardiogram, cardiac catheterization, viral cultures and titers, and PCR of biopsy specimen. Treatment:

- As indicated for underlying cause (such as antibiotics).
- Restriction of activities.
- Careful monitoring for heart failure and medical treatment as indicated (diuretics, digoxin, etc.)
- Oxygen as needed to maintain normal oxygen saturation.
- IV gamma globulin for acute stage.

Acute Pericarditis

Acute pericarditis occurs when the **pericardial sac** becomes inflamed. This is often idiopathic, but is most commonly due to a viral infection. A bacterial, fungal, or a parasitic infection can also cause this condition, as well as tuberculosis. Autoimmune/inflammatory disorders (e.g., lupus, rheumatoid arthritis, rheumatic fever), metabolic disorders (e.g., renal failure/uremia, hypothyroidism), cardiovascular disorders (MI, aortic dissection), drugs (e.g., penicillin, doxorubicin), and cancer can also cause pericarditis. Patients will complain of pleuritic chest pain that is worse upon inspiration and relieved by sitting up and leaning forward. The pain is precordial or substernal and may radiate to the neck or trapezius ridge, usually to the left side. Patients may have dyspnea and a nonproductive cough. A pericardial friction rub is the hallmark finding on exam. *Diagnosis* is based on PE and imaging findings. A CXR may detect a large cardiac silhouette, and an echocardiogram is used to detect a pericardial effusion. An ECG can show serial changes, initially with ST elevation and PR depression. Leukocytosis may be present if viral. *Treatment* is with NSAIDs (typically aspirin), colchicine (which reduces the rate of recurrent pericarditis). and possibly steroids, all used to reduce inflammation. If an effusion is >250 mL, a pericardiocentesis is performed. If severe, a pericardial window may be created surgically to reduce the tension on the pericardial sac or even a pericardiectomy in which the pericardial sac is partially or completely removed. *Complications* include recurrent pericarditis and cardiac tamponade.

Lipid Disorders

Cholesterol/Lipoproteins

The following are **types of cholesterol** and guidelines for lipid control:

- **Chylomicrons**, the least dense lipoprotein; transports dietary triglycerides and cholesterol.
- **Very low-density lipoproteins (VLDL)** are made in the liver and are rich in triglycerides.
- **Intermediate-density lipoproteins (IDL)** result from VLDL and chylomicron metabolism.
- **Low-density lipoproteins (LDL)** are rich in cholesterol and are the most atherogenic.
- **High-density lipoproteins (HDL)** are the smallest and transport cholesterol to the liver.
- **Hyperlipidemias** are classified as primary or secondary. Rule out secondary causes (e.g., DM, sedentary lifestyle, EtOH overuse).
- ***Screening***: Fasting serum lipid profile (total cholesterol, TG, HDL-C, calculated LDL-C, VLDL).

Lipid Disorders

Hypertriglyceridemia

Hypertriglyceridemia is a condition with high levels of triglycerides (fatty molecules).

Patient usually **asymptomatic** until level reaches 1000 mg/dL or greater and some have no obvious symptoms, but others may develop xanthoma, lipemia retinalis, abdominal pain, and hepatosplenomegaly. Increases risk of atherosclerosis, coronary artery disease, metabolic syndrome, as well as pancreatitis.

Diagnosis per triglyceride levels: Normal level is <150 mg/dL.

Treatment include dietary modification (low fat, low carbohydrate), weight loss, and exercise. Medications may include statin, niacin, fibric acid derivative, 3-acid ethyl aster, or HMG-CoA reductase inhibitor.

Chylomicronemia Syndrome

Chylomicronemia syndrome is a genetic disorder in which the body does not break down lipids properly because of the absence of lipoprotein lipase so chylomicrons (lipid particles) accumulate in the blood.

Signs and symptoms include pancreatitis, peripheral nerve damage, memory impairment, xanthomas, and hepatosplenomegaly. Diabetes is common.

Diagnosis includes triglyceride test (>1000 mg/dL) and genetic testing.

Treatment includes fat-free and alcohol-free diet. Patients often take statins and/or fibrates, but benefit is limited.

Hyperlipidemia

The **specific lipid levels** at which to begin treatment can vary depending on the patient, but the following guidelines are usually followed:

- Triglyceride level **150 to 199 (borderline):** Initiate lifestyle changes, including diet, exercise regimen, and weight loss.
- Triglyceride level **200 to 499 (high):** Consider drug therapy in patients with other risk factors for coronary artery disease (CAD).
- Triglyceride level **>500 (very high):** Initiate drug therapy in all patients.

The different classes of drugs used in the treatment of hyperlipidemia include nicotinic acid, statins, bile acid-binding resins, and fibrates. All classes are used for lowering LDL levels. Liver function tests (LFTs) must be monitored in patients on all these drugs except for the bile-acid binding resins.

Current Recommended Guidelines and Goals for LDL Control

Treatment goals for hyperlipidemia are based upon CHD risk. They are as follows:

- **Low risk** (0-1 risk factors): LDL goal is <160. Lifestyle changes should begin with LDL ≥160. Medications should be started with LDL ≥190 (optional if LDL 160-189 mg/dL).
- **Moderate to high risk** (2+ risk factors with 10-year risk ≤20%): LDL goal is <130. Lifestyle changes should begin with LDL ≥130. Medications should be started with LDL ≥130 (if 10-yr. risk 10-20%) or LDL ≥160 (if 10-yr. risk <10%).
- **Highest risk** (10-year risk >20%): LDL goal is <100. Lifestyle changes should begin with LDL ≥100. Medications should be started with LDL ≥130 (optional if LDL 100-129 mg/dL).

Medical Treatments to Control Cholesterol Levels

Medical treatments available to control cholesterol levels:

- **Statins (HMG CoA reductase inhibitors)** are first choice for lowering LDL; have been shown to decrease CV morbidity and mortality. Can decrease LDL-C by 25-50%, TG, apolipoprotein B, and total cholesterol. Recommended if: ASCVD; LDL-C ≥190; age 40-75 if DM and LDL-C 70-189; or if age 40-75 and LDL-C 70-189 and estimated 10-yr. risk of ASCVD ≥7.5%. Side effects include myalgia, myositis, and increased liver enzymes. They are classified as low, medium, and high- intensity.
- **Niacin (nicotinic acid)** decreases LDL, increases HDL, and is very effective at decreasing triglycerides. Also, reduces risk of CVD. Side effects include flushing, itching, gout, and peptic ulcers. Taking with food and 325 mg ASA (30 mins. before) decreases flushing.
- **Bile acid sequestrants** can decrease LDL, can increase HDL, and may or may not be helpful with decreasing triglycerides. Side effects include constipation, gas, and decreased fat-soluble vitamin and drug absorption.
- **Fibrates** can decrease LDL, TG (by 50%), apolipoprotein B, and total cholesterol; and can increase HDL-C (up to 20%). Side effects include myalgia, myositis, hepatitis, gallstones, and potentiate warfarin.
- **Cholesterol absorption inhibitor (Ezetimibe)** can decrease LDL, can lower apolipoprotein B, and may or may not be helpful with decreasing triglycerides. Side effects include increased liver enzymes when used in conjunction with a statin.
- **PCSK9 monoclonal antibodies** are for those with familial hypercholesterolemia.
- **Omega-3-fatty acids** help decrease TGs.

Cardiac Emergencies

Pericardial Effusion

A **pericardial effusion** occurs when an abnormal amount of fluid accumulates within the **pericardial space**. Normal pericardial fluid is about 20-50 mL. It can occur due to a viral infection, tuberculosis, a malignant tumor, radiation to the chest cavity, or trauma. Patients with pericardial effusions do not always complain of chest pain. They can have a cough, SOB, dyspnea, palpitations, and syncope. If the cause is infectious, they may have a fever. On exam, tachycardia may be present, and distant cardiac sounds with a pericardial rub may be heard. An echo is the method of choice for *diagnosing* a pericardial effusion. Early effusions first collect posteriorly. Chest-x-ray will show cardiomegaly with a globular, water-bottle shape. ECG changes will be non-specific and may show a low voltage QRS complex. *Treatment* can include NSAIDs (e.g., ASA, ibuprofen), colchicine, antibiotics, and possibly steroids to treat the inflammation; but a pericardiocentesis is frequently needed to drain off the fluid. In severe cases, the pericardial sac can be partially or completely removed from around the heart. A pericardial biopsy may also be needed to determine the cause of the effusion. *Complications* include cardiac tamponade and death.

Pericardial Effusion

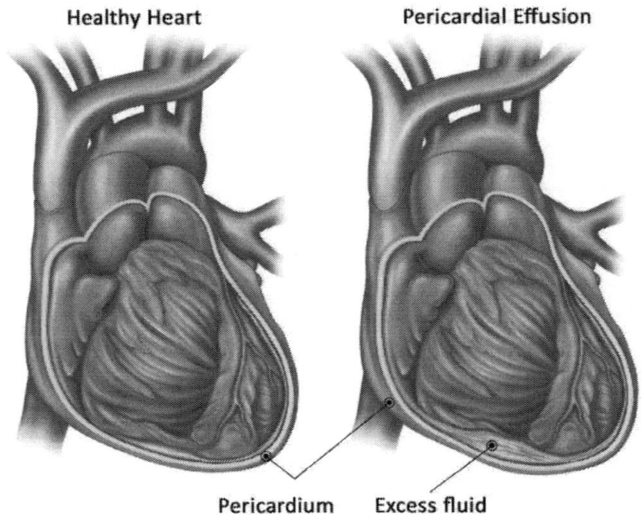

Cardiac Tamponade

Cardiac tamponade is an emergency condition in which fluid accumulates in the **pericardial sac**, leading to cardiac constriction that prevents the ventricles from adequately filling, and thus, decreasing cardiac output. It can occur with malignancy (most common), pericarditis, acute MI, a dissecting thoracic aortic aneurysm, recent cardiac surgery, or trauma. Beck's triad is classic for acute cardiac tamponade: muffled heart sounds, hypotension, and increased jugular venous pressure. Patients may have dyspnea, tachycardia, tachypnea, and chest pain. *Pulsus paradoxus*, which is a >12 mm drop in systolic pressure during inspiration, can be present. Also, the pulse pressure may be narrowed. Cardiac tamponade is a clinical *diagnosis* and prompt diagnosis is key. In patients with suspected cardiac tamponade, perform an immediate echocardiogram. An ECG can show electrical alternans, and a chest x-ray can show a water-bottle-shaped cardiomegaly. A Swan-Ganz catheter to measure pressure within the heart will reveal that all of the pressures are virtually equal. It is an emergency situation, and an immediate pericardiocentesis should be performed to remove the fluid off the heart. Also, a pericardial window or pericardiectomy may be performed. Use inotropes (i.e. dobutamine) and IV fluids as needed to stabilize the patient. *Complications* include death, shock, and pulmonary edema.

Cardiogenic Shock

Cardiogenic shock is a condition of **decreased cardiac output** but with adequate intravascular volume. The heart is not able to supply the body with the necessary blood, O_2, and nutrients that are necessary for proper functioning. It is most often secondary to MI damage that reduces the contractibility of the ventricles, interfering with the pumping mechanism of the heart, and decreasing O_2 perfusion. Cardiogenic shock has 3 characteristics: *Increased preload, increased afterload*, and *decreased contractibility*. Together these result in a decreased cardiac output and an increase in SVR (systemic vascular resistance) to compensate and protect vital organs. This results in an increase of afterload in the left ventricle with increased need for oxygen. As the cardiac output continues to decrease, tissue perfusion decreases, coronary artery perfusion decreases, fluid backs up and the left ventricle fails to adequately pump the blood, resulting in pulmonary edema and left ventricular failure. Decreasing O_2 consumption is a major initial goal of cardiogenic shock.

Symptoms include:

- Hypotension with systolic BP <90 mm Hg
- Tachycardia >100 beats/min with weak, thready pulse and dysrhythmias
- Decreased heart sounds, chest pain
- Tachypnea and basilar rales
- Oliguria
- Cyanotic, cool, clammy skin, pallor, and mottled extremities

Treatment includes:

- IV fluids
- Inotropic agents
- Anti-dysrhythmics
- IABP or left ventricular assist device

STABLE, UNSTABLE, AND PRINZMETAL VARIANT ANGINA PECTORIS

Angina is chest pain due to myocardial ischemia that is usually brought on by stress or exertion and relieved by rest and/or nitrate medications. It can be classified as stable, unstable, or Prinzmetal variant type. **Stable angina** usually lasts <5 minutes. It is increased with activity and decreased with rest and/or nitrates. It is described as a clenching sensation over the chest and the PE is usually normal. **Unstable angina** (also known as preinfarction or crescendo angina) is a progression of coronary artery disease and occurs when there is a change in the pattern of stable angina. The pain may increase, last longer (>5-20 minutes), may not respond to a single nitroglycerin, become more frequent, occur at rest, and may be accompanied by pallor, diaphoresis, and ST-segment depression, but without elevated biomarkers. Unstable angina may indicate an upcoming myocardial infarction. **Prinzmetal variant angina** results from spasms of the coronary arteries, and is often related to stress, cold weather, smoking, or illicit stimulants. Variant angina frequently occurs cyclically, usually at night or the early morning, and at rest. Elevation of ST segments usually occurs with variant angina. Nitroglycerin or calcium channel blockers are used for treatment. Patients presenting with chest pain should be treated with SL nitroglycerin (0.3-0.6 mg every 5 minutes up to 3 times), daily ASA and β-blockers, and an appropriate stress test. It is extremely important to determine the presence of **acute coronary syndrome (ACS)**, which includes unstable angina, NSTEMI, and STEMI, so directed treatment can begin as soon as possible.

ACUTE MYOCARDIAL INFARCTION

Acute myocardial infarction (MI) may be classified as **NSTEMI** (non-ST-segment elevation MI) or **STEMI** (ST-segment elevation MI). Clinical manifestations of MI may vary considerably, with males having the more "classic" symptom of sudden onset of crushing chest pain, and females and those under 55 often presenting with atypical symptoms. Elderly patients and diabetics may have reduced pain sensation, may not have any of the classic symptoms of an acute MI due to neuropathy or dementia (elderly), and may complain primarily of weakness. About two-thirds of patients have prodromal symptoms (chest discomfort, fatigue, SOB) weeks to days preceding the MI, and most MIs occur in the early morning hours. Patients may complain of crushing pressure or pain throughout the chest, radiating into the neck, jaw, or left arm. They may also have epigastric pain or a feeling of weakness or anxiety. Patients may be nauseated, pale, diaphoretic, short of breath, and may appear restless or lethargic. On exam, an S_4 gallop is usually present, blood pressure may be high or low, and acute symptoms of CHF may also be seen. Serial ECGs may show ST elevation, though depression can also be seen. Serial cardiac enzymes(troponin) should be drawn at presentation and 3 hours later. Troponin I or T is a contractile protein that only appears in the serum after cardiac necrosis and is the new standard of measuring cardiac injury. Troponin levels increase within 3-12 hours of cardiac injury, peak at 24-48 hours, and return to normal after 5-14 days. An echocardiogram may show a decreased EF, and cardiac wall stiffness may be seen.

Review Video: Myocardial Infarction
Visit mometrix.com/academy and enter code: 148923

Treatment

The mnemonic MONA stands for immediate acute MI treatment with **morphine**, **oxygen**, **nitrates**, and **aspirin**. Also start β-blockers and heparin (or another anticoagulant). Determine ASAP if chest pain is due to unstable angina, NSTEMI, or STEMI as treatment course is different (Obtain a 12-lead ECG within 10 mins. of arriving to ER). Early reperfusion is key.

For STEMI (ST-segment elevation MI = ECG with ST-elevation not easily reversed with NTG, and elevated troponin I or T):

- Immediate PCI (percutaneous coronary intervention) within 90 mins. **OR** thrombolytics
- CABG if unable to perform PCI

For NSTEMI (non-ST-segment elevation MI = No ST-elevation, but with ST-depression and/or T-wave inversion, and elevated cardiac markers):

- If **unstable**: immediate angiography with PCI or CABG
- If **stable**: PCI or CABG within 24-48 hours

Thrombolytic therapy works best when begun within 12 hours of the onset of chest pain with the goal of starting within 30 min of ER arrival, if that course of reperfusion is chosen. These meds can have serious side effects, so a careful assessment of patient's medical history should be done. Thrombolytics/fibrinolytics are contraindicated with any known intracranial hemorrhage, tumor, or stroke. If STEMI or unstable NSTEMI, ideally, patients should be stabilized and taken for angiography & PCI or CABG within 90 minutes of presenting to the ER. PCI involves PTCA usually with stent placement. The decision to use PCI vs. CABG is based on multiple factors, including availability of PCI, symptoms, comorbidities (e.g., DM), number/location of blocked arteries, and degree of narrowing of arteries. At discharge start lifestyle changes and continue antiplatelets, β-blockers, ACE inhibitors, and statins.

Aortic Aneurysm

An **aortic aneurysm** is a dilation of the aorta ≥50% of normal arterial size. It is usually seen as an **abdominal aortic aneurysm** (AAA) >3cm at a level below the renal arteries, but can be common in the **thoracic aorta** in patients who have connective tissue disorders (e.g., Marfan syndrome). High risk patients for developing an aortic aneurysm are men >65-y/o who smoke, have HTN, and atherosclerosis. Many aortic aneurysms are found incidentally during an imaging study. Most are asymptomatic, but patients may have complaints of vague back pain before dissection or rupture occurs. An abdominal pulsatile mass may be felt or a bruit heard, and if dissection or rupture occurs, there will be hypotension and decreased pulses below the level of the aneurysm. A dissected AAA classically present with abdominal pain, a pulsatile abdominal mass, and hypotension and requires immediate emergency surgery without imaging studies. If *diagnosis* is unclear, ultrasound or CT will visualize the aneurysm. CT angiography or MRA can confirm the diagnosis in patients who have not ruptured. If a patient has a known but asymptomatic aneurysm, an annual ultrasound should be done to monitor its growth. The risk of surgical repair typically outweighs the risk of aneurysm rupture until the ascending aorta reaches >5-6cm, the descending aorta is >6-7cm, and the abdominal aneurysm is >5-5.5 cm. Patients with Marfan syndrome require surgery when it reaches ≥4.5-5cm in any location. *Repair* is with endovascular stent grafting or open surgery for more complicated cases. In the asymptomatic patient, medical management includes aggressive control of blood pressure with β-blockers, serial imaging, smoking cessation, and patient education of signs of complications (sudden intense back or abd pain). *Complications* include thrombus/embolus, dissection, rupture, or death.

DISSECTING AORTIC ANEURYSM

A **dissecting aortic aneurysm** occurs when the wall of the aorta is torn and blood flows in the channel created between the intima and media, dilating and weakening it until it risks rupture (which has 90% mortality). This most often occurs in the proximal ascending aorta.

DeBakey classification uses anatomic location as the focal point:

- **Type I** begins in the ascending aorta but may spread to include the aortic arch and the descending aorta (50%). (AKA *Stanford type A*)
- **Type II** is restricted to the ascending aorta (35%). (AKA *Stanford type A*)
- **Type III** is restricted to the descending aorta (15%). (AKA *Stanford type B*)

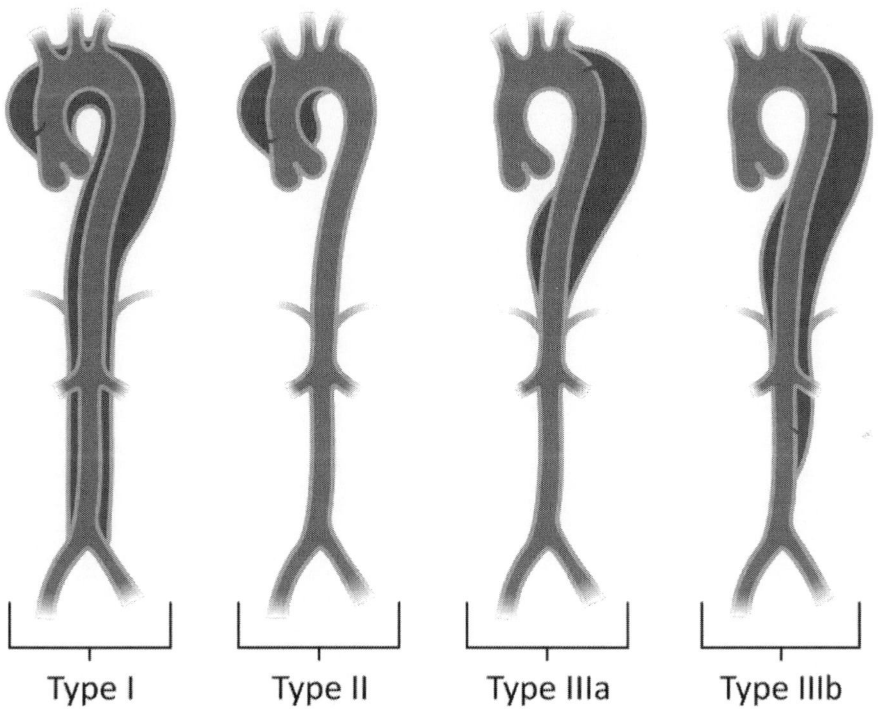

DeBakey classification

Patients will describe a fairly sudden onset of mid-abdominal pain or back pain that is ripping or tearing in quality. This pain may be aggravated by taking a deep breath or by performing any activities. Hip pain may also be present if blood is pooling in the lower abdominal cavity. Clinically, a pulsatile mass may or may not be palpated. It is advised that no hard palpation be performed on the abdomen until an aneurysm is ruled out because of fear of causing sudden rupture if the dissection is advanced. *Diagnosis* is with immediate TEE, CT with angiography, or MRA. *Treatment* consists of open surgery or endovascular methods. However, in patients that present with a descending aortic dissection, medical management using β-blockers to control BP is sometimes chosen. *Complications* include pericardial tamponade, shock, organ failure or death.